# BASIC MEDICAL LABORATORY TECHNIQUES

Mary Ann
Reinert

# BASIC MEDICAL LABORATORY TECHNIQUES

NORMA J. WALTERS, R.N., PH.D.
TEACHER EDUCATOR AND COORDINATOR
HEALTH OCCUPATIONS EDUCATION
CENTER FOR VOCATIONAL AND ADULT EDUCATION
COLLEGE OF EDUCATION
AUBURN UNIVERSITY
AUBURN, ALABAMA

BARBARA H. ESTRIDGE, B.S., MT(ASCP)
ANNA P. REYNOLDS, B.S., MT(ASCP)
LABORATORY AND MEDICAL TECHNOLOGY
DEPARTMENT OF CHEMISTRY
COLLEGE OF SCIENCES AND MATHEMATICS
AUBURN UNIVERSITY
AUBURN, ALABAMA

DELMAR PUBLISHERS INC.®

**DEDICATION**

*To our teachers, students, and families*

**Delmar Staff:**

Administrative Editor: Leslie F. Boyer
Production Editor: Carol Micheli

For information address Delmar Publishers Inc.
2 Computer Drive West, Box 15015
Albany, NY 12212-9985



10 9 8 7 6

Printed in the United States of America
Published simultaneously in Canada
by Nelson Canada,
a division of International Thomson Limited

**Library of Congress Cataloging in Publication Data**

Walters, Norma J.
Basic medical laboratory techniques.

Bibliography: p.
Includes index.
1. Diagnosis, Laboratory. 2. Medical technology.
I. Estridge, Barbara H. II. Reynolds, Anna P.
III. Title. [DNLM: 1. Diagnosis, Laboratory.
2. Technology, Medical. QY 25 W235b]
RB37.W25 1986 616.07'5 85-12885
ISBN 0-8273-2511-8
ISBN 0-8273-2512-6 (instructor's guide)

# Contents

# List of Color Plates



Color Plates 1–8 and 11. Courtesy of John Estridge

Color Plate 20. Courtesy of Ames Division of Miles Laboratories, Inc., Elkhart, IN. From *Modern Urine Chemistry*, 1982.

Color Plates 21, 22, 23. Courtesy of W.B. Saunders Co., Philadelphia, PA. From *Clinical Diagnosis by Laboratory Methods*, 17th Ed., 1984.

# List of Figures and Tables

## UNIT 1: INTRODUCTION TO THE MEDICAL LABORATORY

Figures



Tables

## UNIT 2: BASIC HEMATOLOGY

Figures



Tables

**UNIT 3: ADVANCED HEMATOLOGY**

Figures



Tables



**UNIT 4: INTRODUCTION TO SEROLOGY**

Figures

Tables



**UNIT 5: URINALYSIS**

Figures



Tables

## UNIT 6: INTRODUCTION TO BACTERIOLOGY

Figures



Table

# Preface

*Basic Medical Laboratory Techniques* was written in response to a need to provide students and prospective teachers with a text which combines both theory and techniques of basic medical laboratory procedures.

### Educational Challenges

Individuals interested in pursuing careers in health fields such as clinical laboratory medicine, nursing, pharmacy, dental assisting, respiratory therapy, or medical records can no longer acquire mastery of the chosen field by learning only on the job. Even though on-the-job training remains important, training in the various health care skills must also be taught in the classroom and laboratory. There is a need for well-trained personnel prepared to teach these skills.

Educators have encountered many challenges in trying to provide well-designed materials for training personnel for the various health careers and have been handicapped by a lack of appropriate textbooks. Students being introduced to health careers in laboratory medicine have found it very difficult to obtain fundamental information in one text written in a concise, sequential, and clear manner to meet their needs. In addition, personnel already employed in a health career have not been able to obtain educational materials concerning clinical laboratory procedures which provide a basic review or supplement their knowledge and experience.

In order to respond to the needs of teacher educators, teachers and students, the authors conducted workshops for health occupations teachers in which basic medical laboratory procedures were taught. As a result of the positive response to these workshops, the idea of a textbook of *Basic Medical Laboratory Techniques* and the *Basic Medical Laboratory Techniques Instructor's Guide* was conceived. *Basic Medical Laboratory Techniques* incorporates the workshop materials and evaluations from workshop participants as well as reviewers. The performance-based text and guide have been carefully designed to promote learning and to aid teaching in group sessions and individualized study.

## ACKNOWLEDGMENTS

The authors wish to express their appreciation to all who gave freely of their time, despite busy schedules, in the development of the book including:

John A. Estridge
Illustrations and photographs

Student assistants

Johnny deGuzman
Donda Huett
Kathy Kirby
Susan McDonald
Kelley Patterson
Howard Scott
Carol Stewart
Pamela White
Dottie Whitehead

Health Occupations teachers and students
Participants in workshops

The authors also wish to thank the following companies and institutions for providing some of the information and photographs:

Ames Company, Division of Miles Laboratories, Inc.
Becton-Dickinson Labware
Clay-Adams Division, Becton-Dickinson and Company
Drake Student Health Center, Auburn University, AL
East Alabama Medical Center, Opelika, AL
Fisher Scientific Company
General Diagnostics, Division of Warner Lambert Company
International Equipment Company, Division of Damon Corporation
Marion Laboratories, Inc., Marion Scientific Division
Ortho Diagnostics Systems, Inc.
Reichert Scientific Instruments
W. B. Saunders Company

# About the Book

*Basic Medical Laboratory Techniques* has been specifically designed for maximum use by the health occupations teacher educators in training prospective student teachers for teaching in a cluster or a specific program. The book may also be used by teachers and students in other allied health training programs, such as the medical laboratory technician programs and the medical laboratory assistant programs. In addition, persons already employed in the medical field may use the book as a reference to augment or supplement their knowledge and experience.

The content and organization of the book provides for unlimited flexibility in the teaching and learning processes. The book has been written emphasizing many basic manual laboratory procedures which illustrate fundamental principles and are taught in most training programs, even though larger hospitals and laboratories use automation for most procedures.

The topics of the six units in the text are: Introduction to the Medical Laboratory, Basic Hematology, Advanced Hematology, Introduction to Serology, Urinalysis, and Introduction to Bacteriology. An overview precedes each unit and includes a list of unit objectives. Each lesson in the units contain objectives, glossary terms, and basic information. Precautions, student activities, lesson reviews, and worksheets, and student performance guides are included where appropriate. Figures, tables, and photographs are incorporated to aid in understanding and interpreting the information and procedures. Color plates are also included to assist the student to identify blood cells, components of urine sediment, and bacteria. In addition, a glossary and list of references has been provided to supplement the text.

The appendices contain important information which is easily located. These include abbreviations, prefixes, suffixes and stems, tables of normal values, metric and temperature conversion charts, %T–A conversion chart, and samples of hematology and urinalysis report forms. Helpful information on preparation of reagents, examples of preparing solutions and dilutions and sources of laboratory supplies is also included. In addition, a safety agreement form has been included which should be read and completed by each student and filed before any laboratory procedure is performed.

An instructor's guide is also available to assist the teacher in teaching various procedures. The guide includes self-contained lesson plans for each lesson in the student text. These contain objectives, glossary terms, introduction, lesson content, method of teaching, resources, student learning activities, equipment and materials, a method of evaluation, summary of lesson, test, test key and a final performance check sheet and worksheets, as appropriate. After Unit 1 has been completed, Units 2, 4, 5 or 6 may be studied in the order of preference of the instructor, depending on the availability of time, laboratory space, and equipment. Unit 3 should be used as a sequel to Unit 2.

Educators and students should find this book

an essential aid in understanding and teaching basic laboratory techniques. The book can be used as a methodology text and as a valuable reference book.

## TO THE STUDENT

*Basic Medical Laboratory Techniques* was written primarily to introduce the prospective teacher or student to the basic principles and techniques of some commonly performed medical laboratory procedures. The information is presented in a brief and interesting manner to facilitate learning.

The book is divided into six units, each containing a list of objectives of the unit and an introduction to the unit. The units are divided into lessons with each procedure in the unit represented by a lesson.

Each lesson begins with the objectives followed by a list of glossary terms, words which may be unfamiliar or need further explanation. Basic theoretical concepts are briefly presented along with clinical information. Figures, tables, photographs, and color plates are included where appropriate to clarify points and expand your understanding. Precautions which should be observed, both for safety and for technical reasons, are emphasized in each procedure and restated in the "Precautions" sections. Review questions and learning activities have been included to test and reinforce understanding of the material.

*Basic Medical Laboratory Techniques* is performance-based and includes Student Performance Guides which allow you to practice a procedure to become proficient before evaluation. Where appropriate, worksheets have been included for calculations and the recording of results. Care must be taken in each procedure to read and follow the instructions given in the text and any additional ones the instructor may add. All parts of the lesson must be completed before attempting to practice the procedure. If there are any questions regarding content or procedure, the instructor should be consulted.

The performance guide has been designed to allow you to practice a procedure and judge individual performance. The Student Performance Guide includes instructions, a materials and equipment list, a step-by-step procedure with a satisfactory and unsatisfactory check column and a comment section for you and the instructor to note errors or positive comments, and the date and the signature of the instructor to verify practice performance. Once you feel a specific procedure has been mastered, the instructor can observe your performance and complete the final performance evaluation.

The final evaluation is based on two components: 1) results of a written examination, and 2) completion of a final performance of the procedure using the instructor's Performance Check Sheet. The format of the final Performance Check Sheet includes the same step-by-step procedure as the Performance Guide.

By using the Student Performance Guide and the instructor's Performance Check Sheet, you will be able to achieve higher standards of performance and learn to master all steps of the procedures. Repetition of the procedures is an important requirement in the development of technique. Thus, the more you practice the methods and procedures, the more proficient you will become in terms of speed and accuracy. This also provides an opportunity for you to develop confidence in performance capabilities. You must always remember that all laboratory tests must be performed in an exacting manner and with the highest accuracy since the results submitted are relied upon by the physician in the diagnosis and prognosis of disease and in charting a course of treatment for a patient.

The authors hope that through the performance of the procedures and the completion of the lessons you will obtain much self-satisfaction in becoming knowledgeable and proficient in laboratory procedures. It is also hoped that you will come to realize the special qualities that are required of the person who works in the medical laboratory.

Norma J. Walters
Barbara H. Estridge
Anna P. Reynolds

# UNIT 1

# Introduction to the Medical Laboratory

## UNIT OBJECTIVES

After studying this unit, you should be able to:

- Discuss the organization and function of the medical laboratory.
- Discuss the qualifications and functions of medical laboratory personnel.
- List laboratory safety rules for chemical, physical, and biological hazards.
- Identify and use laboratory glassware.
- Use the compound microscope.
- Identify prefixes, stems, and suffixes in selected medical terms.
- Perform measurements and conversions using the metric system.
- Perform common laboratory mathematical calculations.

## OVERVIEW

The medical laboratory is a place where body fluids and blood specimens are tested, analyzed, or evaluated. It is where precise measurements are made and the results are calculated and interpreted. The observations may be macroscopic or microscopic. The tests may be performed manually or by using specialized instruments. Because of this, laboratory workers must have the skills needed to perform or master a variety of tasks.

This unit is an introduction to the laboratory environment as a work place. Also introduced are key procedures or concepts that a laboratory worker may need to know. This unit discusses the organization and function of the laboratory. Qualifications and job functions of laboratory personnel are also reviewed. A lesson on laboratory safety is included because anyone working in the laboratory must be thoroughly aware of potential hazards. The person must also be familiar with safety practices before any laboratory exercises can be conducted.

The care, use, and cleaning of frequently used laboratory glassware is also introduced. This includes pipets, beakers, test tubes, and flasks. The proper care and use of the microscope is also included since it is required in the bacteriology, hematology, and urinalysis units.

Since most laboratory analyses use the metric system and require some calculations, there is a brief introduction to the metric system. Simple calculations such as percentages and ratios are also presented. The principles of the metric system and laboratory mathematics which are covered in this unit will be expanded upon in Units 2 and 3. To learn the structure of medical terms, medical terminology is included in one lesson. As other units are studied, additional vocabulary terms will be introduced and defined.

Unit 1 is an introduction to the techniques, rules, and skills that are needed to perform the exercises in Units 2–6. Unit 1 may also be used alone as an introduction to the laboratory. After Unit 1 has been completed, Units 2, 4, 5, or 6 may be studied in the order of the instructor's preference. This usually depends on the availability of time, laboratory space, and equipment. Unit 3 is a sequel to Unit 2, and should be studied only after finishing Unit 2.

# LESSON 1-1

## The Medical Laboratory

### LESSON OBJECTIVES

After studying this lesson, you should be able to:

- Draw an organizational chart of a typical medical laboratory.
- List the major departments of a medical laboratory and name a test which might be performed in each department.
- List locations of non-hospital medical laboratories.
- Define the glossary terms.

### GLOSSARY

**hematology** / the science concerned with the study of blood and blood-forming tissues

**immunohematology** / blood banking; the study of blood group antigens and antibodies

**microbiology** / the scientific study of microorganisms such as bacteria

**pathologist** / a physician specially trained in the nature and cause of disease

**phlebotomist** / one trained to draw blood

## INTRODUCTION

Many medical (clinical) laboratories are located in a hospital. Others are found in clinics, group practices, public health departments, physicians' offices, and reference laboratories.

The type of laboratory facility found in a hospital depends on the hospital's size. A small hospital, under 100 beds, may have the ability to perform only very routine test procedures. More complicated or seldomly requested tests are sent out to reference laboratories. In a medium-size hospital, up to 300 beds, routine tests and some of the more complicated test procedures may be performed. Only the most recently developed tests or ones with complicated procedures need to be sent to a reference laboratory. The laboratories in most larger hospitals, over 300 beds, can handle large volumes of work and most test procedures.

## ORGANIZATION OF THE LABORATORY

Although the details may vary, the organization of most hospital laboratories follows a general outline (Figure 1–1). Usually the head of the laboratory is a **pathologist,** a physician who is specially trained in the nature and cause of disease. Directly under the pathologist's authority is the laboratory manager. This is usually someone with an education in the medical laboratory sciences and a business or management degree. In addition, some laboratories have a chief or head technologist. The heads of the various departments report to this person. The department heads are responsible for the quality and quantity of work performed. The number of major departments in laboratories varies. Chemistry, hematology, microbiology, and the blood bank usually operate as independent units, each with its own department head. The subdivisions within each department may differ from one laboratory to another.

### Chemistry

In the chemistry department, test procedures are usually performed on *serum,* the liquid part of blood left after a clot has formed. Tests may also be performed on urine. Although urine and serum are the most frequently used specimens, spinal fluid, joint fluid and other body fluids are tested also. The more commonly performed procedures in this department include blood glucose content, assays of enzymes to determine if heart damage has occurred, and the electrolytes—a set of tests which determine the chloride, bicarbonate, potassium, and sodium levels in the blood. The chemistry department usually has one or more subdivisions. One common subdivision is special chemistry. In this department, a patient's blood may be analyzed to discover what drug is involved in an overdose. The level of prescribed drugs may also be monitored.

The number of instruments available for chemistry analysis has grown rapidly in the last 20 years. Thus, it is possible for almost every laboratory to have instruments capable of performing most routine test procedures.

### Microbiology

The **microbiology** department is responsible for growing and identifying the organisms obtained from a patient's blood, urine, sputum, or wound. After the organism is grown out, susceptibility testing can be performed. Susceptibility testing involves exposing the organism to different antibiotics. This helps to determine which antibiotic is most effective against the organism. The microbiology department usually deals with bacteria and fungi. Many hospital laboratories also test for tuberculosis.

The parasitology laboratory is often included as a part of the microbiology department. This department examines patient specimens for parasites. The patient's blood may be examined for evidence of the blood parasite which causes malaria. Or, the stools may be examined for evidence of intestinal parasites such as tapeworms or hookworms.

The microbiology department has been where procedures were performed manually. However, that is rapidly changing. Automated systems are now widely used. These systems can identify the organism and determine which antibiotic would be most effective in treating an infection.

### Hematology

In the **hematology** laboratory, whole blood is used for the majority of test procedures. Hematology procedures can be qualitative or quantitative. The quantitative procedures include actual counts of the various blood components. For example, the number of leukocytes (white blood cells), erythrocytes (red blood cells), and platelets in a blood sample can be determined. All of these counts can now be performed using automated systems. The qualitative procedures are ones in which the various blood components are observed for qualities such as cell size,

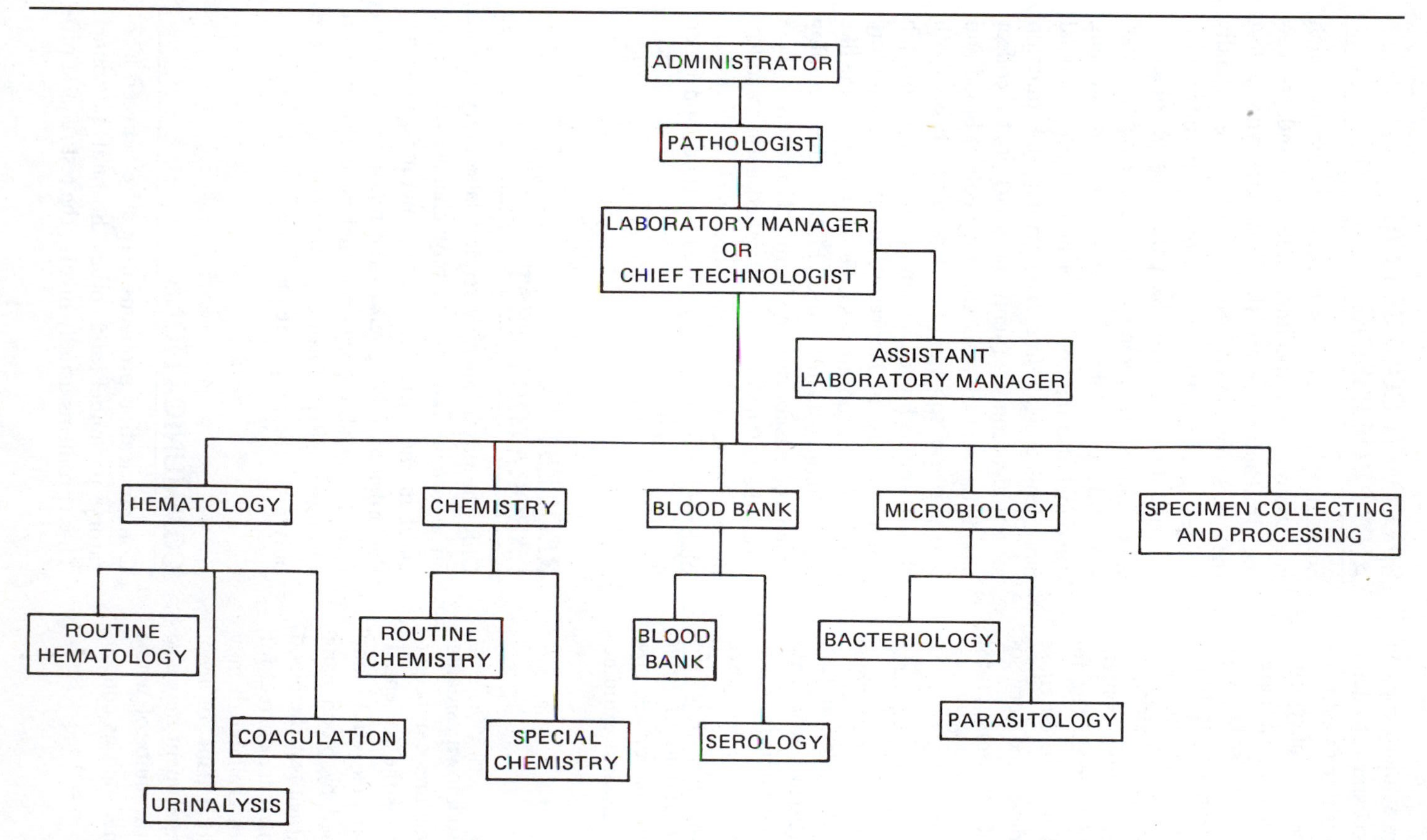


**Figure 1-1.** Organizational chart of a typical medical laboratory

shape, and maturity level. Using a microscope, a laboratory worker can view a blood smear to determine the types of leukocytes present or to estimate the size, shape, and hemoglobin content of erythrocytes. The number of platelets can also be estimated. The presence of any abnormalities can also be noted during the microscopic examination of the blood smear. This may include identifying immature leukocytes or erythrocytes. The microhematocrit, the blood indices, and the blood hemoglobin content are additional tests commonly performed. The results of these three tests can be used to diagnose anemias. Some companies have developed very sophisticated instruments capable of performing most or all of the routine hematology procedures.

***Coagulation and Urinalysis.*** In some laboratories, coagulation tests and urinalyses are also performed in the hematology department. Coagulation tests help to diagnose and monitor patients who have defects in their blood clotting mechanism. Automated systems for coagulation tests have been used for several years. Urinalysis includes physical, chemical, and microscopic examinations of urine specimens. Several methods of automation are now being used for the physical and chemical examination of urine.

### Blood Bank

The blood bank department is also known as **immunohematology.** Here, several procedures can be performed, depending on the needs of the patient. If a transfusion is required, the patient's ABO blood type and Rh type are determined by blood bank technologists. The technologists then test the blood units in storage to determine which are correct for the patient. If suitable blood is not available, it may be obtained from a regional blood bank or from blood donors. The blood bank department may also have the capability to process the units of whole blood into specialized components such as concentrated red blood cells.

## SPECIMEN COLLECTING AND PROCESSING

Some hospitals have a separate department which is responsible for specimen collecting and processing. **Phlebotomists** are the personnel who collect the necessary blood specimen. They are specially trained to efficiently obtain a blood specimen with as little discomfort to the patient as possible. In other laboratories, some or all of the regular staff share this responsibility. In some instances, nursing personnel also may be responsible for all or partial blood collecting. (Note: The primary job function of a phlebotomist (venipuncturist) is to collect blood. Laboratory assistants may collect blood and also perform some routine laboratory tasks, both clerical and technical. Technologists can do any job a phlebotomist or laboratory assistant can do and much more. Laboratories differ in policy—some like for technologists to collect blood, others employ phlebotomists for most collecting. However, in these cases, the technologist is still called upon to collect the specimens which require special skills or responsibility, for example Ivy bleeding time, and blood for cross match.)

## REQUESTING A LABORATORY TEST

Only the physician may request laboratory testing on a patient. Usually the physician writes the request in the patient's chart. Sometimes, however, the order may be given to the registered nurse to record. The laboratory personnel can collect a blood specimen and perform a particular test procedure only after the proper request has been received.

## COMMUNICATIONS

Communication problems may arise between laboratory personnel and other hospital personnel. These problems usually involve the test request procedure and/or the delivery of the test results to the physicians. Following the health agency's procedure manual will eliminate many of these problems. All laboratory personnel must strive to perform the test procedures as efficiently and accurately as possible. They must insure that emergency requests are treated as such and that the test results are reported as soon as possible. Likewise, other departments in the hospital must realize that only a physician can designate a test as "stat." This means there is an emergency and the test must be performed immediately. Other hospital personnel must carry out their responsibilities to see that test requests and specimens are transported to the laboratory as quickly as possible. A breakdown in communication causes stress and bad feelings among all personnel involved. Health care employees must remember that the welfare of the patient is of uppermost importance.

## NON-HOSPITAL MEDICAL LABORATORIES

Non-hospital medical laboratories may be associated with a group practice, such as internal medicine specialists. These laboratories may also be located in the office of a physician who has a specialty such as hematology. A physician with a general practice may have laboratory facilities to perform some of the more routine procedures. State Public Health Departments may have medical laboratory facilities; these laboratories perform a variety of medical tests such as those for venereal and viral diseases. Additional procedures can include tests for water and milk purity.

*Reference laboratories* are regional laboratories which do high volume testing and offer a wide variety of procedures. Large hospitals use reference laboratories primarily to perform complicated or seldom-ordered tests. Small hospitals or doctors' offices may use them for a wide range of tests.

A recent development is the walk-in medical facility, usually located near shopping centers. Routine laboratory procedures such as blood counts, throat cultures, and urine tests are performed in these offices. As a greater number of patients use these facilities, the laboratories in these facilities will grow and new or additional tests will be added as necessary.

## *LESSON REVIEW*

1. Draw an organizational chart of a typical medical laboratory.
2. Name five major departments a hospital medical laboratory might have.
3. Name two procedures which are performed in a hematology department.
4. Name one procedure performed in the chemistry department.
5. Why is cooperation between laboratory personnel and other hospital personnel so important?
6. List three locations of medical laboratory facilities other than in a hospital.
7. Define hematology, immunohematology, microbiology, pathologist, and phlebotomist.

## *STUDENT ACTIVITIES*

1. Re-read the information on the medical laboratory.
2. Review the glossary terms.
3. Interview an employee of a medical laboratory in a health agency. Inquire about the organization of the laboratory and the types of tests which are performed. Obtain various laboratory test report forms.

# LESSON 1-2

## The Medical Laboratory Professional

### LESSON OBJECTIVES

After studying this lesson, you should be able to:

- Give a brief history of medical technology.
- List five qualities which are desirable in a medical laboratory professional.
- Describe the educational requirements for medical technologists and medical laboratory technicians.
- Discuss the relationship between laboratory personnel and the patient.
- Name five areas of employment for laboratory personnel other than in a hospital laboratory.
- Define the glossary terms.

### GLOSSARY

**certified medical laboratory technician** / a professional who has completed a minimum of two years of specific training in an accredited program, consisting of one year of college and one year of clinical training, and has passed a national certifying examination

**certified medical technologist** / a professional who has a bachelor's degree from an accredited college or university, has completed one year of clinical training, and has passed a national certifying examination

**medical technology** / the health profession concerned with the performance of laboratory analyses used in the diagnosis and treatment of disease as well as in health maintenance

## MEDICAL TECHNOLOGY

**Medical technology** is the health profession concerned with performing laboratory analyses. The analyses are used to diagnose and treat disease as well as maintain good health. The tests are performed by trained, skilled medical technologists and technicians, or by other medical laboratory or allied health personnel. The laboratory tests are standardized and controlled. This insures reliable and accurate results.

## History of Medical Technology

Medical technology can be traced back several centuries. Papyrus writings dated before 1000 B.C. record descriptions of intestinal parasites. Such is an early example of parasitology. Before medieval times, Hindu doctors performed crude urinalyses when they observed that some urines had a sweet taste and attracted ants. With the invention and improvement of the microscope in the seventeenth century, the study of biological specimens progressed from simple visual examination to microscopic examination.

The first clinical laboratories in the United States appeared in the late nineteenth century and were very crude. Some consisted of only a table and a microscope. They were staffed mostly by doctors who showed special interest in "laboratory medicine." The U.S. census of 1900 listed only one hundred laboratory technicians, all male.

After World War I, laboratories grew in size and in number. This is when schools to train laboratory workers were organized. Since World War II, the technology for laboratory testing has become more complex. At that time, laboratory tests began to play an important role in medicine. Today's technology allows us to provide a level of health care which was only imagined a few years ago.

Presently, there are thousands of medical laboratories, both large and small. Laboratories are highly sophisticated and offer many complex tests. The technologists and technicians staffing these laboratories are highly skilled professionals who perform complicated analyses. They may also serve as laboratory managers, teachers, supervisors, and administrators.

## Educational Requirements for Medical Laboratory Professionals

Soon after the emergence of medical laboratories, it was clear that there was a need for (1) educating laboratory workers, (2) defining educational requirements, and (3) identifying adequately trained persons. By the 1930s, schools of medical technology were training laboratory workers and basic educational requirements were established. At that time, certifying examinations were being given to measure the knowledge and ability of workers. Trained workers now comprise most of the work force in the medical laboratory. The two most common levels of professionals in the medical laboratory are the technician and the technologist.

*Medical Laboratory Technician.* The **medical laboratory technician** is a worker who has two years of training after high school—one year of college and one year of clinical training. After the clinical training has been completed satisfactorily, the worker takes a national certifying examination. Upon receiving satisfactory scores on the exam, the medical laboratory technician is certified.

*Medical Technologist.* The **medical technologist** is a laboratory worker who has a bachelor's degree from a college or university and one year of clinical training. To become a certified medical technologist, the individual must also pass one of the national certifying exams for medical technologists. These examinations are administered by agencies such as the American Society of Clinical Pathologists (ASCP), the National Certification Agency for Medical Laboratory Personnel (NCAMLP), the American Medical Technologists (AMT) and the International Society for Clinical Laboratory Technology (ISCLT). Certified medical technologists are qualified to perform analyses in all departments of the laboratory. These individuals may be supervisors or department heads. They may also work in other leadership positions in the laboratory.

## Areas of Specialization

Some laboratory workers may specialize in one area of laboratory work such as chemistry or microbiology. Usually, these workers have a four-year degree in the area of specialization and are certified by examination in the specialty area. Laboratories may also employ laboratory assistants and phlebotomists, or venipuncturists, who are responsible for collecting blood specimens.

Laboratory managers oversee the day-to-day management of the laboratory. They are usually medical technologists who have some additional educational training in business, management, or other health-related field. With the increasing cost of health care and the emphasis on cost containment, efficient medical laboratory management is becoming more important.

## Qualities of Laboratory Workers

Dedication, cooperation, neatness, and a caring attitude are essential qualities of the health care professional. In addition, there are special characteristics needed in persons performing laboratory analyses. The workers in each department need to be knowledgeable of the procedures performed in that department. They must be able to perform accurate, precise manipulations and calculations. Communication skills, reliability, honesty, and the ability to relate well to fellow workers are important qualities for laboratory workers. Organizational skills must also be developed. To function professionally in any laboratory, the personnel must learn how to prioritize laboratory requests and schedules.

## Responsibilities of Laboratory Workers

Set rules and regulations govern health care in all states. Most health care agencies have very specific standards, rules, and regulations governing the responsibilities of various health care employees. Each health care worker should assume the responsibility of learning exactly what activities are allowed in their position. They should understand their job responsibilities fully for their protection, the protection of their employer, and the safety of the patient.

## The Patient and the Laboratory Professional

The field of medical technology exists for the patient, as do all other fields of health care. In order for a patient to receive the best possible care, a physician must make the proper diagnosis. To make this diagnosis, the physicians rely on laboratory analyses along with information gained from the medical history, physical examination and clinical symptoms. For this reason, it is important that the laboratory analyses are performed carefully and accurately, using the best techniques available.

The only contact patients may have with the laboratory is through the lab assistant, technologist, or phlebotomist who collects a blood sample from them for testing. At best, it is not pleasant to have blood taken from a vein or finger. At all times, the technologist needs to be aware of the stress the patient is feeling when hospitalized. The technologist must be professional, courteous, and considerate when obtaining the specimen.

## Professionalism

Laboratory workers should consider themselves health care professionals and should conduct themselves ethically. Patient information is confidential. It should only be discussed with health care workers who are directly related to the case and who have a need to know. Test results should not be discussed with the patients, their relatives, or other inappropriate persons. The results should be reported only to the physician or other appropriate designated employee.

## Professional Organizations

Laboratory personnel usually have a choice of membership in one or more professional societies. These societies provide opportunities for professional growth and continuing education by offering workshops and seminars, and by publishing journals. Membership in a national society usually also includes membership in the state affiliate. It is important for all laboratory professionals to be active in one or more of these organizations.

## Licensing

Although certification is usually sufficient to meet most employment requirements, some states regulate laboratory personnel by requiring state licensure. Licensing laws vary from state to state and are nonexistent in some. The state may require a fee to obtain a license, or it may require that a test be taken before the license is issued; many states require both.

## Employment Opportunities

There are many employment opportunities for medical laboratory workers. Most of the nation's laboratory workers are employed in hospitals. However, some are employed in public health agencies, reference laboratories, the military, research, veterinary medicine, and in sales or product development for medical suppliers.

## *LESSON REVIEW*

1. What is medical technology?
2. Describe the beginnings of medical technology.
3. What educational requirements are required for medical technologists—for medical technicians?
4. List five qualities that a laboratory worker should possess.
5. What is the obligation of the medical laboratory professional to the patient?
6. List five places of employment for laboratory personnel other than in hospitals.
7. Define certified medical laboratory technician, certified medical technologist, and medical technology.

## *STUDENT ACTIVITIES*

1. Re-read the information on the medical laboratory professional.
2. Review the glossary terms.
3. Complete a Career Information Fact Sheet on the medical laboratory technician and the medical laboratory technologist. This should include the educational training, cost of program, nature of job, advantages and disadvantages, employment opportunities, and salary range of the occupation.
4. Interview a laboratory worker using the fact sheet format provided by the instructor. Be sure to consider the following areas: his or her job functions, relationships with co-workers and patients, advantages and disadvantages, satisfactions, dissatisfactions, salary range, and opportunities for advancement with appropriate educational training. Describe the benefits of talking to the laboratory worker in person rather than reading the information in a book.

# Career Information Fact Sheet

NAME ______________________________ DATE __________

## LESSON 1–2 THE MEDICAL LABORATORY PROFESSIONAL

Title:

Legal Requirement:

Length of Program:

Educational Institution:

Cost of Program:

Admission Requirements:

Nature of the Job:

Earnings:

Advancement:

Related Occupation(s):

Advantages:

Disadvantages:

# Interview Fact Sheet

NAME ______________________________ DATE ______________

## LESSON 1–2 THE MEDICAL LABORATORY PROFESSIONAL

Title of Career:

Educational Preparation:

Approximate Cost of Education Program:

Job Functions:

Approximate Salary:

Job Satisfaction:

Job Dissatisfaction:

Opportunities for Advancement:

Options Available to Broaden Employment Opportunities:

# LESSON 1-3

## Laboratory Safety

### LESSON OBJECTIVES

After studying this lesson, you should be able to:

- Identify the three major types of laboratory hazards.
- Give an example of each type of hazard.
- List one way to prevent or correct each type of hazard.
- List thirteen basic rules of laboratory safety.
- Define the glossary terms.

### GLOSSARY

**acid** / a substance which liberates hydrogen ions in solution; turns litmus paper red

**autoclave** / a device for sterilization by steam pressure

**base** / a substance which accepts hydrogen ions; turns litmus paper blue

**carcinogenic** / having the ability to produce or cause cancer

**fume hood** / a device which draws contaminated air out of an area and either cleanses and recirculates it or discharges it to the outside

## INTRODUCTION

To avoid injury to anyone in the laboratory and to prevent equipment damage, certain basic safety rules must be observed. Before any laboratory procedures are performed, the laboratory supervisor should explain the safety rules. The supervisor should require the worker to sign a safety agreement form (Appendix A). There are constant hazards in most laboratories, regardless of the type of work being performed. Any accidents which may occur must be reported immediately to the laboratory supervisor. The hazards in a medical or clinical laboratory can be classified as either physical, chemical, or biological.

## PHYSICAL HAZARDS

Physical hazards may be present in what is thought of as ordinary equipment or surroundings. Electrical equipment is one major source of physical hazards. All electrical equipment must be properly grounded following the manufacturer's instructions. When even minor repair is undertaken, such as replacing a bulb in a microscope, the electrical supply must be disconnected before work is begun. All electrical cords and plugs must be kept in good repair. There must be no frayed cords or exposed wires.

Fire is another danger in the laboratory. Everyone working in the laboratory should know the location of the fire extinguisher. They must also know the fire escape route and how to use the fire extinguishers properly. A fire blanket should also be readily available. If Bunsen burners or other open flames are used, care must be taken to insure that loose clothing and long hair do not catch fire.

All equipment must be used only as the instructions dictate. Any equipment with moving parts must be used with care. A centrifuge lid should not be opened until the centrifuge has completely stopped. **Autoclaves,** which use pressurized steam to sterilize materials, present special laboratory hazards. Instructions for their use should be followed carefully.

## CHEMICAL HAZARDS

Chemicals may cause burns, or may be poisonous or **carcinogenic.** Some of the chemicals used in laboratory work are strong **acids** or **bases** which are capable of causing severe skin burns. They must be used with great caution to avoid splashes which could damage the eyes or burn the skin. Any chemicals which contact the skin should be washed off immediately with water for approximately five minutes unless the label says otherwise. Many suppliers now label their chemical containers with information listing the hazards the chemical presents, the procedure to follow if an accident occurs, and the proper storage and disposal of the chemical. Toxic fumes are produced by some laboratory chemicals and these should be used only in a **fume hood.**

Chemicals should be disposed of properly. Some laboratory chemicals can be safely poured into the sink, followed by lots of water. However, it is very important that explicit directions are provided and followed for the disposal of each chemical. Some chemicals may require special disposal by toxic waste personnel.

Mouth pipetting can be very dangerous. In most laboratories, mouth pipetting is not allowed. Generally, safety bulbs must be used. These are available in various sizes and types. If mouth pipetting is necessary, special filters are available which can be placed on the mouthpiece of the pipet.

## BIOLOGICAL HAZARDS

Biological specimens and reagents present a special problem because they may contain agents which are potentially harmful but are not readily evident. Commercial plasmas, sera, and other reagents derived from blood products may be capable of transmitting hepatitis. The blood-derived reagents are screened for evidence of the agent by the manufacturer. However, a negative result does not guarantee that the reagent cannot transmit hepatitis.

The laboratory work area should be disinfected before and after each use. An appropriate solution might include a 10% solution of chlorine bleach or a good commercial disinfectant such as Amphyll®. Eating, drinking, or smoking should not be allowed in the laboratory. Mouth pipetting of biological specimens is not allowed. Plastic gloves should be worn if there are cuts or open wounds on the hands. A laboratory coat or apron is recommended to prevent contamination of the clothing by microorganisms or stains.

The bacteriology laboratory presents additional hazards and special precautions are necessary. All organisms must be handled as if they can cause disease.

Biological specimens and any contaminated articles such as used lancets and tubes must be placed in special biohazard bags or containers. These must be disposed of by incineration or sterilized by autoclave before disposal.

Hands must be washed before and after each procedure using biological materials. Easily obtainable disinfectants for the hands are Hibiclens® by Stuart Pharmaceuticals or a dilute solution of tincture of green soap. Both can be purchased at medical supply and drug stores.

## LABORATORY CLOTHING

It is important that proper clothing be worn when working in the laboratory. This includes a laboratory coat, jacket, or apron to protect clothing and skin from chemicals, stains, and biological specimens. If strong chemicals are being handled, laboratory safety glasses should be worn. Long hair should be pinned back to prevent contact with open flames or equipment with moving parts. Loose jewelry, such as long chains and bracelets, may get caught in equipment and should not be worn. Shoes should be comfortable. They should have a closed toe to protect feet from spills or broken glass.

## LABORATORY RULES

Although there are many hazards present in the laboratory, it is possible for the laboratory to be a safe environment for all workers. Each worker must make it his or her responsibility to observe all safety rules, whether or not they are posted. The laboratory can provide a safe, pleasant environment for all concerned.

No set of rules can cover all the hazards that may be present in a laboratory setting. Also, nothing can replace the use of good common sense. However, there are several good, general principles which should always be observed:

1. Avoid eating, drinking, smoking, or gum chewing.
2. Wear a laboratory jacket or coat.
3. Pin long hair away from face and neck to avoid contact with chemicals, equipment, or flames.
4. Wear closed-toe shoes.
5. Avoid wearing chains, bracelets, rings, or other loose, hanging jewelry.
6. Use gloves if cuts or open sores are present on hands.
7. Clean work area properly before beginning laboratory procedures and at the end of each period.
8. Wash hands before and after laboratory procedures and any other time that it is necessary.
9. Wipe up spills promptly and appropriately.
10. Follow manufacturer's instructions for operating equipment.
11. Handle equipment with care.
12. Store equipment properly.
13. Report any accident to the instructor immediately.
14. Refrain from horseplay.
15. Allow visitors only in nonwork area of the laboratory.

## *LESSON REVIEW*

1. Name the three classifications of laboratory hazards.
2. Give an example of each type of hazard and how it might be prevented or corrected.
3. Why must safety rules be strictly observed?
4. What is the major hazard present when blood or blood-derived products are used?
5. What precaution is taken by the manufacturers of blood-derived products to protect laboratory workers?
6. What should be done if an accident occurs in the laboratory?
7. Define acid, autoclave, base, carcinogenic, and fume hood.

## *STUDENT ACTIVITIES*

1. Re-read the information on laboratory safety.
2. Review the glossary terms.
3. Make a poster warning of a laboratory hazard or listing basic safety rules.
4. Make a safety check of the laboratory. Check for frayed cords, exposed wires, fire extinguishers, safety posters, etc.
5. Inspect the chemicals present in the laboratory. Note the procedure to follow for storage and disposal. Note procedure to follow in case of skin contact or chemical spill.
6. Practice the laboratory procedure for fire and the use of fire extinguishers; learn the fire escape route.

# LESSON 1-4
## Laboratory Glassware

### LESSON OBJECTIVES

After studying this lesson, you should be able to:

- Identify five basic types of glassware used in the laboratory and explain one use of each.
- Identify two types of pipets and explain one use of each.
- Describe the proper care and cleaning procedures for laboratory glassware.
- List precautions to be observed in the use of laboratory glassware.
- Define the glossary terms.

### GLOSSARY

**critical measurements** / measurements made when accuracy of the concentration of a solution is important; measurements made using glassware which is manufactured to strict standards

**meniscus** / the curved surface of a liquid in a container

**noncritical measurements** / measurements which are estimated; measurements made in containers (such as the Erlenmeyer flask) which estimate volume

**reagents** / substances which are used in laboratory analyses

**solute** / a liquid, gas, or solid which is dissolved in a liquid to make a solution

**solvent** / that liquid into which the solute is dissolved

**TC** / to contain

**TD** / to deliver

## INTRODUCTION

The use of laboratory glassware is necessary to perform many laboratory procedures. The glassware may be used in a specific procedure or in the preparation of **reagents** for a test. Basic laboratory glassware consists of beakers, flasks, pipets, test tubes, and graduated cylinders.

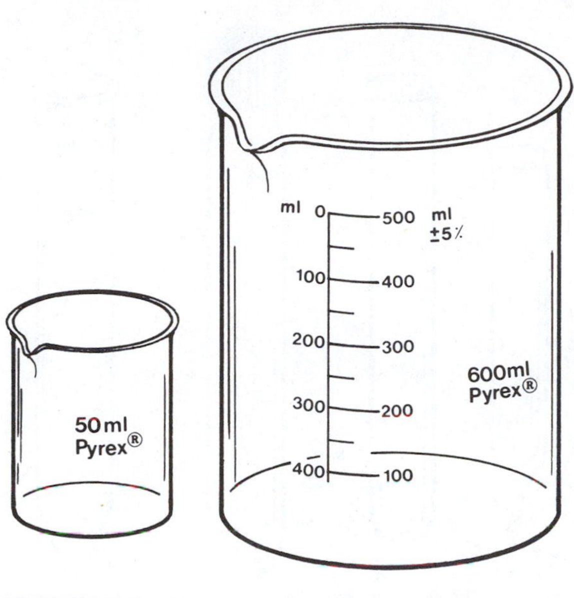


Figure 1-2. Beakers with markings

## Beakers

Beakers are wide-mouthed, straight-sided jars which have a pouring spout formed out of the rim (Figure 1–2). They are useful for estimating the amount of liquids or mixing solutions, or for simply holding liquids. On the side of each beaker are markings. These indicate the total capacity in milliliters (ml). Many beakers have additional markings to indicate volume increments of 50 ml to 100 ml. Beakers have many functions in a laboratory, but they must not be used when **critical measurements** are needed.

## Flasks

Three commonly used flasks are the Erlenmeyer, Florence, and volumetric flasks (Figure 1–3). The Erlenmeyer flask has a flat bottom and sloping sides which gradually narrow in diameter so that the top

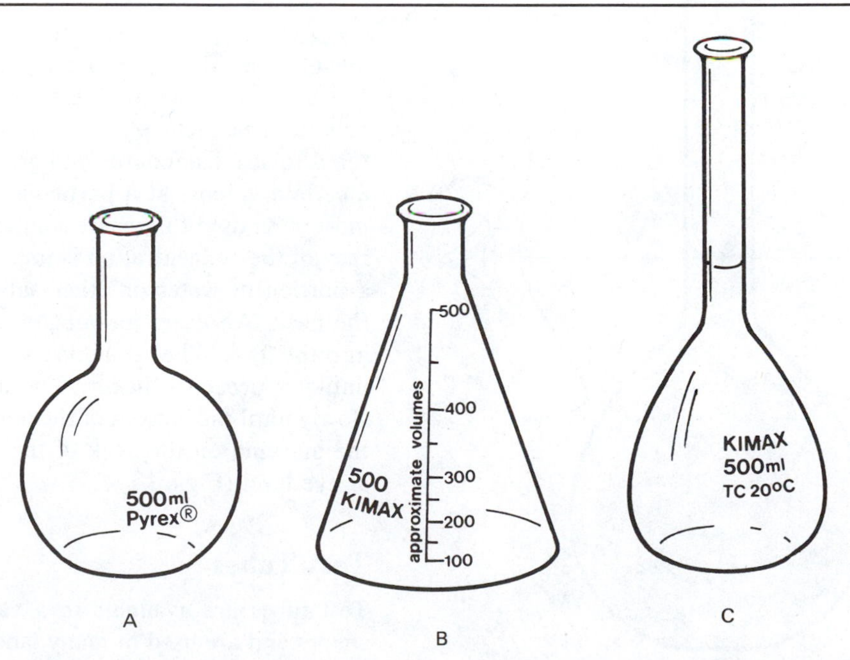


Figure 1-3. Flasks A) Florence flask, B) Erlenmeyer flask, and C) Volumetric flask

opening is bottle-like. The opening may be plain, to be stoppered with a cork, or it may have threads for a cap. Erlenmeyer flasks range from 50 ml capacity to 2000 ml capacity. They may be used to hold liquids, to mix solutions, or to measure **noncritical** volumes. Markings on the side indicate the total capacity in mls. In addition, some also have 50 ml to 100 ml increment marks. These are called *graduated flasks* and are convenient for estimating volumes. However, they should not be used for making critical measurements.

The Florence flask has a flat bottom and rounded sides which give rise to a long cylindrical neck. The only markings are the total capacity in milliliters. These flasks usually range in size from the 50 ml to the 2000 ml capacity. The uses of the Florence flask are similar to those of beakers and Erlenmeyer flasks. Only noncritical measurements are made in a Florence flask.

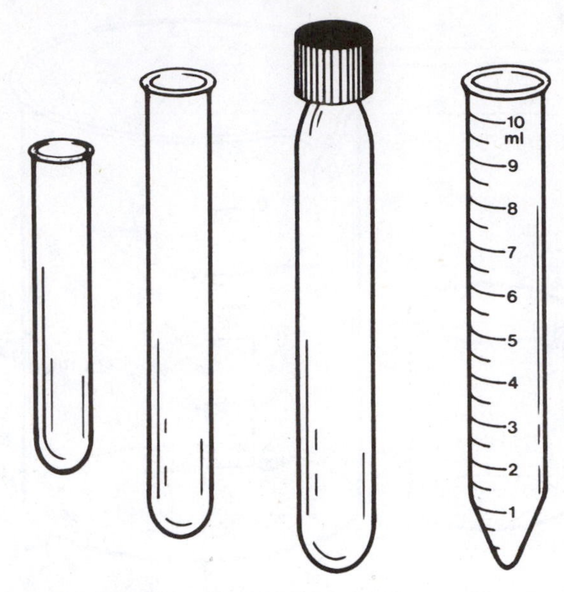

**Figure 1-5.** Test tubes

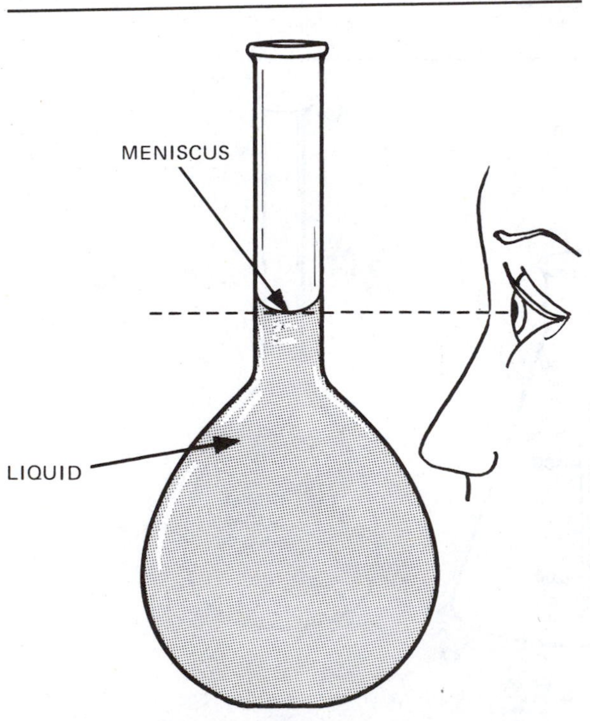

**Figure 1-4.** Meniscus

The volumetric flask is the one to be used when volume measurements are critical. It is manufactured to strict standards and guaranteed to contain a certain volume at a particular temperature. It is most often used to prepare solutions when the accuracy of the concentration is important. When used, a portion of water or other **solvent** is placed into the flask. An exact amount of **solute** is measured into the flask. The remaining solvent is then added until it approaches the line. The last portion is added slowly until the bottom of the **meniscus** is level with the marking on the neck of the flask when viewed at eye level (Figure 1–4).

## Test Tubes

Test tubes are available in a variety of sizes and shapes and are used in many laboratory procedures (Figure 1–5). They may function as containers for liquid samples such as blood, urine, or serum. In

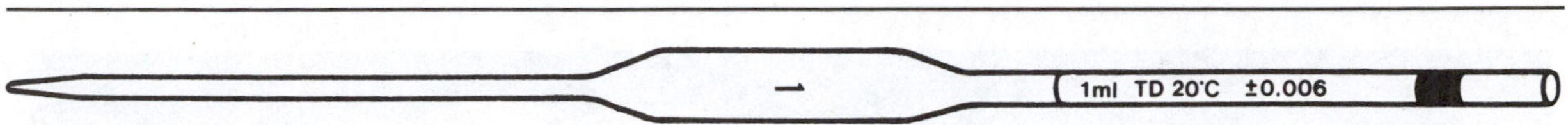


**Figure 1-6.** Volumetric pipet

some procedures, the reaction may take place in the test tube itself. Sometimes a test method requires that the contents be heated in the test tube. This should be done with caution after checking to insure that the test tube is made of heat-resistant glass.

## Pipets

Pipets are used often in laboratory work to measure and transfer liquids. There are two basic types of pipets, volumetric or transfer (Figure 1–6) and graduated or measuring (Figure 1–7). Volumetric pipets are tubes with a mouthpiece on one end, a round or oval bulb in the center, and a tapered tip on the other end. These are usually labeled **TD** which indicates that they are manufactured to deliver a specified volume of liquid in a certain time period. They are used whenever the accuracy of a transferred volume is critical. To use a volumetric pipet, a pipet bulb is attached to the mouthpiece. The liquid is suctioned up into the pipet to the marking on the stem above the center bulb. The outside of the pipet stem is wiped dry with tissue. The pipet is held nearly vertical, and the tip is placed on the surface of the container into which the liquid is to be transferred. The suction is released and the liquid is allowed to flow into the container. The tip is left in contact with the container surface a few seconds to completely drain the pipet. (A small drop will remain in the pipet tip.)

Graduated pipets are long tubes with a total capacity marking near the mouthpiece. Graduated pipets are usually labeled TD. They may have a frosted band around the top indicating that the last drop of liquid is blown out after the contents are drained. Pipets without a frosted band (non blow-out) are used as described in volumetric pipets. Graduated pipets are graduated to the tip with markings indicating uniform increments. One commonly used graduated pipet is the serological pipet. Graduated pipets may be used to transfer their total capacity or a partial volume. To use a serological pipet, a pipet bulb is attached. The liquid is suctioned up to the line as for the volumetric pipet. The outside stem of the pipet is wiped dry with tissue. To deliver the total volume from the pipet, the liquid is allowed to drain out while the pipet is held almost vertically. The last remaining drops are forced out by using the bulb.

In laboratory work, it is often necessary to accurately measure or transfer very small volumes. Micropipets, which can be calibrated for 0.5 ml or less, are available for this purpose (Figure 1–8). Micropipets may be of a semi-automated type. These can be pre-set to draw up and dispense a specific volume. They may also be of the manual type in which the sample is drawn up to a certain mark. An example is the Sahli pipet (0.02 ml) which is used for hemoglobin determinations. Micropipets are often labeled **TC** (to contain). This means that they must be rinsed in order to dispense the stated volume of the pipet.

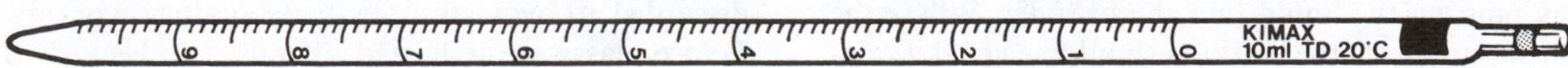

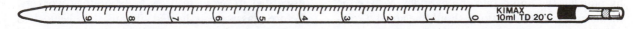

**Figure 1-7.** Serological pipet

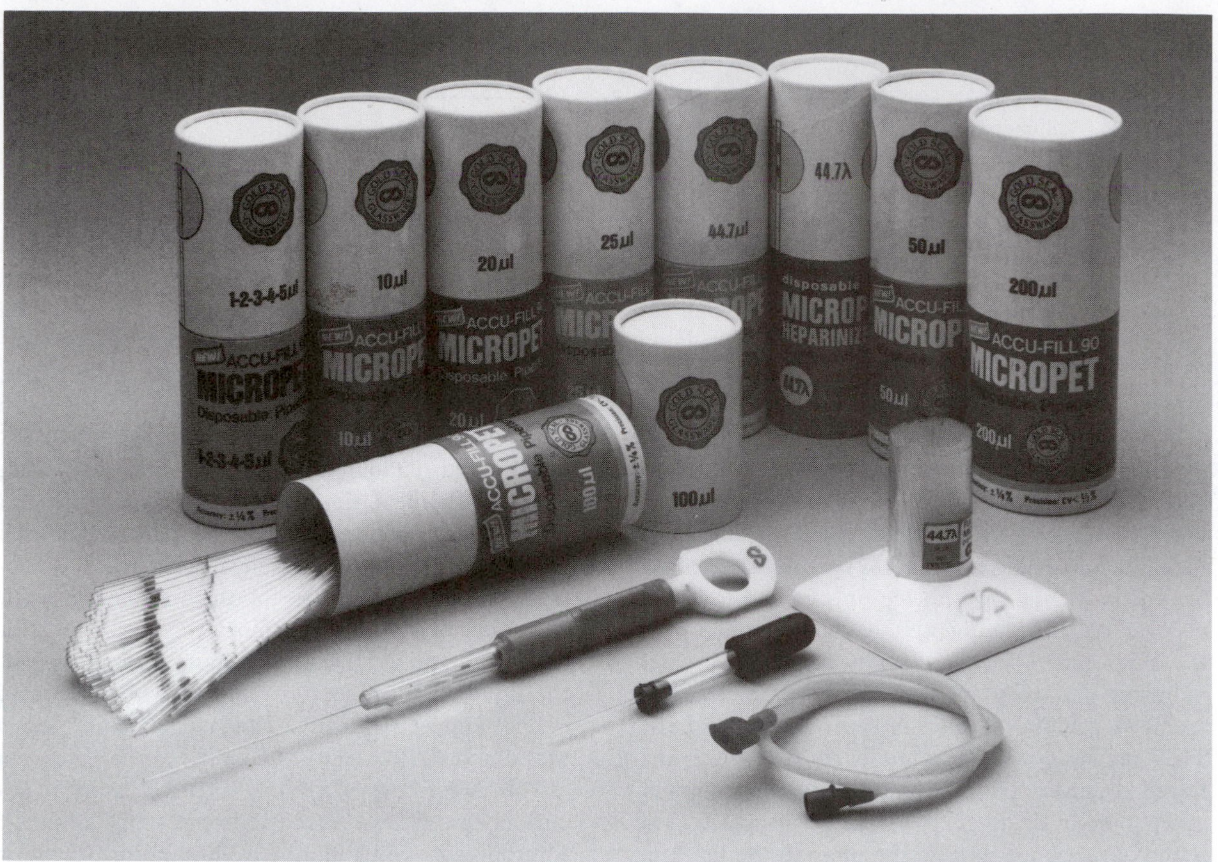


**Figure 1-8.** Micropipets (*Photo courtesy of Becton Dickinson & Co.*)

## Graduated Cylinders

Graduated cylinders are upright, straight-sided tubes with a flared base to provide stability. They are used in the laboratory to make noncritical volume measures (Figure 1–9). In size they range from 10 ml to 2000 ml capacity. Markings on the side indicate the total capacity and various increments in ml. Liquids are measured in a graduated cylinder by pouring the liquid into the cylinder. Where the meniscus meets the marking should be noted. Graduated cylinders are commonly used to measure the volume of 24-hour urines.

## CARE AND CLEANING OF GLASSWARE

Good quality laboratory glassware is expensive and must be handled with care. Glassware should be stored in a place which offers protection from dust and accidental breakage. Pipets with tips which have been chipped or broken are no longer accurate. Glassware which is chipped or cracked should be discarded to avoid injuries to laboratory workers. Before glassware is heated, it must be checked to insure that it is heat-resistant. Pyrex® and Kimax® are two types of heat-resistant glassware.

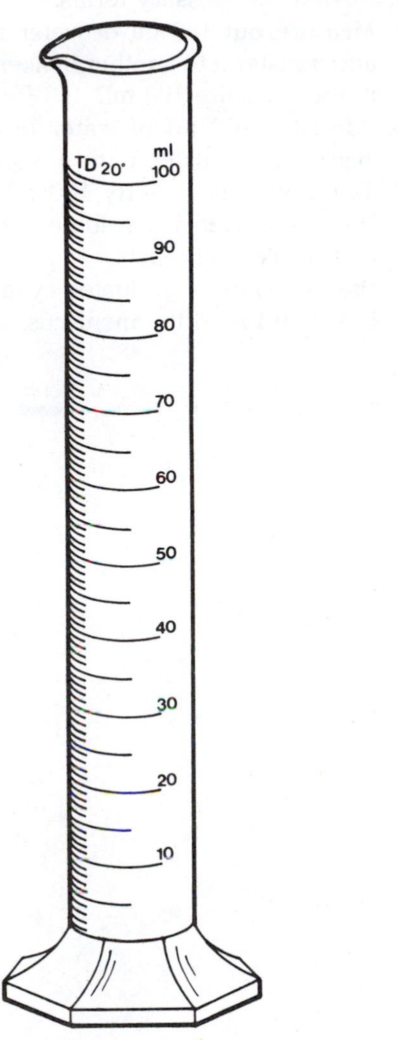


**Figure 1-9.** Graduated cylinder with markings

Glassware should be washed in a good laboratory detergent and rinsed thoroughly. Residues of detergent left in glassware are detrimental to laboratory results. A tap-water rinse followed by a distilled-water rinse is sufficient in most instances. However, rinsing up to twelve times with distilled water is required for some glassware used in delicate procedures.

Stubborn deposits can usually be removed by soaking the glassware in laboratory detergent overnight. More persistent problems may require the use of an acid cleaning solution. This can be a dangerous procedure and must not be attempted by a student. The majority of cleaning problems can be avoided if glassware is rinsed with water immediately after it is used. If liquids are allowed to dry in the glassware, cleaning is difficult. Larger pieces of glassware may be inverted and allowed to air dry. Smaller pieces, such as pipets and test tubes, are dried by placing them inverted into a drying oven.

### *Precautions*

- Insure that the correct glassware is being used for the task.
- Check pipets for broken or chipped tips.
- Check beakers, flasks, and cylinders for chips and cracks to avoid cuts and other injuries.
- Rinse glassware with water after use.
- Always use a clean pipet for each measurement.
- Use clean glassware for measurements.

## *LESSON REVIEW*

1. Name three types of laboratory flasks.
2. Name three pieces of glassware which may be used to hold liquids.
3. Which pieces of glassware are used to make critical volume measurements?
4. Do broken pipet tips affect the accuracy of the pipet?
5. Name two types of pipets and explain the differences in them.
6. The last drop is forced out of which type pipet?
7. Why is immediate rinsing of glassware important after use?

8. Why must glassware be handled with care?
9. Why is it important that glassware be rinsed free of detergent?
10. What is the major use for volumetric flasks?
11. Define critical measurement, meniscus, non-critical measurement, reagents, solute, solvent, TC, and TD.

## *STUDENT ACTIVITIES*

1. Re-read the information on laboratory glassware.
2. Review the glossary terms.
3. Measure out 100 ml of water in one beaker and transfer it to another beaker or flask. Does it also measure 100 ml?
4. Measure 100 ml of water in a Erlenmeyer flask and transfer it to a volumetric flask. Is the volume exactly 100 ml?
5. Practice dispensing volumes from volumetric and serological pipets.
6. Practice filling a graduated cylinder to various levels and read the meniscus.

# LESSON 1–5

## The Microscope

### LESSON OBJECTIVES

After studying this lesson, you should be able to:

- Locate and name the parts of a microscope and explain the function of each.
- Explain the use of the coarse and fine adjustments.
- Use the low power objective to view an object.
- Use the high power objective to view an object.
- Use the oil immersion objective to view an object.
- Adjust the condenser and diaphragm.
- Clean the oculars and objectives.
- Explain the proper care and storage of the microscope.
- Define the glossary terms.

### GLOSSARY

**binocular** / having two oculars or eyepieces

**coarse adjustment** / adjusts position of microscope objectives; used to initially bring objects into focus

**condenser** / apparatus located below the microscope stage which directs light into the objective

**eyepiece** / ocular

**fine adjustment** / adjusts position of microscope objectives; used to sharpen focus

**iris diaphragm** / regulates the amount of light which strikes the object being viewed through the microscope

**lens** / a transparent material curved on one or both sides which spreads or focuses light

**lens paper** / a special nonabrasive material used to clean optical lenses

**microscope arm** / the portion of the microscope which connects the lenses to the base

**microscope base** / the portion of the microscope which rests on the table and supports the instrument
**monocular** / having one ocular
**nosepiece** / revolving unit to which microscope objectives are attached
**objective** / magnifying lens which is closest to the object being viewed with a microscope
**ocular** / eyepiece of the microscope; contains a magnifying lens
**stage** / platform on which object to be viewed microscopically is placed
**working distance** / distance between the microscope objective and the slide when the object is in sharp focus

## INTRODUCTION

The microscope is an indispensable instrument which is used in many laboratory departments. By using the microscope, it is possible to view structures or cells which are too small to be seen with the naked eyes. The microscope is used to evaluate stained blood smears and tissue sections, perform cell counts, examine urine sediment, observe cellular reactions, and observe and interpret smears containing microorganisms.

The microscopist must be skilled in using the microscope if maximum information is to be gained from studying prepared slides. Because the microscope is a delicate, expensive instrument, special care must be taken in its use, cleaning, and storage.

## TYPES OF MICROSCOPES

The microscope used most in clinical laboratories is the compound microscope, which has two lens systems. The **lens** system nearest the eye is in the ocular (eyepiece). The other system is in the objectives, which are close to the object being viewed.

A microscope may be monocular or binocular. A **monocular** microscope has only one eyepiece for viewing objects. It is used frequently in schools because of its low cost. A **binocular** microscope has two eyepieces. It is used in most laboratories because both eyes are used to view an object, which reduces eyestrain.

## PARTS OF THE MICROSCOPE

Microscopes may differ slightly from one model to another. However, there are some parts which may be found on all microscopes. Figure 1–10 shows a binocular microscope and Figure 1–11 shows a monocular microscope. The parts of a microscope are shown in Figure 1–12. Note: The microscopes have basic similarities, but since the binocular microscope is slightly more complex, that one has been used to identify the various components.

### Magnification

Located at the top of the microscope are the **oculars** or **eyepieces.** They are attached to a barrel or tube that is connected to the **microscope arm.** The oculars, through which the object is viewed, contain magnifying lenses which magnify objects. The usual magnification is ten times (10×), but oculars are also available in 15× and 20×. The underside of the arm contains a revolving **nosepiece** to which the objectives are attached. Most microscopes have three **objectives** or magnifying lenses: the low power objective which magnifies × 10; the high power objective which magnifies × 40, 43, or 45; and the oil immersion objective which magnifies × 95, 97, or 100. Each objective is marked with color-coded bands and the degree of magnification.

### Light

The arm of the microscope connects the objectives and eyepiece(s) to the **microscope base** which supports the microscope. The base also contains the

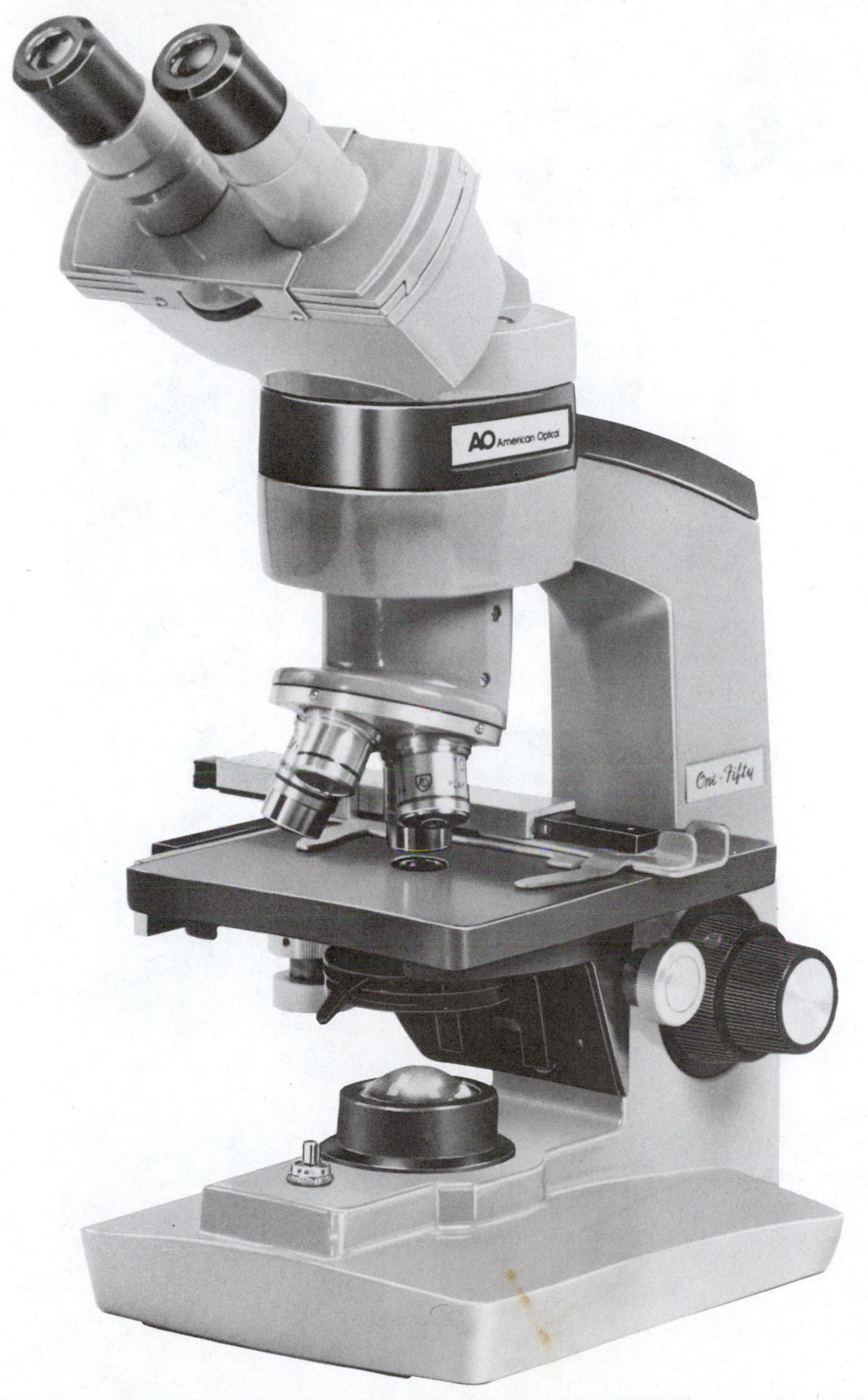


**Figure 1-10.** Binocular microscope (*Photo courtesy of Reichert Scientific Instruments*)

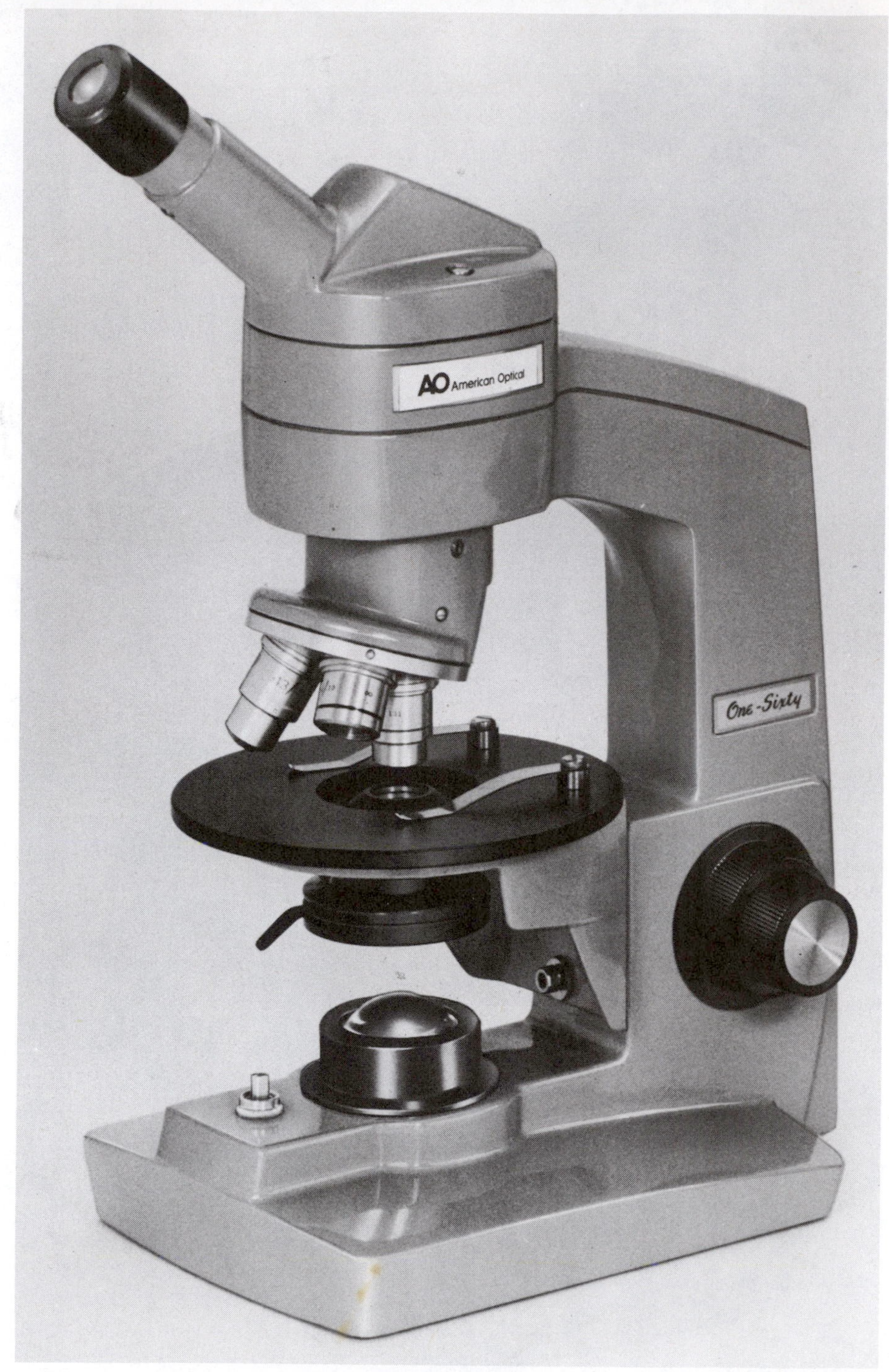


**Figure 1-11.** Monocular microscope (*Photo courtesy of Reichert Scientific Instruments*)

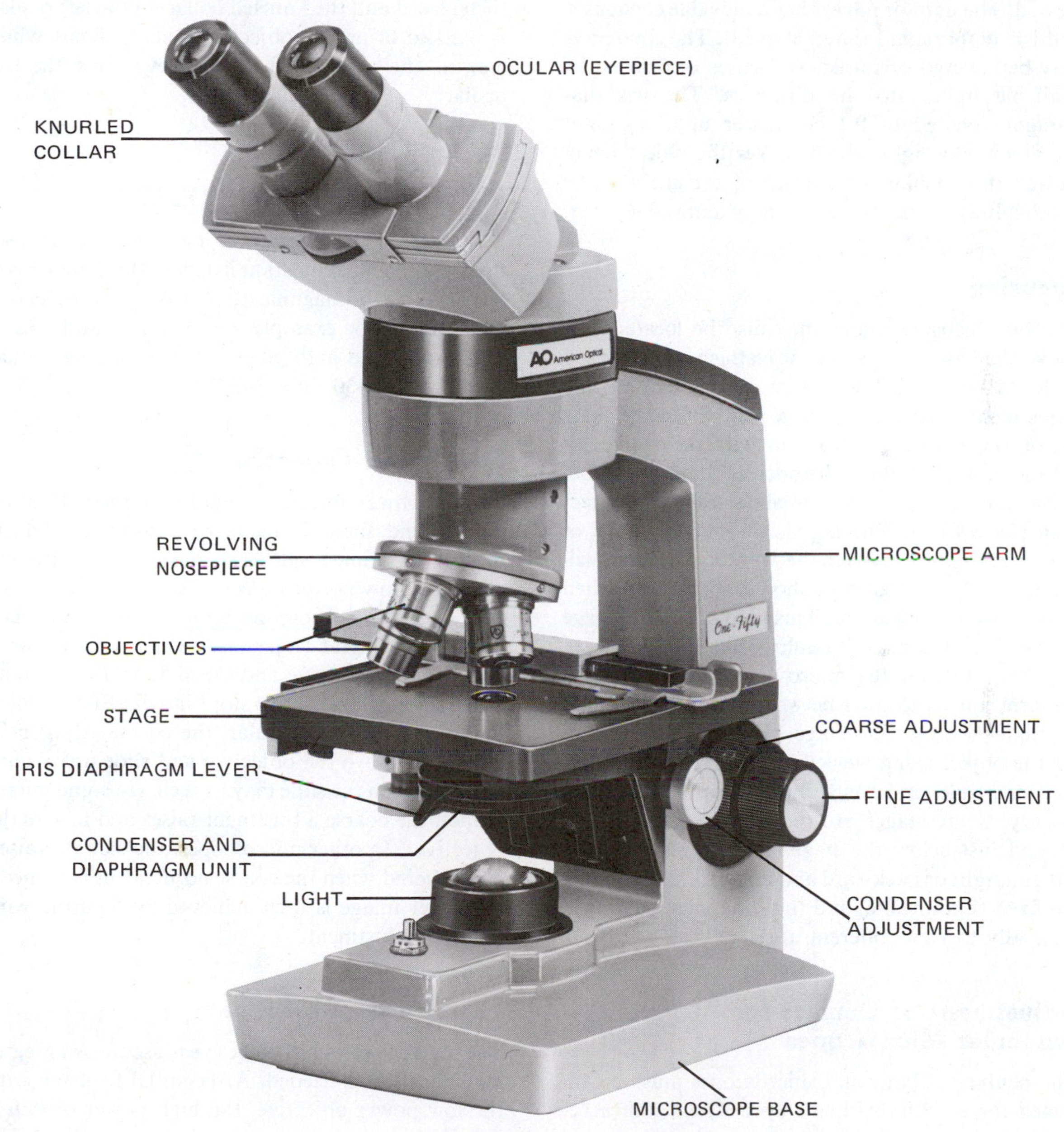


**Figure 1-12.** Parts of a microscope (*Photo courtesy of Reichert Scientific Instruments*)

light or mirror which supplies light to the object viewed. The light or mirror has a movable **condenser** and **iris diaphragm** located above it. The condenser may be lowered or raised. It focuses or directs the available light into the objective. The iris diaphragm, located in the condenser unit, regulates the amount of light which strikes the object being viewed (much like the shutter of a camera). The iris diaphragm may be adjusted by a movable lever.

### Focusing

The two focusing knobs may also be located just above the base. The **coarse adjustment** is only used to focus with the low power objective. The **fine adjustment** is used to give a sharper image after the object is brought into view with the coarse adjustment. The **working distance** is the distance between the objective and the slide when the object is in sharp focus. The higher the magnification of the objective, the shorter the working distance will be. The coarse adjustment should not be used when using high magnification. This is to prevent damage to the objective since it could strike the slide.

The **stage** of the microscope is supported by the arm and is located between the nosepiece and the light source. The stage serves as the support for the object being viewed, usually a prepared microscope slide, and has a clip to keep the slide stationary. Some stages are movable by using knobs located just below the stage. This moves the stage left and right or backward and forward. Other stages are fixed (immovable) and the slide must be moved manually to view different areas.

### Adjustment of Oculars for Binocular Microscopes

The oculars of binocular microscopes must be adjusted for each individual's eyes. The distance between the oculars should be adjusted (as when using binoculars) so that one image is seen. The object is then brought into sharp focus with the coarse and fine adjustments, while looking through the right ocular with the right eye. The right eye is then closed and the knurled collar on the left ocular is used to bring the object into sharp focus while viewing the object with the left eye using the left ocular.

## MAGNIFICATION OF OBJECTS

To determine the degree of magnification in use, multiply the magnification listed on the ocular (usually 10×) by the magnification listed on the objective being used. For example, an object viewed with a 10× ocular and high power (43×) objective would be magnified 430 times (430×).

### Low Power Objective

The low power objective is used for initially locating objects and for viewing large objects. A slide is secured, specimen side up, on the stage with the clips. The low power objective is rotated into position, and the microscope light is turned on. The coarse adjustment is used to decrease the distance between the objective and the slide while watching to see when the objective stops moving. Then, while looking through the ocular, the coarse adjustment is used to move the objective and slide apart until the objects on the slide may be seen. (In some microscopes, the coarse adjustment raises and lowers the objectives. In other microscopes, the stage is raised and lowered when the coarse adjustment is turned.) A clearer image is then achieved by focusing with the fine adjustment.

### High Power Objective

The high power (43×) objective is used when greater magnification is needed. After initial focusing with the low power objective, the high power objective is used by carefully rotating it into position. The fine adjustment is used to bring the objects into sharp focus. Most microscopes are parfocal and therefore require only slight changes in the fine adjustment. The coarse adjustment should not be used when the high power objective is in position. The high power objective is used in procedures such as cell counts and viewing urine sediments.

### Oil Immersion Objective

The oil immersion objective is used to identify stained blood cells, tissue sections, and stained slides containing microorganisms. After initial focusing with low power, the objective is slightly rotated to the side. A drop of immersion oil is placed on the slide directly over the condenser. The oil immersion objective is then carefully rotated into the drop of oil. Be careful not to allow any other objective to contact the oil. The fine adjustment is used to focus the object. The coarse adjustment should not be used when the oil immersion objective is in position. Immersion oil should never be used on any objective other than the one marked oil immersion.

When examination of the slide is completed, the low power objective is rotated into position and the slide is removed from the stage. All oil should be cleaned from the objective with **lens paper.**

### Variations in Light

The condenser and diaphragm must be adjusted according to the objective being used and the type of specimen being observed. When viewing objects with the oil immersion lens, the condenser should be raised until it is almost touching the slide. The diaphragm should be completely open to give maximum light. When looking at objects with low power, the condenser may need to be lowered somewhat to reduce the brightness of the light. The condenser should be raised and diaphragm opened when viewing most stained preparations with high power. However, the condenser may need to be lowered somewhat when viewing unstained fluids, such as urine sediments or cell dilutions for counting. This gives more contrast between the constituents being viewed and the background.

## CARE OF THE MICROSCOPE

### Care of Lenses

The microscope should be stored in a plastic dust cover when not in use. The lenses should be cleaned before and after each use with lens paper. Any other material such as laboratory tissue will scratch the lenses. It is especially important that lenses never be left with oil on them. Oil will soften the cement (glue) which holds the lens in the objective.

### Transporting the Microscope

A microscope should be left in a permanent position on a sturdy lab table in an area where it will not get bumped. However, if the microscope must be moved, it should be held securely with one hand supporting the base and the other hand holding the arm (Figure 1–13). The microscope should be placed gently on tabletops, to avoid jarring.

### Storage of Microscope

When the microscope is not being used, it should be left with the low power objective in position and the nosepiece in the lowest position. The stage should be centered so that it does not project from either side of the microscope.

#### *Precautions*

- Avoid jarring or bumping the microscope.
- Use the coarse adjustment only with low power objective.
- Use oil each time the oil immersion lens is used.
- Use immersion oil on the oil immersion objective only.
- Move or transport the microscope with one hand under the base and the other hand gripping the arm.
- Clean all oculars and objectives with lens paper after each use.
- Store microscope covered in a protected area.

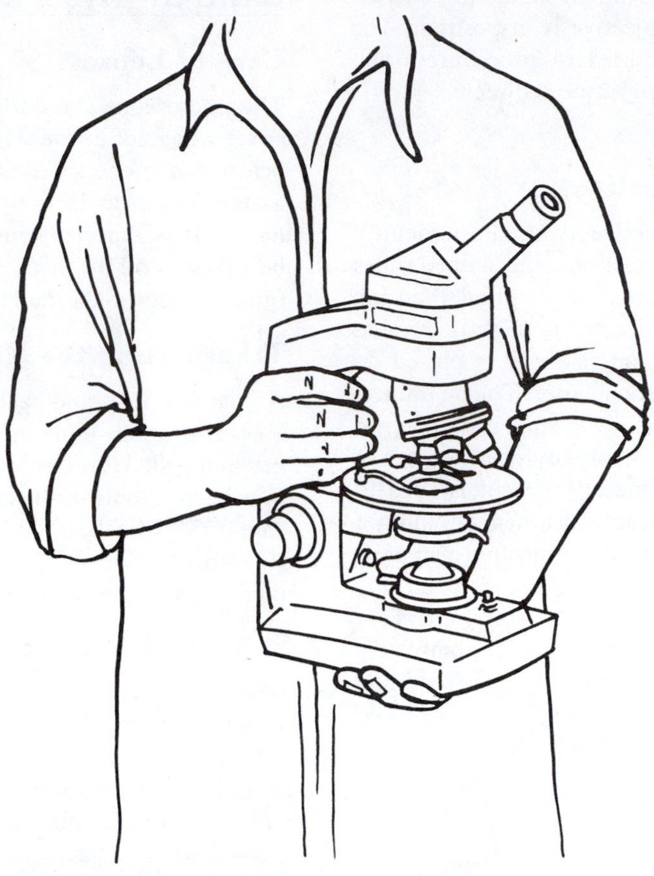

**Figure 1-13.** Transporting the microscope

## *LESSON REVIEW*

1. Explain the functions of the iris diaphragm and condenser.
2. Name the three objectives on a microscope.
3. Explain the difference in the use of the coarse and fine adjustments.
4. What is the proper method of cleaning a microscope after use?
5. How should a microscope be stored when not in use?
6. When is the oil immersion lens used?
7. When is immersion oil used on a slide?
8. Define binocular, coarse adjustment, condenser, eyepiece, fine adjustment, iris diaphragm, lens, lens paper, microscope arm, microscope base, monocular, nosepiece, objective, ocular, stage, and working distance.

## *STUDENT ACTIVITIES*

1. Re-read the information on the microscope.
2. Review the glossary terms.
3. Locate and identify the parts of a microscope.
4. Practice using a microscope using the procedure as outlined in the Student Performance Guide.

# Student Performance Guide

NAME ______________________

DATE ______________________

## LESSON 1–5
## THE MICROSCOPE

### Instructions

1. Practice using the microscope.
2. Demonstrate the proper use of the microscope satisfactorily for the instructor. All steps must be completed as listed on the instructor's Performance Check Sheet.
3. Complete a written examination satisfactorily.

### Materials and Equipment

- hand disinfectant
- microscope (monocular or binocular)
- lens paper
- prepared slides
- immersion oil
- surface disinfectant

*Note:* Procedure will vary slightly according to microscope design. Consult operating procedure in microscope manual for specific instructions.

| **Procedure** | | | S = Satisfactory<br>U = Unsatisfactory |
|---|---|---|---|
| **You must:** | **S** | **U** | **Comments** |
| 1. Wash hands | | | |
| 2. Assemble equipment and materials | | | |
| 3. Clean the ocular(s) and objectives with lens paper | | | |

| You must: | S | U | Comments |
|---|---|---|---|
| 4. Use the coarse adjustment to raise the nosepiece unit | | | |
| 5. Raise the condenser as far as possible by turning the condenser knob | | | |
| 6. Rotate the 10×, or low power, objective into position, so that it is directly over the opening in the stage | | | |
| 7. Turn on the microscope light. If using a mirror, position the light about ten inches in front of the microscope so that it shines directly on the mirror. Adjust the mirror position so that a bright light is reflected upward into the center of the condenser | | | |
| 8. Open the diaphragm until maximum light comes up through the condenser | | | |
| 9. Place slide on stage and secure with clips. The condenser should be positioned so that it is almost touching the bottom of the slide | | | |
| 10. Locate the coarse adjustment | | | |
| 11. Look directly at the stage and 10× objective and turn the coarse adjustment until the objective is as close to the slide as it will go. Stop turning when the objective no longer moves. *Note:* Do not lower any objective toward a slide while looking through the ocular(s) | | | |
| 12. Look into the ocular(s) and slowly turn the coarse adjustment in the opposite direction (as step 11) to raise the objective until the object on the slide comes into view | | | |
| 13. Locate the fine adjustment | | | |
| 14. Turn the fine adjustment to sharpen the image | | | |
| *Note:* If a binocular microscope is used, the oculars must be adjusted for each individual's eyes.<br>a. Adjust distance between oculars so that one image is seen (as when using binoculars) | | | |
| b. Use coarse and fine adjustments to bring object into focus while looking through the right ocular with right eye | | | |
| c. Close the right eye, look into the left ocular with left eye, and use the knurled collar on the left ocular | | | |

| You must: | S | U | Comments |
| --- | --- | --- | --- |
| to bring the object into sharp focus. (Do not turn coarse or fine adjustment at this time.) | | | |
| d. Look into oculars with both eyes to observe that object is in clear focus. If not, repeat the procedure | | | |
| 15. Scan the slide by either method: a. Use the stage knobs to move the slide left and right and backward and forward while looking through the ocular(s), or | | | |
| b. Move the slide with the fingers while looking through the ocular(s) (for microscope without movable stage) | | | |
| 16. Rotate the high power (40×) objective into position while observing the objective and the slide to see that the objective does not strike the slide | | | |
| 17. Look through the ocular(s) to view the object on the slide; it should be almost in focus | | | |
| 18. Locate the fine adjustment | | | |
| 19. Look through the ocular(s) and turn the fine adjustment until the object is in focus. Do not use the coarse adjustment | | | |
| 20. Scan the slide as in step 15, using the fine adjustment if necessary to keep the object in focus | | | |
| 21. Rotate the oil immersion (100×) objective into position while looking directly at the objective to see that it does not strike the slide | | | |
| 22. Locate the fine adjustment | | | |
| 23. Look through the ocular(s) and turn the fine adjustment until the object is in focus | | | |
| 24. Rotate the oil immersion objective to the side slightly (so that no objective is in position) | | | |
| 25. Place one drop of immersion oil on the portion of the slide which is directly over the condenser | | | |
| 26. Rotate the oil immersion objective back into position being careful not to rotate the 40× objective through the oil | | | |

| You must: | S | U | Comments |
|---|---|---|---|
| 27. Look to see that the oil immersion objective is touching the drop of oil | | | |
| 28. Look through the ocular(s) and slowly turn the fine adjustment until the image is clear. Use only the fine adjustment to focus the oil immersion objective | | | |
| 29. Scan the slide using the procedure in step 15 | | | |
| 30. Rotate the 10× objective into position (do not allow 40× objective to touch oil) | | | |
| 31. Remove the slide from the microscope stage and gently clean the oil from the slide with lens paper | | | |
| 32. Clean the oculars, 10× objective, and 40× objective with clean lens paper | | | |
| 33. Clean the 100× objective to remove all oil | | | |
| 34. Clean any oil from the microscope stage and condenser | | | |
| 35. Turn off the microscope light and disconnect | | | |
| 36. Position the nosepiece in the lowest position using the coarse adjustment | | | |
| 37. Center the stage so that it does not project from either side of the microscope | | | |
| 38. Cover the microscope and return it to storage | | | |
| 39. Clean work area | | | |
| 40. Wash hands | | | |

Comments:

Student/Instructor:

Date: ______________________ Instructor: ______________________

# LESSON 1-6

## Introduction to Medical Terminology

### LESSON OBJECTIVES

After studying this lesson, you should be able to:

- Define stem words from a selected list.
- Define prefixes from a selected list.
- Define suffixes from a selected list.
- Identify some common abbreviations of medical laboratory terms from a selected list.
- Pronounce some commonly used medical terms.
- Define the glossary terms.

### GLOSSARY

**prefix** / modifying word or syllable(s) placed at the beginning of a word
**stem** / main part of a word; root word
**suffix** / modifying word or syllable(s) placed at the end of a word
**terminology** / special terms used in any specialized field

### INTRODUCTION

Most specialized fields have a unique vocabulary or **terminology.** Medical terminology is the study of terms or words used in medicine. It is necessary for health care workers to know, understand, and be able to use medical terms in order to carry out instructions and to communicate effectively.

This lesson is only an introduction to the structure of medical terms and to abbreviations that are frequently used in the medical laboratory. Learning medical vocabulary is a long process. Knowledge of medical terms will evolve and expand as the terms are used while working in health care delivery systems. The proper use of medical terminology is as much a part of the job of laboratory and health care workers as other job functions. Each individual will gain confidence in using medical terminology by using the terms in daily activities.

### STRUCTURE OF MEDICAL TERMS

Most medical terms are a combination of word parts—prefixes, suffixes, and stems—which are clues to the meaning of the word. A **prefix** is a word or syllable(s) which modifies the stem and is placed at the beginning of the word. A **suffix** is a word or syllable(s) placed at the end of the word and usually describes what happens to the stem. The **stem** or root is the main part of the word. These word parts are usually connected by a vowel such as "o" or "a."

Most of the stems, prefixes, and suffixes are derived from Latin or Greek words and have a specific meaning. By combining various prefixes, stems, and suffixes, many medical terms with precise meanings may be formed. Not all terms will have all three word parts. Some words may have only a prefix and a stem or a stem and suffix. All terms, though, will have a stem or root word. If the meanings of commonly used word parts are known, then a new term can often be analyzed to determine the general idea of its meaning. For example, hyperproteinuria can be broken into three word parts: hyper, protein, uria. "Hyper" means an increased amount. "Uria" refers to "in the urine." Therefore, the term means a condition with an increased amount of protein in the urine. By combining these parts to make a word, a medical shortcut has been created. One word can describe what would normally take a sentence or sometimes a paragraph. These medical terms, although shorter than sentences, have precise meanings. Sometimes a slight modification, such as alteration of one or two letters, can change the meaning of a word. For example, a macrocyte is a cell larger than normal while a microcyte is a cell smaller than normal. It is very important to spell, pronounce, and use medical terms correctly so that the intended meaning is conveyed.

## Prefixes

Prefixes, placed before stem words, give more information about the stem, such as location, time, size, or number. For example, *intra*vascular means inside the vessel, and *pre*natal refers to something that happens before birth. A list of commonly used prefixes and the definition of each is given in Table 1–1. A sample term using the prefix is also given.

**Table 1-1.** Selected Prefixes Commonly Used in Medical Terminology

| Prefix | Definition | Example of Term | Prefix | Definition | Example of Term |
|---|---|---|---|---|---|
| a, an | absent, deficient | anemia | dia | through | dialysis |
| ab | away from | absent | dipl | double | diplococcus |
| ad | toward | adrenal | dis | apart, away from | disease |
| ambi | both | ambidextrous | dys | bad, difficult, improper | dysphagia |
| aniso | unequal | anisocytosis | | | |
| ante | before | antenatal | e, ecto, ex | out from | ectoparasite |
| ant(i) | against | antibiotic | end(o) | inside, within | endoparasite |
| auto | self | autograft | enter(o) | intestine | enterotoxin |
| baso | blue | basophil | epi | upon, after | epidermis |
| bi | two | binuclear | equi | equal | equilibrium |
| bio | life | biology | hemi | half | hemisphere |
| brady | slow | bradycardia | hyper | above, excessive | hyperglycemia |
| circum | around | circumnuclear | hypo | under, deficient | hypoventilation |
| co, com, con | with, together | concentrate | infra | beneath | infracostal |
| contra | against | contraception | inter | among | intercostal |
| de | down, from | decay | intra | within | intracranial |
| di | two | dimorphic | iso | equal | isotonic |

Table 1-1 (*Cont.*)

| Prefix | Definition | Example of Term | Prefix | Definition | Example of Term |
|---|---|---|---|---|---|
| macr | large | macrocyte | poly | many | polyuria |
| mal | bad, abnormal | malformation | post | after | post-op |
| medi | middle | median | pre, pro | before | prenatal |
| mega | huge, great | megaloblast | pseudo | false | pseudoappendicitis |
| melan | black | melanoma | psych(o) | mind | psychology |
| meta | after, next | metamorphosis | py(o) | pus | pyuria |
| micro | small | microscope | quad(r) | four | quadrant |
| mon(o) | one, single | monoxide | retro | backward | retroactive |
| morph | shape | morphology | semi | half | semiconscious |
| neo | new | neoplasm | steno | narrow | stenosis |
| necro | dead | necropsy | sub | under | subcutaneous |
| neutro | neutral | neutrophil | super, supra | above | superinfection |
| olig | few | oliguria | syn | together | synergistic |
| orth | straight, normal | orthopedic | tachy | swift | tachycardia |
| pan | all | pandemic | tetra | four | tetramer |
| para | beside | paraplegic | therm | heat | thermometer |
| per | through | percolate | trans | through | transport |
| peri | around | pericardium | tri | three | trimester |
| phago | to eat | phagocyte | uni | one | unicellular |

## Stems

The stem gives the major subject of the term. For example, in the term *appendi*citis, the stem is appendix. Therefore, appendicitis means an inflammation of the appendix. In the term endo*card*itis, the root or stem is "card," referring to heart; the term literally means an inflammation within the heart. A list of commonly used stem words and the meaning of each is given in Table 1–2.

## Suffixes

Suffixes are attached to the end of a stem. Suffixes usually tell what is happening to the subject of the stem. They often indicate a condition, operation, or symptom. For example, in the term appendec*tomy,* "ectomy" is a suffix which means to cut out or remove by excision. Therefore, an appendectomy is the surgical removal of the appendix. A list of commonly used suffixes and their definitions is given in Table 1–3.

# PRONUNCIATION

It is not enough to just understand written medical terms. You also need to pronounce them correctly to communicate effectively with others. Correct pronunciation may be easy for some frequently used terms or short terms, but more difficult for some of the longer terms. Although most terms are derived from Greek and Latin, the Latin and Greek pronouncing rules cannot always be relied on for the proper pronunciation. Your medical dictionary can give you a guide to common usage but even authors disagree on some standard pronunciations. By listening to others who work with you, you can learn how words are commonly pronounced in your area. Pronunciation will be improved and confidence will be gained by practicing the pronunciation of terms.

**Table 1-2.** Selected Stems Commonly Used in Medical Terminology

| Stem | Definition | Example of Term | Stem | Definition | Example of Term |
|---|---|---|---|---|---|
| adeno | gland | lymphadenitis | lip | fat | lipoma |
| alg | pain | analgesic | lith | stone | cholelithiasis |
| arter | artery | arteriogram | mening | membrane covering brain | meningitis |
| arthr | joint | arthritis | | | |
| audio | hearing | auditory | myel | marrow | myelogram |
| brachi | arm | brachial | myo | muscle | myositis |
| bronch(i) | air tube in lungs | bronchitis | nephro | kidney | nephron |
| cardi | heart | myocardium | neur | nerve | neurectomy |
| calc | stone | calcify | noct | night | nocturia |
| carcin | cancer | carcinogen | onc | tumor | oncology |
| caud | tail | caudate | oo | egg | oogenesis |
| ceph(al) | head | encephalitis | ophthal | eye | ophthalmologist |
| chol | bile, gall bladder | cholesterol | os, osteo | bone | osteosarcoma |
| chondr | cartilage | chondroplasia | oto | ear | otitis |
| chrom | color | chromogen | path | disease | pathogen |
| cran | skull | craniotomy | ped | child | pediatrician |
| cut | skin | subcutaneous | phleb | vein | phlebitis |
| cyan | blue | cyanosis | phob | fear | phobia |
| cyst | bladder, bag | cystocele | phot | light | photosensitive |
| cyt(o) | cell | monocyte | pneum | air | pneumonitis |
| dactyl | finger | arachnodactyly | pod | foot | pseudopod |
| dent, dont | teeth | orthodontist | pulm | lung | pulmonary |
| derm | skin | dermatitis | ren | kidney | adrenal |
| edema | swelling | edematous | rhin | nose | rhinoplasty |
| erythro | red | erythrocyte | scler | hard | sclerosis |
| febr | fever | afebrile | sep | poison | septic |
| gastr(o) | stomach | gastritis | soma(t) | body | somatic |
| genito | reproductive | genital | sperm | seed | spermatogenesis |
| gloss | tongue | glossitis | stoma | mouth, opening | stomatitis |
| glyco | sweet | glycosuria | therm | temperature | thermometer |
| gran | grain | granulocyte | thorac | chest | thoracotomy |
| hem(a), haem, | blood | hematology | thromb | clot | thrombocyte |
| hepat(o) | liver | hepatitis | tome | knife | microtome |
| histo | tissue | histology | tox | poison | toxin |
| hydro | water | hydrocephalic | ur(o), uria | urine | hematuria |
| hystero | uterus | hysterectomy | vas | vessel | intravascular |
| iatro | physician | podiatrist | ven | vein | intravenous |
| leuk | white | leukocyte | | | |

**Table 1-3.** Selected Suffixes Commonly Used in Medical Terminology

| Suffix | Definition | Example of Term | Suffix | Definition | Example of Term |
|---|---|---|---|---|---|
| algia | pain | neuralgia | osis | state, condition, increase | leukocytosis |
| blast | primitive, germ | erythroblast | | | |
| centesis | puncture, aspiration | amniocentesis | ostomy | create an opening | ileostomy |
| cide | death, killer | bacteriocide | otomy | cut into | phlebotomy |
| ectomy | excision, cut out | gastrectomy | opathy, pathia | disease | adenopathy |
| emesis | vomiting | hematemesis | penia | lack of | leukopenia |
| emia | in the or of the blood | bilirubinemia | phil | affinity for, liking | eosinophil |
| ferent | carry | afferent | phyte | plant | dermatophyte |
| genic | origin, producing | pyogenic | plastic, plasia | to form or mold | hyperplasia |
| ia, iasis | state, condition | iatrogenic | pnea | breathing | apnea |
| iole | small | bronchiole | poiesis | to make | hemopoiesis |
| itis | inflammation | pharyngitis | rrhage | excessive flow | hemorrhage |
| lysis | free, breaking down | hemolysis | rrhea | flow | diarrhea |
| oid | resembling, similar to | blastoid | scope, scopy | view | arthroscope |
| (o)logy | study of | pathology | stasis | same, standing still | hemostasis |
| oma | tumor | hepatoma | troph(y) | nourishment | hypertrophy |

## ABBREVIATIONS

Abbreviations are used commonly in medicine to avoid having to repeatedly write or say several syllables. A short list of common abbreviations used in the medical laboratory is shown in Table 1–4. This does not include abbreviations used in prescriptions, nursing care, and other areas of health care. A worker should be familiar with abbreviations so that physician's orders or instructions can be carried out correctly.

**Table 1-4.** Abbreviations Commonly Used in a Medical Laboratory

| | | | |
|---|---|---|---|
| BP | blood pressure | $CO_2$ | carbon dioxide |
| BUN | blood urea nitrogen | CSF | cerebral spinal fluid |
| C | Centigrade, Celsius | E.U. | Ehrlich units |
| CBC | complete blood count | F | Fahrenheit |
| cc, ccm | cubic centimeter | FUO | fever of unknown origin |
| cm | centimeter | g, gm | gram |
| CNS | central nervous system | GI | gastrointestinal |
| CO | carbon monoxide | GU | genitourinary |

**Table 1-4** (*Cont.*)

| | | | |
|---|---|---|---|
| Hb | hemoglobin | MLT | medical laboratory technician |
| HCl | hydrochloric acid | mm | millimeter |
| Hct | hematocrit | MT | medical technologist |
| Hgb | hemoglobin | NaCl | sodium chloride, saline |
| $H_2O$ | water | nm | nanometer |
| HPF | high power field | O.D. | optical density |
| IM | infectious mononucleosis | pH | a number indicating the relative acidity of a solution |
| IU | international unit | RBC | red blood cell |
| IV | intravenous | S.I. | Le Système International d'Unités (International System of Units) |
| L | liter | sp. gr. | specific gravity |
| LPF | low power field | Staph | *Staphylococcus* |
| MCH | mean corpuscular hemoglobin | stat | immediately |
| MCHC | mean corpuscular hemoglobin concentration | Strep | *Streptococcus* |
| MCV | mean corpuscular volume | UA | urinalysis |
| mg | milligram | WBC | white blood cell |
| MI | myocardial infarction | | |
| mL, ml | milliliter | | |

## *LESSON REVIEW*

1. What is a prefix?
2. What is a suffix?
3. What is a stem?
4. Name the stems used for cell, heart, head, skin, chest, kidney, muscle, liver, stomach.
5. Name ten common suffixes and give a meaning for each.
6. Name ten common prefixes and give a meaning for each.
7. List ten abbreviations frequently used in the medical laboratory.
8. Define prefix, stem, suffix, and terminology.

## *STUDENT ACTIVITIES*

1. Re-read the lesson on medical terminology.
2. Review the glossary terms.
3. Practice pronouncing the word parts and medical terms in Tables 1–1 through 1–3. Look up pronunciations of ten terms and practice saying them out loud.
4. Study the definitions for prefixes, suffixes, and stems listed in the tables.
5. Study the abbreviations listed in Table 1–4.
6. Use each of the prefixes, suffixes, or stems in a word not on the list.
7. Look up the meanings of the examples of medical terms listed in Tables 1–1 through 1–3.

# LESSON 1–7

## The Metric System

### LESSON OBJECTIVES

After studying this lesson, you should be able to:

- Discuss the importance of the proper use of metric units.
- Name prefixes commonly used to denote smaller or larger metric units.
- Convert English units to metric units.
- Convert metric units to English units.
- Convert units within the metric system.
- Perform measurements of distance, volume, and weight using metric units.
- Define the glossary terms.

### GLOSSARY

**gram** / basic metric unit of weight or mass
**liter** / basic metric unit of volume
**meter** / basic metric unit of distance or length
**S.I. units** / standardized units of measure; international units

## INTRODUCTION

The metric system is the system of measurements used internationally for scientific work. In European countries, the metric system is also used in everyday life. Milk is purchased by the liter. Body weight is measured in kilograms. If the weather report predicts a high of 34°C for the day, the European knows not to wear a coat because it will be a hot day. This is because the temperature is measured on the centigrade or Celsius scale.

In the United States, use of the metric system is encouraged. However, the English system is still used for most measurements and observations made in everyday life. We drive our cars at fifty-five miles per hour. We report our weight in pounds and our height in feet and inches. We cook using measures such as teaspoon, cup, and pint. However, the English system is not accurate enough for most scientific measurements. Therefore, a student of science must know and be able to use the metric system in laboratory observations and measurements.

## IMPORTANCE OF MEASUREMENTS

Units of measurements are used frequently in medicine. They are used to measure vital statistics such as height, weight, and temperature; the amount of fluid intake and output; and dosages of medication. In the laboratory, measurements are used to indicate numbers of cells or quantities of substances in a patient's blood, serum, or other body fluids. Very small quantities can be measured accurately and easily using the metric system. These measurements are then compared to normal values and the patient's condition is assessed. The results may be used to establish a diagnosis and to prescribe therapy. Therefore, it is important that all measurements are made correctly and accurately.

## COMMON MEASUREMENTS

Measurements that are commonly determined include the:

- weight of a substance or object
- volume of a solution or object
- size or length of an object
- temperature
- time

The weights, volumes, and sizes or lengths of objects can be most accurately measured using the metric system. In the United States, body temperatures are commonly measured on the Fahrenheit scale. Laboratory temperatures are measured on the centigrade or Celsius scale. Fortunately, laboratory time is measured in seconds, minutes, and hours as is the time of day.

## THE METRIC SYSTEM

The metric system is named because it is based on a fundamental unit of distance, the **meter.** In the metric system, the meter (m) is the basic unit used to measure distance. The **gram** (g) is the basic unit used to compare mass or weight. And, the **liter** (l) is the basic unit used to measure volume.

The metric system uses decimal notations and the units are divided into increments of ten. This means that units larger or smaller than the basic units (meter, liter, and gram) can be obtained by multiplying or dividing by increments of ten (or by a power of ten).

Prefixes may be added to the basic units to indicate larger or smaller units (Table 1–5). For example, "kilo" means 1,000. Therefore, a kilometer (km) is 1,000 meters or $10^3$ meters; a kilogram (kg) is 1,000 grams, and a kiloliter (kl) is 1,000 liters. Although "kilo" is the prefix most commonly used for large units, "deca" may be used to indicate the unit times ten, as in decaliter. Or, "hecto" may indicate the unit times one hundred. The prefixes and their definitions are the same for the three basic units.

In laboratory analyses, it is more common to measure units smaller than the basic units. Table 1–5 lists the prefixes and the multiple of the basic unit which each represents. Two common prefixes used are "milli," which means one-thousandth (.001 or $10^{-3}$), and "centi," which means one-hundredth (.01 or $10^{-2}$). A milliliter is .001 liter or $10^{-3}$ liter. In chemistry, solutions may be made by adding milligrams (mg) of substances to milliliters (ml) of solvent. Substances such as glucose may be measured in mg per 100 ml of serum. In hematology, blood cells are counted per cubic millimeter (cu mm or $mm^3$) of blood.

Other prefixes commonly used to denote size are "micro," which denotes one millionth or $10^{-6}$, and "nano" which is $10^{-9}$. (See Table 1–5 for abbreviations and prefixes.) Small samples are measured in microliters ($\mu$l) or $10^{-6}$ liter. Wavelengths of light are measured in nanometers (nm) or $10^{-9}$ meter.

### Converting Units

It may be necessary to convert units within the metric system or to convert English units to metric or metric units to English units. For this reason,

**Table 1-5.** Commonly Used Prefixes in the Metric System

| Abbreviation | Prefix | Meaning | Multiple of Basic Unit | Weight Gram (g) | Length Meter (m) | Volume Liter (L) |
|---|---|---|---|---|---|---|
| k | kilo | 1000 | $10^3$ | kg | km | kl |
| h | hecto | 100 | $10^2$ | hg* | hm* | hl* |
| da | deca | 10 | $10^1$ | dag* | dam* | dal* |
| d | deci | .1 | $10^{-1}$ | dg* | dm* | dl |
| c | centi | .01 | $10^{-2}$ | cg* | cm | cl* |
| m | milli | .001 | $10^{-3}$ | mg | mm | ml |
| μ | micro | .000001 | $10^{-6}$ | μg | μm | μl |
| n | nano | | $10^{-9}$ | ng | nm | nl* |
| p | pico | | $10^{-12}$ | pg | pm* | pl* |

* Units not commonly used in the laboratory

it is helpful to have a general idea of the metric equivalents of commonly used English measures. Equivalents are listed in Tables 1–6 and 1–7. To convert units from one system to another, simply multiply by the factor listed. For example, since one inch is equal to 2.54 centimeters (cm), twelve inches would equal 12 × 2.54, or 30.48 cm. To convert metric units to English units, use Table 1–7 in the same manner. Since one kg equals 2.2 pounds, the weight in pounds of a patient weighing 70 kg may be determined by multiplying 70 × 2.2 to equal 154 pounds.

In laboratory work, it is more common to need to convert units within the metric system. To make these conversions, the worker needs to know equivalents, such as how many milliliters or microliters are in a liter, or how many milligrams are in a gram. These conversions can be made by using the information in Table 1–8.

Metric units may be converted to larger units

**Table 1-6.** Conversion of English Units to Metric Units

| | English Unit | English Abbreviation | | Multiply By | To Get Metric Unit | Metric Abbreviation |
|---|---|---|---|---|---|---|
| **Distance** | 1 mile | mi | = | 1.6 | kilometers | km |
| | 1 yard | yd | = | 0.9 | meters | m |
| | 1 inch | in | = | 2.54 | centimeters | cm |
| **Mass** | 1 pound | lb | = | 0.454 | kilograms | kg |
| | 1 pound | lb | = | 454 | grams | g |
| | 1 ounce | oz | = | 28 | grams | g |
| **Volume** | 1 quart | qt | = | 0.95 | liters | l |
| | 1 fluid ounce | fl. oz. | = | 30 | milliliters | ml |
| | 1 teaspoon | tsp | = | 5 | milliliters | ml |

**Table 1-7.** Conversion of Metric Units to English Units

| | Metric Unit | Metric Abbreviation | | Multiply By | To Find English Unit | English Abbreviation |
|---|---|---|---|---|---|---|
| **Distance** | 1 kilometer | km | = | 0.6 | miles | mi |
| | 1 meter | m | = | 3.3 | feet | ft |
| | 1 meter | m | = | 39.37 | inches | in |
| | 1 centimeter | cm | = | 0.4 | inches | in |
| | 1 millimeter | mm | = | .04 | inches | in |
| **Mass** | 1 gram | g | = | .0022 | pounds | lb |
| | 1 kilogram | kg | = | 2.2 | pounds | lb |
| **Volume** | 1 liter | 1 | = | 1.06 | quarts | qt |
| | 1 milliliter | ml | = | .03 | fluid ounces | fl. oz. |

**Table 1-8.** Common Metric Equivalents

| | | | | |
|---|---|---|---|---|
| **Mass** | $10^{-3}$ kg | = 1 gram | = $10^3$ mg | = $10^6$ μg |
| | $10^{-3}$ g | = 1 mg | = $10^3$ μg | = $10^6$ ng |
| | $10^{-9}$ g | = 1 ng | = $10^3$ pg | |
| **Volume** | $10^{-3}$ kl | = 1 liter | = $10^3$ ml | = $10^6$ μl |
| | $10^{-3}$ l | = 1 ml | = $10^3$ μl | = $10^6$ nl |
| | $10^{-1}$ l | = 1 dl | = $10^2$ ml | |
| **Length** | $10^{-3}$ km | = 1 meter | = $10^3$ mm | = $10^6$ μm |
| | $10^{-3}$ m | = 1 mm | = $10^3$ μm | = $10^6$ nm |
| | $10^{-2}$ m | = 1 cm | = 10 mm | = $10^4$ μm |
| | $10^{-3}$ mm | = 1 nm | = 10 Å | |

such as grams to kilograms or milliliters to liters; the decimal in the original unit is moved to the left for the appropriate number of spaces. Example: To convert 50 g to kg, multiply by .001 or move the decimal to the left three places: 50 g = .050 kg. To convert centimeters to meters, multiply by .01 or move the decimal two places to the left: 160 cm = 1.6 meters.

Metric units may be converted to smaller units, such as g to mg or liters to microliters; the decimal in the number is moved to the right the appropriate number of spaces. To convert 5 g to mg, multiply by 1000 or move the decimal to the right three places: 5 g = 5000 mg. Scientific notation is often used to make the numbers less bulky and easier to compute. For example, five grams equals 5,000,000 μg or $5.0 \times 10^6$ μg.

## S.I. UNITS

Even though the metric system is used internationally to attain laboratory measurements, the method of reporting results differs from country to country or even within countries. This can be confusing when one is trying to compare laboratory data. For example, the concentration of protein may be expressed as g/L in some laboratories or g/dl in others.

An effort is being made to standardize the reporting of laboratory values by using an International System of Units called **SI units** (Table 1–9). Blood cell counts have traditionally been expressed as the number of cells per cubic millimeter (cu mm) of blood. In the SI system, however, they are expressed as number of cells per liter of blood. Chemical substances such as bilirubin or glucose

**Table 1-9.** International System of Units (SI Units)

| Common Usage | SI Equivalent |
|---|---|
| micron (μ) | micrometer (μm; $10^{-6}$ meter) |
| cubic micron ($\mu^3$) | femtoliter (fl; $10^{-15}$ liter) |
| micromicrogram (μμg) | picogram (pg; $10^{-12}$ gram) |
| microgram (mcg) | microgram (μg; $10^{-6}$ gram) |
| Angstrom (Å) | nm $\times$ $10^{-1}$ |
| millimicron (mμ) | nanometer (nm; $10^{-9}$ meter) |
| lambda (λ) | microliter (μl; $10^{-6}$ liter) |

| Test | Old Unit | S.I. Unit |
|---|---|---|
| Cell counts | cells/mm³ or cells/cumm | cells/μl or cells/liter |
| Hematocrit | % (Ex: 41%) | Percent expressed as decimal (Ex: 0.41) |
| Hemoglobin | g/dl | g/liter |
| MCV | $\mu^3$ | fl |
| MCH | μμg | pg |
| MCHC | % | g/dl (or g/l) |

which were expressed as mg per deciliter (dl) or per 100 ml, are now expressed as mg or g per liter or as micromoles (μmol) or millimoles (mmol) per liter. It is imperative that the proper units of measurement be included with all laboratory results. For example, a glucose reported simply as 5.6 would cause great concern in a lab that measures blood glucose in mg/dl. The normal value should be around 80–100 mg/dl and 5.6 would be extremely low. However, in labs where blood glucose is measured in mmol/liter, 5.6 would be a normal finding.

### Common Equivalents

There are a few units which have been commonly used in the laboratory but are being phased out in favor of more appropriate terms. Since these units are still used by some laboratories and appear in older books or manuals, one needs to understand the equivalents of these units. A milliliter (ml) may also be called a cc (cubic centimeter), especially when referring to dosages. A cubic centimeter may be written as cc, cu cm, or cm³. A microliter (μl), which is one-thousandth of a ml, may also be called a cubic millimeter (cu mm or mm³). Micron is the old term referring to micrometer. Lambda (λ) is the old term referring to microliter or wavelength of light (nanometer).

## TEMPERATURE CONVERSIONS

The two temperature scales used in medicine are the Fahrenheit scale and the Celsius or centigrade scale. The Fahrenheit scale is used for measuring body temperature. The Celsius scale is used in the laboratory for measuring temperatures of reaction and incubation and boiling points. The method of converting from one temperature scale to another is discussed in Lesson 1–8, Laboratory Math.

## *LESSON REVIEW*

1. What is the basic metric unit of distance or length?
2. What is the basic metric unit of volume?
3. What is the basic metric unit of weight?
4. What are the meanings of kilo, micro, milli, nano, centi?
5. Why is the metric system preferred over the English for scientific measurements?
6. Convert the following English measurements to metric units:

   3 inches = _____ cm or _____ mm
   5 qt. = _____ liters or _____ ml
   64 oz. = _____ g or _____kg or _____mg

7. Convert the following units:

   12 mg = _____μg or _____g
   50 ml = _____μl or _____cc or _____dl

8. Define gram, liter, meter, and S.I. units.

## *STUDENT ACTIVITIES*

1. Re-read the information on the metric system.
2. Review the glossary terms.
3. Practice measuring metric volumes, lengths, and weights and converting metric units using the worksheets.

# Metric Worksheet–Distance

NAME ______________________________ DATE ____________

## LESSON 1–7 THE METRIC SYSTEM

Obtain a meter stick or metric ruler and an English ruler from the instructor. Use the information in Tables 1–5 through 1–9 to answer the questions below.

1. Look at the meter stick. Locate the cm and mm divisions. How many centimeters are in a meter? _____ How many mm in a cm? _____ How many mm in a meter? _____

2. Draw the indicated length of line beside each number beginning at the dot.

   35 mm •
   6 cm •
   83 mm •
   1.2 dm •

3. Measure the lines above using a ruler marked in English units (inches):

   35 mm = ____________ inches
   6 cm = ____________ inches
   83 mm = ____________ inches
   1.2 dm = ____________ inches

   Which of the measurements (English or metric) do you feel is the most accurate? ____________

4. How many mm in one inch? ____________ One mm = ____________ inch
   How many cm in one inch? ____________ One cm = ____________ inch

   Convert the following units:

   4 inches = ____________cm
   0.5 inches = ____________cm

   What number did you multiply by to obtain the answers? ____________

   38 cm = ____________in.
   7 cm = ____________in.

   What number did you multiply by to obtain the answers? ____________

   3.5 inches = ____________mm
   35 mm = ____________in.

5. How many inches are in a meter? _______What English unit of measure is the closest in size to the meter? _______

6. Measure your height or the height of another student using the meter stick. What is the height in cm? _______in meters? _______Convert the height in cm to inches:___________ Now measure the height in inches and compare the results.

# Metric Worksheet–Weight

NAME ______________________________ DATE ____________

## LESSON 1–7 THE METRIC SYSTEM

Use Tables 1–5 through 1–9 to answer the questions below.

1. What is the basic metric unit of weight? ____________________

2. How many mg in a g? __________
   How many μg in a g? __________
   How many g in a kg? __________

3. Convert the following units:

   300 mg = _____g = _____kg
   50 mg = _____g = _____kg
   4000 mg = _____g = _____kg
   200 μg = _____g
   750 μg = _____mg
   80 g = _____kg

   What decimal rule did you follow to make the conversions? ____________________
   ________________________________________

4. Convert the following units:

   0.4 kg = __________mg = __________μg
   9.2 g = __________mg = __________μg
   0.6 g = __________μg
   10 mg = __________μg = __________pg
   280 mg = __________μg = __________pg

   What decimal rule did you follow in making the conversions? __________
   ________________________________________

5. Weigh yourself or another student. What is the weight in g? __________
   in kg? __________

6. A man who weighs 165 pounds would weigh __________kg.

7. A child who weighs 32 pounds would weigh __________kg or __________ g.

8. Is a man who is 178 cm tall and weighs 135 kg overweight, underweight, or of normal weight? __________

9. If scales are available, weigh 10 ml of water in a container. How much does the water weigh? __________
   Does one milliliter of water weigh approximately 1 gram?
   Yes _____ No _____

# Metric Worksheet–Volume

NAME ______________________________ DATE ____________

## LESSON 1–7 THE METRIC SYSTEM

Obtain a medicine cup, a 50 ml graduated cylinder, and a 50 ml beaker from the instructor. Use Tables 1–5 through 1–9 to answer the questions below.

1. What is the basic unit of volume in the metric system? __________

2. How many ml in a liter? _____ dl in a liter? _____ µl in a liter? _____

3. Convert the following units:

   45 cc = _____ liter = _____ ml
   550 ml = _____ liter
   4 dl = _____ liter
   60 µl = _____ liter = _____ ml
   0.1 dl = _____ liter
   6,700 ml = _____ liter

   What decimal rule did you follow to make the conversions? ____________

   ______________________________________________

4. Convert the following units:

   0.3 liter = _____ dl = _____ ml
   5 liters = _____ ml
   7 ml = _____ µl
   3 dl = _____ ml = _____ µl
   0.1 dl = _____ ml

   What decimal rule did you follow to make the conversions? ____________

   ______________________________________________

5. What English unit is closest in volume to the liter? ____________

6. Convert the following English units:

   3.5 pints = _____ ml = _____l
   3 quarts= _____ ml = _____l
   5 fl. oz. = _____ ml = _____l

7. If gasoline is $1.20 per gallon at station A and 30 cents a liter at station B, which has the cheapest gasoline? ____________________

8. Fill the medicine cup to the one ounce mark with water. Transfer the water to a 50 ml graduated cylinder. How many milliliters of water was in the one fluid ounce? ____________________
   Fill the medicine cup again with water and transfer the one fl. oz. to a 50 ml beaker. Which gives the most accurate measurement, the beaker or the graduated cylinder? ____________________

# LESSON 1-8

## Laboratory Math

## LESSON OBJECTIVES

After studying this lesson, you should be able to:

- Convert Celsius temperatures to Fahrenheit.
- Convert Fahrenheit temperatures to Celsius.
- Prepare percent solutions.
- Prepare laboratory dilutions.
- Use proportions to prepare laboratory solutions.

## GLOSSARY

**Celsius** / temperature scale having the freezing point of water at zero (0°) and the boiling point at one hundred (100°); indicated by "C"; also called centigrade

**distilled water** (dist. $H_20$) / the condensate collected when water has been boiled to remove impurities

**Fahrenheit** / a temperature scale having the freezing point of water at 32° and the boiling point at 212°; indicated by "F"

**ratio** / relationship in degree or number between two things

**saline** / an isotonic solution of sodium chloride in distilled water; usually made in either a 0.85 or 0.9% concentration for use in medical laboratory procedures; may be referred to as normal or physiological saline

## INTRODUCTION

Some form of math is used in most laboratory exercises no matter how simple the procedure. The math principles may be used directly in the procedure. Or, math may be used indirectly, as in the preparation of test reagents and in the research and development of the procedures themselves. It is not sufficient just to understand the fundamentals of laboratory math. One must also be able to use math principles correctly if laboratory results are to be accurate.

### The Direct Use of Math

The direct use of math in a procedure could involve making a dilution of the blood or serum being analyzed. For example, to do a white blood cell count,

**Problem:** Convert 98.6° F (normal body temperature) to Celsius (C) degrees.

**Formula:** $C = \frac{5}{9}(F-32)$

**Solution:** $C = \frac{5}{9}(98.6-32)$

$C = \frac{5}{9}(66.6)$

$C = 36.99$ or 37

**Answer:** 98.6° F is equal to 37° C

**Figure 1-14.** Example of Fahrenheit temperature converted to Celsius

the blood must first be diluted to a 1/20 concentration.

## Indirect Uses of Math

In some instances, math is not obviously used in a laboratory procedure, but is used indirectly. One example is in the preparation of the reagents. The concentration of laboratory reagents is often expressed as a percentage (%). An example is the 2% solution of acetic acid which is combined with a blood sample to perform one type of white blood cell count. A 70% solution of ethyl alcohol is used to cleanse the skin at the site of puncture before blood collection. A solution of 0.85% **saline** is widely utilized in medical laboratory procedures. In serology and blood banking, a reagent commonly used is a 2% concentration of red blood cells. The directions for some reagents may also express the concentration as a proportion, such as two parts of Solution "A" to three parts of Solution "B."

# TEMPERATURE CONVERSION

Converting temperatures from Celsius (C) to Fahrenheit (F), or vice versa, also employs math. The temperature scale most widely used in laboratory work is **Celsius** (centigrade). In scientific work, the required temperature for a specific reaction is almost always expressed in Celsius degrees. There are, however, instances in which one might need to convert Celsius to **Fahrenheit** or vice versa. Normal human body temperature is usually stated as 98.6° Fahrenheit. A laboratory procedure may require that a test be run at normal body temperature, but the equipment in the laboratory is calibrated in Celsius degrees. This makes it necessary that the 98.6°F be converted to Celsius degrees (Figure 1–14). This can be accomplished by the use of the formula:

$$\text{Celsius degrees} = 5/9(F-32)$$

The normal body temperature may then be expressed as 37°C. Conversely, the normal body temperature, 37°C, can be converted to Fahrenheit degrees (Figure 1–15) by using the formula:

$$\text{Fahrenheit degrees} = 9/5(C) + 32$$

**Problem:** Convert 37° C to Fahrenheit (F) degrees.

**Formula:** $F = \frac{9}{5}(C) + 32$

**Solution:** $F = \frac{9}{5}(37) + 32$

$F = 66.6 + 32$

$F = 98.6$

**Answer:** 37° C is equal to 98.6° F

**Figure 1-15.** Example of Celsius temperature converted to Fahrenheit

**Problem:** A buffer is made by adding 2 parts of "solution A" to 5 parts of "solution B." How much of solution A and solution B would be required to make 70 ml of the buffer?

**Formula:** $\dfrac{\text{Total volume required (C)}}{\text{parts of "A"} + \text{parts of "B"}} = \text{volume of one part (V)}$

**Solution:** $\dfrac{\text{70 ml required}}{\text{2 parts "A"} + \text{5 parts "B"}} = \text{volume of one part}$

$\dfrac{70}{7} = 10 \text{ ml} = \text{volume of one part (V)}$

2 parts of solution "A" $= 2 \times 10 = 20$ ml
5 parts of solution "B" $= 5 \times 10 = 50$ ml

**Answer:** The buffer would be made by mixing 20 ml of solution A with 50 ml of solution B to give a total volume of 70 ml.

**Figure 1-16.** Preparing a solution using proportions

## PROPORTION

Proportion is used when reagents are prepared by adding together a specific amount of one solution with a specific amount of another solution. An example would be instructions which direct that two parts (measures) of solution "A" be added to three parts (measures) of solution "B" to prepare the final solution, "C." The formula to determine the actual volumes required of solutions "A" and "B" is:

$$\frac{(C)}{(A) + (B)} = V$$

where: C = Total volume of final solution
A = Total parts of solution A
B = Total parts of solution B
V = Total volume of one part

When doing the bilirubin level in serum, a Diazo reagent is used. This reagent is prepared by adding 0.3 parts of Diazo reagent B to ten (10) parts of Diazo reagent A. Buffer solutions are also often prepared using proportions. An example is illustrated in Figure 1–16.

Proportion can also be used to determine how much of a solution of a specific concentration is required to prepare a second solution of a lower concentration. The 2% solution of acetic acid used in white blood cell counts can be prepared using proportions. If a 10% solution of acetic acid is available, the 2% solution can be prepared from that concentration (Figure 1–17). The general formula is:

$$C_1 \times V_1 = C_2 \times V_2$$

In this formula $C_1$ refers to the concentration of solution one and $V_1$ to its volume. The $C_2$ and $V_2$ refer to the concentration and volume of solution two.

## PERCENTAGE SOLUTIONS

The concentrations of many laboratory reagents are expressed in percentage. Percentage solutions may be made by weighing out a specific amount of a solute for each 100 ml of solvent, usually **distilled water.** This is called a weight to volume percentage (w/v). One example of this type is the 0.85% saline (sodium chloride) solution which is used in many serological and bacteriological procedures. One hundred ml of 0.85% saline can be prepared by placing about 50 ml of distilled water into a 100 ml volumetric flask, adding 0.85 grams of sodium chloride and then adding the water up to 100 ml; thus 100 ml of 0.85% saline contain 0.85 g sodium

**Problem:** Prepare 100 ml of a 2% solution of acetic acid using a 10% acetic acid solution.

**Formula:** $C_1V_1 = C_2V_2$

$C_1$ = concentration of first solution
$C_2$ = concentration of second solution
$V_1$ = required volume of first solution
$V_2$ = required volume of second solution

**Solution:**

$$(2)(100 \text{ ml}) = (10)(V_2)$$
$$200 \text{ ml} = 10(V_2)$$
$$\frac{200}{10} \text{ ml} = V_2$$
$$20 \text{ ml} = V_2$$

**Answer:** Twenty ml of 10% acetic acid are added to 80 ml of distilled water to make 100 ml of a 2% solution of acetic acid.

**Figure 1-17.** Using the formula: $C_1 \times V_1 = C_2 \times V_2$ to prepare a solution

chloride. In a similar manner 500 ml of 0.85% saline could be prepared (Figure 1–18).

Another type of percentage is called volume to volume (v/v), in which a certain volume of one liquid is added to a specific volume of another. A 1% solution of hydrochloric acid can be prepared by adding one ml of the concentrated acid to 99 ml of water. Another example is the preparation of one liter of 2% acetic acid (Figure 1–19).

## RATIOS

A **ratio** is the relationship in number or degree between two things. Dilutions, which are ratios, express the relationship between a part of a solution and the total solution. Dilutions are used frequently in the laboratory, especially in hematology and serology (Figure 1–20). One procedure for performing the white blood cell count requires that a 1 to 20

**Problem:** Prepare 500 ml of 0.85% saline.

**Solution:**
1. A 0.85% solution contains 0.85 g of the solute in every 100 ml of solution.
2. Therefore, to prepare 500 ml, 5 × 0.85 g or 4.25 g of sodium chloride (NaCl) must be used.
3. To prepare the solution:
   a. Weigh out 4.25 g of NaCl
   b. Fill a 500 ml volumetric flask approximately half full with distilled water
   c. Add 4.25 g of NaCl and swirl gently to dissolve
   d. Fill the flask to the line with distilled water

**Figure 1-18.** Preparation of a weight to volume (w/v) percentage solution

**Problem:** Prepare one liter of 2% acetic acid from concentrated (glacial) acetic acid.

**Solution:**
1. A 2% solution of acetic acid contains 2 ml of acetic acid in each 100 ml of solution.
2. Therefore, one liter of 2% acetic acid contains 2 ml × 10, or 20 ml of acetic acid.
3. To prepare the solution:
   a. Fill a one-liter volumetric flask approximately half full of distilled water
   b. Add 20 ml of concentrated acetic acid and swirl to mix
   c. Fill the flask to the line with distilled water

**Figure 1-19.** Preparation of a volume to volume (v/v) percentage solution

**Problem:** Prepare 10 ml of a 1:10 dilution of serum using saline as the diluent.

**Solution:**
1. A 1:10 dilution contains one part of a substance combined with 9 parts of a diluent to give a total of 10 parts.
2. Add 1 ml of serum to 9 ml of saline to form 10 ml of a 1:10 dilution of the serum.
3. If 50 ml were required, 5 ml of serum would be added to 45 ml saline.

**Figure 1-20.** Preparation of a 1:10 dilution

(1:20) dilution of the blood be made in order to count the cells. This is accomplished by adding 0.5 units of blood to 9.5 units of the diluting fluid. The total volume is equal to 0.5 plus 9.5 (0.5 + 9.5) or 10 parts. The relationship between the 0.5 and the total volume is expressed as the ratio of $\frac{10}{.5}$, a dilution factor of 20, or a dilution of 1:20.

## *LESSON REVIEW*

1. Give an example of a percentage solution used in the laboratory.
2. Why are temperature conversions sometimes necessary?
3. What is the total of the parts in a 1:10 dilution?
4. What are the two formulas used to solve proportion problems?
5. How is a 1% (v/v) solution prepared?
6. How is a 5% (w/v) solution prepared?
7. Define Celsius, distilled water, Fahrenheit, ratio, and saline.

## *STUDENT ACTIVITIES*

1. Re-read the information on laboratory math.
2. Review the glossary terms.
3. Find examples of temperature in Celsius degrees, percent solutions, and dilutions or ratios in a chemistry or similar textbook.
4. Practice preparing solutions in the laboratory as instructed by the teacher.
5. Practice the calculations for percentage solutions, proportions, and ratios using the worksheets.

# Laboratory Math Worksheet–Proportions

NAME ______________________________ DATE __________

## LESSON 1–8 LABORATORY MATH

1. In the lab a procedure calls for 200 ml of a 2% solution of red cells. A 50% solution is available. How much of the 50% solution is needed? How would the solution be prepared?

2. A 1% solution of hydrochloric acid is required for a procedure. A 5% solution is available. How much of the 5% will be required to make 500 ml of a 1% solution?

3. A procedure calls for acetic acid and water with the proportions being two parts of acetic acid to three parts of water. One hundred ml are needed. How much acetic acid and how much water are required?

4. One liter of 70% alcohol is needed. How much 95% alcohol is required?

5. Two hundred ml of 2% acetic acid are needed. How many ml of 5% acetic acid are required?

HEMATOLOGY

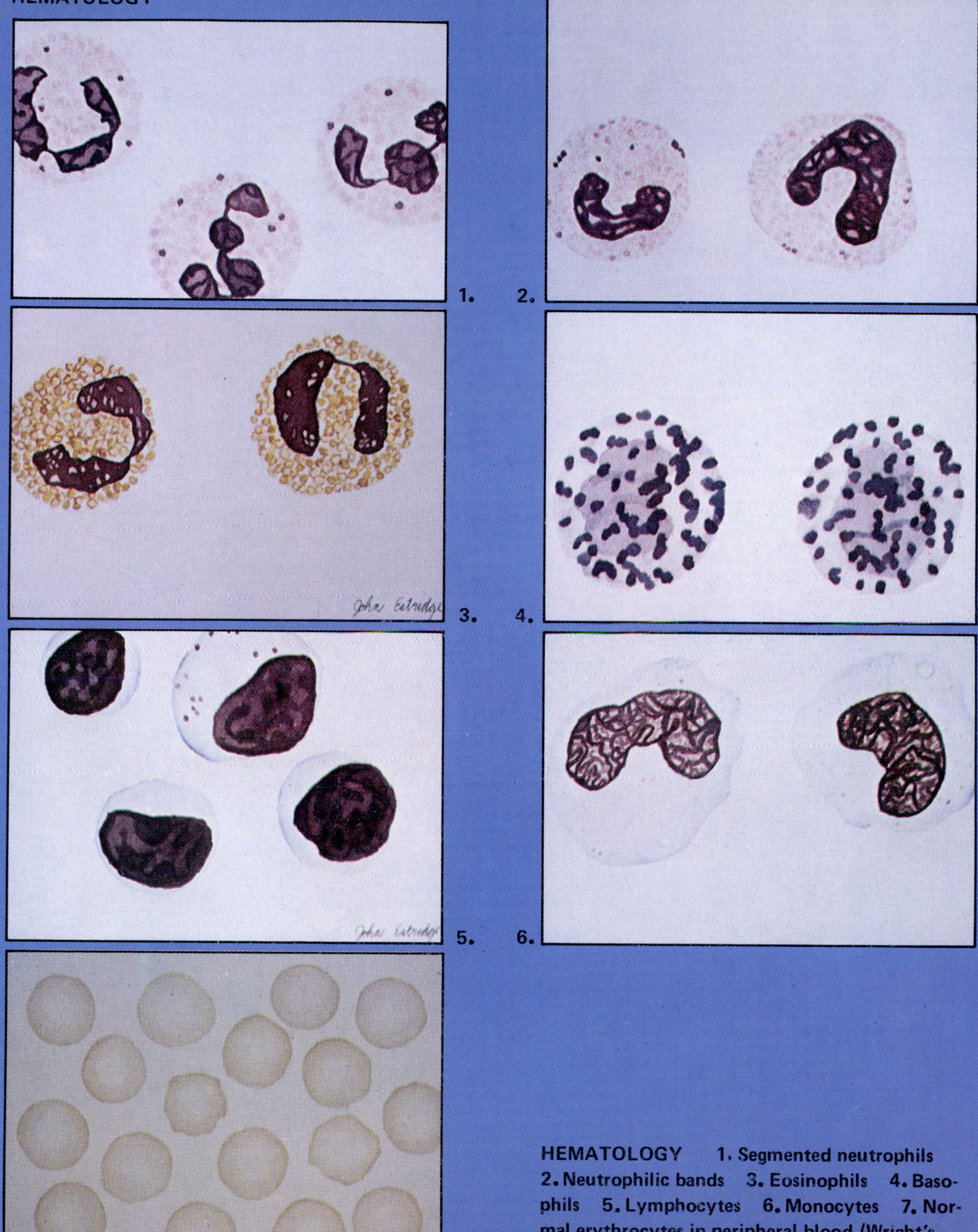


HEMATOLOGY 1. Segmented neutrophils 2. Neutrophilic bands 3. Eosinophils 4. Basophils 5. Lymphocytes 6. Monocytes 7. Normal erythrocytes in peripheral blood (Wright's stain)

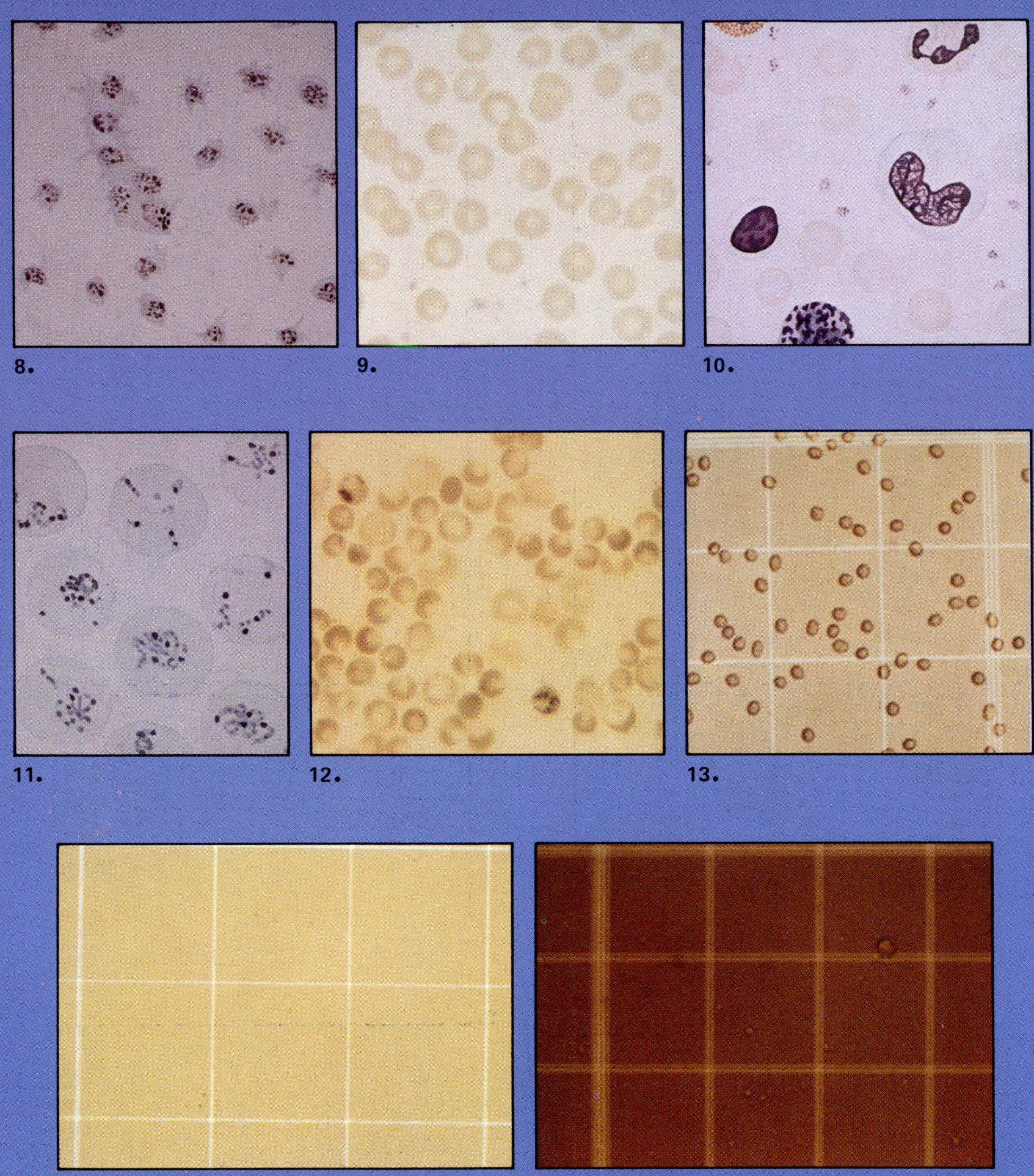


**8.** Platelets in peripheral blood (Wright's stain) **9.** Photomicrograph of Wright's stained erythrocytes and platelets in peripheral blood (1000X) **10.** Examples of blood cells seen in peripheral blood smear from a normal individual (Wright's stain) **11.** Drawing of reticulocytes showing stained reticulum (new methylene blue preparation) **12.** Photomicrograph of reticulocytes stained with new methylene blue (1000X) **13.** Photomicrograph of erythrocytes as they appear in an RBC count (400X) **14.** Photomicrograph of leukocytes as they appear in a WBC count (100X) **15.** Photomicrograph of platelets as they appear in a platelet count (400X)

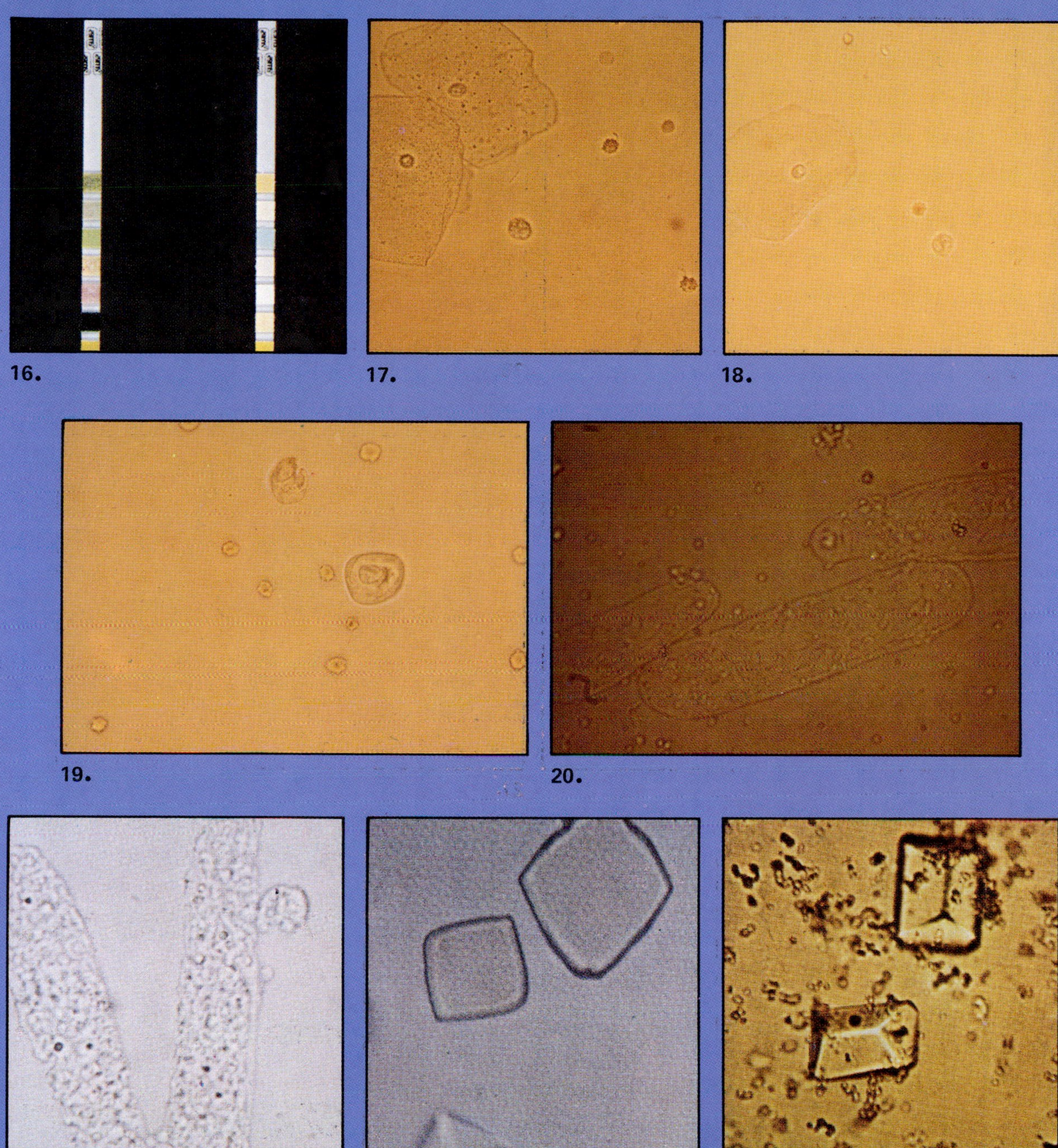

21. 22. 23.

**URINALYSIS** 16. Reagent strips used for chemical analysis of urine 17. Squamous epithelial cells, red blood cells, leukocyte 18. Squamous epithelial cell, red cell and white cell 19. Renal epithelial cell and erythrocytes 20. Hyaline cast 21. Granular casts and a leukocyte 22. Two uric acid crystals and part of a calcium oxalate crystal 23. Two ammonium magnesium phosphate crystals (triple phosphate) with amorphous phosphate granules

## BACTERIOLOGY

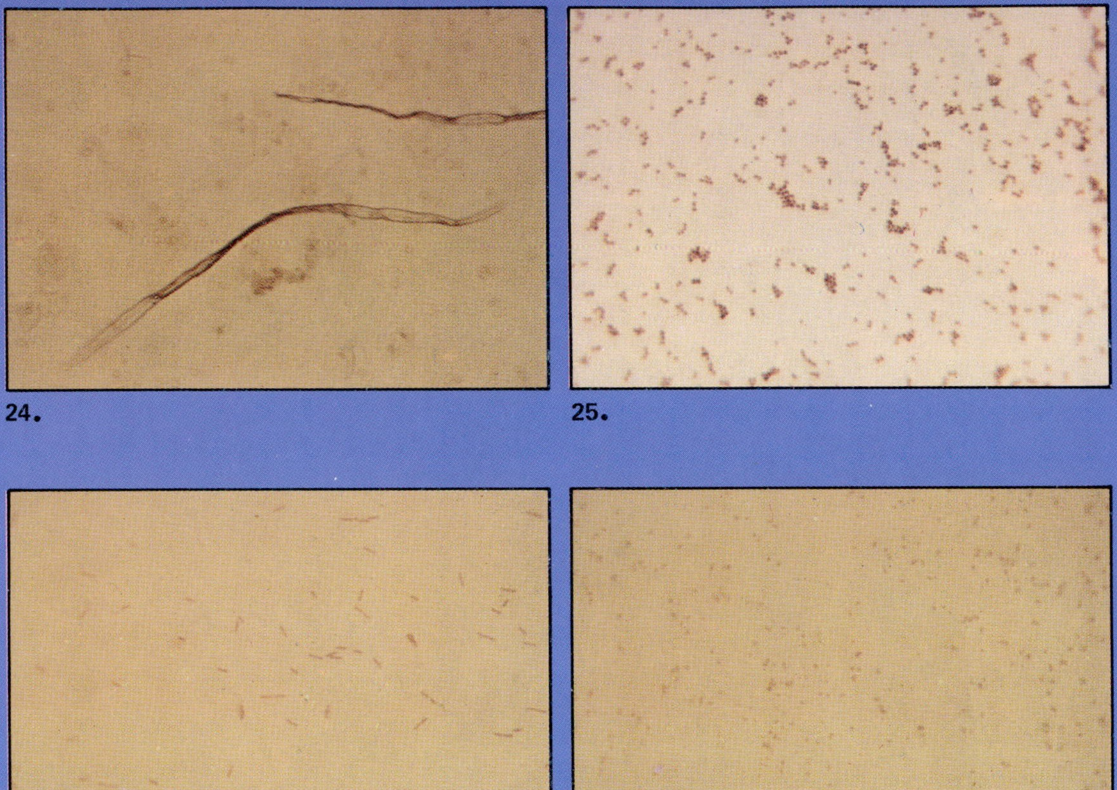

24. 25.

26. 27.

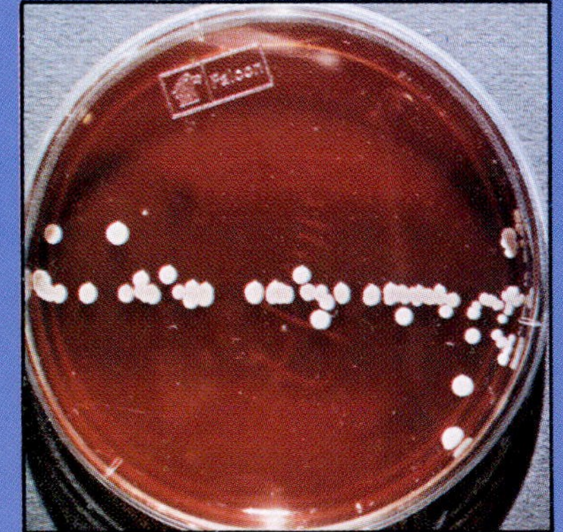

28.

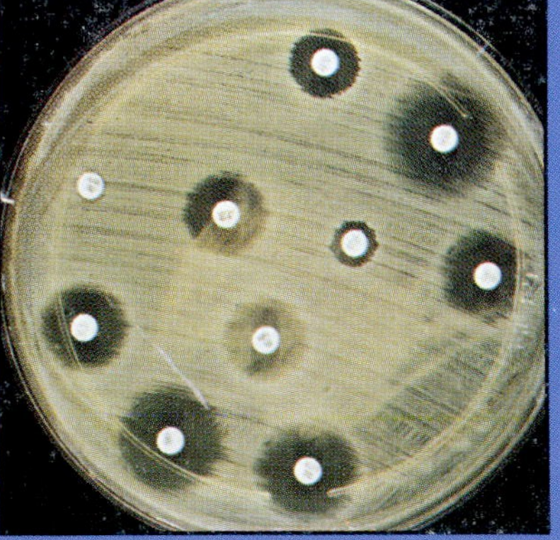

29.

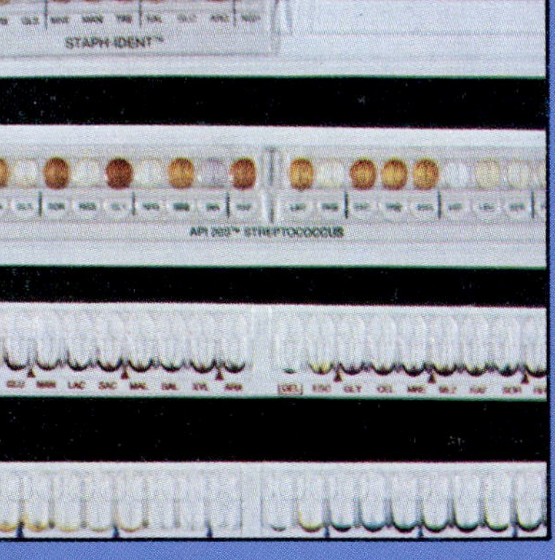

30.

**24.** Artifacts  BACTERIOLOGY  **25.** Gram positive coccus from a pure culture  **26.** Gram negative rod from a pure culture  **27.** Gram negative diplococcus from a pure culture  **28.** A blood agar plate showing isolated colonies of bacteria  **29.** Antibiotic susceptibility test plate  **30.** Biochemical strip tests

# Laboratory Math Worksheet–Percentage Solutions

NAME ______________________________ DATE ______________

## LESSON 1–8 LABORATORY MATH

1. How would 100 ml of a 10% solution of sodium chloride be prepared?

2. For a lab procedure, 50 ml of a 2% solution of red cells are needed. How is the solution prepared?

3. Give the instructions for the preparation of 300 ml of a 5% solution of acetic acid.

4. If 250 ml of a 4% solution of hydrochloric acid are needed for a procedure, how could it be prepared?

5. Give the instructions for preparing one liter of a 3% solution of sodium chloride.

# Laboratory Math Worksheet–Ratios

NAME ______________________________ DATE ____________

## LESSON 1–8 LABORATORY MATH

1. A 1 to 25 dilution of blood is required for a procedure. How is it prepared?

2. The red blood cell count requires that blood be diluted so that 0.5 parts are diluted to a total of 100 parts. What is the dilution?

3. How could a 1:10 dilution of serum be prepared?

4. If 0.5 ml of serum is added to 4.5 ml of saline, what is the dilution?

5. If 0.5 ml of blood is added to 9.5 ml of saline, what is the dilution?

# UNIT 2
# Basic Hematology

## UNIT OBJECTIVES

After studying this unit, you should be able to:

- Perform a capillary puncture.
- Perform a microhematocrit.
- Perform blood dilutions using blood diluting pipets.
- Use a hemacytometer.
- Perform a manual red cell count and calculate the results.
- Perform a manual white cell count and calculate the results.
- Make a blood smear.
- Stain a blood smear.
- Identify blood cells from a stained smear.
- Perform a differential leukocyte count.

## OVERVIEW

Blood is composed of formed elements suspended in a fluid called plasma. These formed elements include erythrocytes (red blood cells), leukocytes (white blood cells), and thrombocytes (platelets). These cellular elements are produced and mature in the bone marrow. They are then released into the bloodstream where they play important roles in oxygen transport, blood clotting and providing immunity.

Hematology is the study of the formed elements of blood and the blood-forming tissues. The cellular elements of blood may be studied by counting the cells, as in red cell and white cell counts. Cellular elements may also be studied from stained blood smears. From these smears, the percentages of cell types and the morphology (the structure and form) of cells can be determined.

A blood sample adequate for most hematological tests may be obtained from capillaries by finger puncture. If a larger sample is required, blood is obtained from a vein by venipuncture. Venous blood samples are usually collected in a tube containing an anticoagulant which prevents clotting. When a blood sample has had anticoagulant added, the liquid portion is called plasma. When blood is collected without an anticoagulant, it forms a clot and the liquid portion remaining is called serum. Anticoagulated blood is used for most hematological tests.

One of the most frequently requested tests in the hematology laboratory is the CBC, or complete blood count. The CBC is a combination of tests that usually includes a red cell count, white cell count, hemoglobin, hematocrit, differential count, estimation of platelet numbers, and observation of blood cell morphology. In this unit, you will be introduced to basic procedures. These will include performing a CBC, collecting a capillary blood specimen, and using medical laboratory instruments and equipment.

The examination of blood can provide important information. It can help in the diagnosis and treatment of many blood diseases such as the leukemias and anemias. It also aids in the diagnosis and management of diseases that originate in other body systems.

Test results are relied upon for the diagnosis and treatment of disease. Therefore, it is vital that the tests are performed with accuracy, precision, and utmost attention to proper procedure. It takes practice and skill to become proficient and perform most of the basic hematology procedures in a reliable manner.

# LESSON 2–1

## Capillary Puncture

## LESSON OBJECTIVES

After studying this lesson, you should be able to:

- Identify sites for capillary punctures.
- Perform a capillary puncture.
- Collect a blood specimen from a capillary puncture.
- List the precautions to be observed when performing a capillary puncture.
- Define the glossary terms.

## GLOSSARY

**anticoagulant** / agent which prevents blood coagulation

**capillary** / a minute blood vessel which connects the smallest arteries to the smallest veins

**capillary tube** / a glass tube of very small diameter used for laboratory procedures

**heparin** / an anticoagulant used in certain laboratory procedures

**lancet** / a sterile, sharp-pointed blade used to perform a capillary puncture

**lateral** / toward the side

## INTRODUCTION

A **capillary** is a small blood vessel connecting the small arteries (arterioles) to the small veins (venules). Because of the capillary's small diameter, the capillary puncture is an efficient means of collecting a blood specimen when only a small amount of blood is required. It may also be used when the patient has a condition which would make venipuncture difficult. Capillary blood is an ideal specimen because the cell distribution resembles that normally found in the circulating blood. Blood cell counts, the microhematocrit, and the blood smear are some of the procedures which can be performed using a capillary blood sample.

## PUNCTURE SITES

The puncture sites used to obtain capillary blood are the finger, heel, and ear lobe. In adults and children, the usual puncture site is the ring finger because it usually is not calloused. The puncture is made at the tip of the fleshy pad and slightly to the side (Figure 2–1) using a sharp-pointed blade called a **lancet.** If the tips of the fingers are heavily calloused or thickened, a special lancet may be used. Although the ear lobe may be used as a puncture site, the blood from there may not have normal cell distribution. In infants, the **lateral** portion of the heel pad is usually used. If possible, previous puncture sites should always be avoided.

### Preparation of Puncture Site

The area selected for a capillary puncture must be carefully prepared. The puncture site will be warm if circulation is adequate. Coolness of the skin indicates decreased circulation. If this is so, the patient's hands may be gently massaged or placed in warm water for a few minutes. Alcohol-soaked gauze or cotton should be used to cleanse and disinfect the puncture site. The site should then be allowed to air dry or should be wiped dry with sterile gauze. This allows the blood to form a well-rounded drop—something it will not do on moist skin.

*Capillary Tubes.* **Capillary tubes** which contain **heparin,** an **anticoagulant,** are used to collect capillary samples. Tubes which are heparinized have a red ring on one end. Pre-calibrated tubes are usually also heparinized. Plain capillary tubes are non-heparinized. These tubes have a blue ring and are used for blood already containing an anticoagulant.

## PERFORMING THE PUNCTURE

The patient's hand and finger should be held **laterally** so that the puncture site is readily accessible (Figure 2–1). The skin near the chosen site should be pulled taut. A sterile lancet is then used to pierce the site to a depth of 3–4 mm. The puncture should be performed in one quick, steady motion. The first

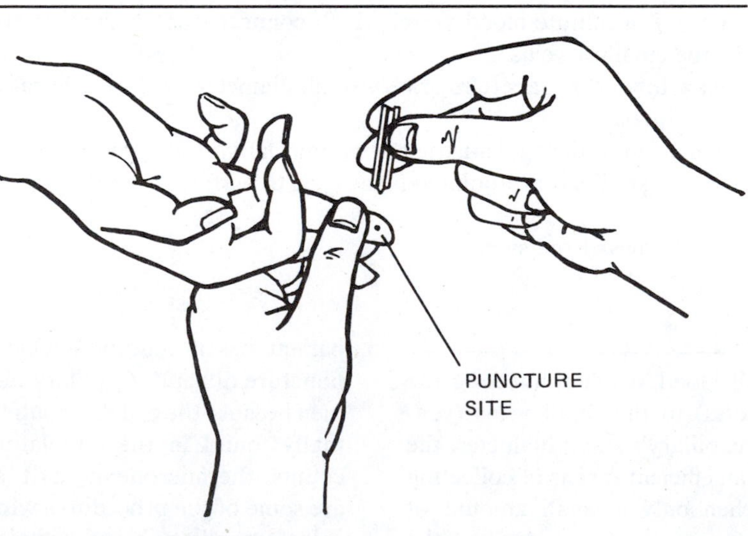


**Figure 2-1.** Capillary puncture

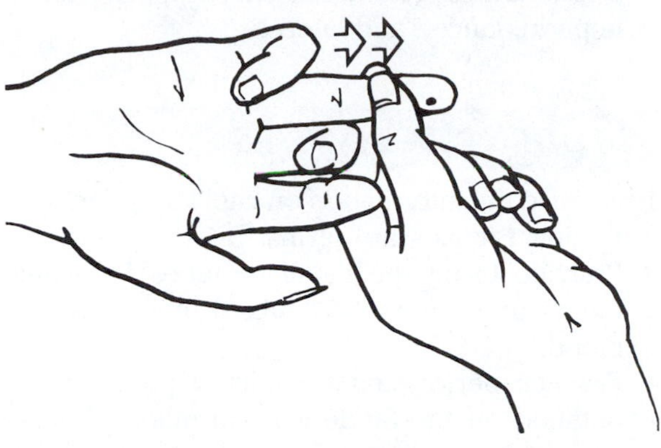

**Figure 2-2.** Massaging the finger gently to increase blood flow

drop of blood that appears is wiped away because it contains tissue fluid.

The second and following drops of blood are used for samples. Depending on the tests to be performed, the blood may be collected in blood-diluting pipets or in capillary tubes. It may be necessary to massage the finger to increase blood flow. However, pressure should not be applied near the puncture site (Figure 2–2). Squeezing the finger will force tissue fluid into the blood sample and dilute it. The capillary tube should be held in an almost horizontal position and should be filled ⅔ to ¾ full. Heparinized capillary tubes should always be used when collecting capillary blood samples. The samples must be collected quickly to avoid blood clotting (Figure 2–3). Capillary punctures may also be performed using semi-automated devices such as the Autolet®.

### *Precautions*

- Circulation around the puncture site must be adequate.
- The puncture site should be cleansed thoroughly.
- The puncture site must be dry because blood will spread and will not form a drop on moist skin.
- The puncture should be performed quickly and to a depth of 3–4 mm to assure good blood flow.
- The finger should not be squeezed; tissue fluid will dilute the blood sample.
- Capillary samples must be collected quickly to prevent blood clotting.

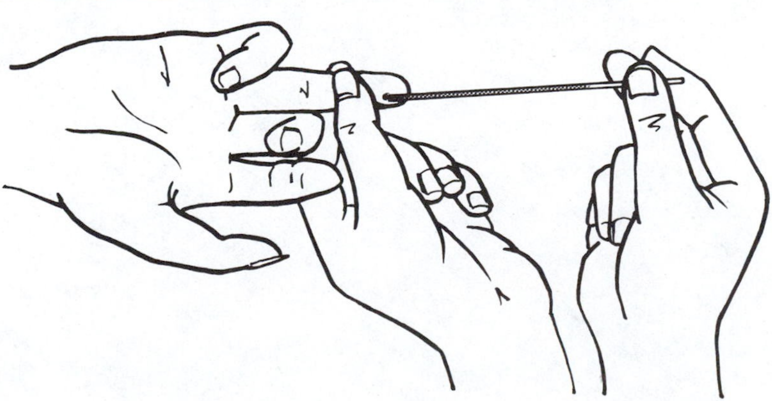

**Figure 2-3.** Collecting capillary blood into a capillary tube

## *LESSON REVIEW*

1. Why would a capillary puncture be performed?
2. Why is the ring finger usually used?
3. What is a capillary vessel?
4. What are the usual puncture sites for adults—for infants?
5. What should be done if the patient has cold hands?
6. Why is the first drop of blood wiped away?
7. What procedure is followed if the patient has very calloused fingers?
8. List three precautions that should be observed when performing a capillary puncture.
9. Define anticoagulant, capillary, capillary tube, heparin, lancet, and lateral.

## *STUDENT ACTIVITIES*

1. Re-read the information on capillary puncture.
2. Review the glossary terms.
3. Practice using the capillary tubes by filling them from a tube of well-mixed anticoagulated blood.
4. Practice performing a capillary puncture as outlined on the Student Performance Guide.

# Student Performance Guide

NAME ______________________________

DATE ______________________________

## LESSON 2–1 CAPILLARY PUNCTURE

### Instructions

1. Practice the procedure for performing a capillary puncture.
2. Demonstrate the procedure for a capillary puncture satisfactorily for the instructor. All steps must be completed as listed on the instructor's Performance Check Sheet.
3. Complete a written examination successfully.

### Materials and Equipment

- hand disinfectant
- lancets (sterile, disposable)
- sterile cotton balls or gauze squares
- 70% alcohol
- capillary tubes (heparinized)
- sealing clay for capillary tubes
- pre-calibrated capillary tubes (optional)
- surface disinfectant
- biohazard container

**Procedure**

S = Satisfactory
U = Unsatisfactory

| You must: | S | U | Comments |
|---|---|---|---|
| 1. Wash hands with hand disinfectant | | | |
| 2. Assemble equipment and materials | | | |
| 3. Explain the procedure to the patient | | | |
| 4. Select and warm the puncture site | | | |
| 5. Cleanse the puncture site with alcohol-soaked gauze or cotton | | | |

| You must: | S | U | Comments |
|---|---|---|---|
| 6. Allow the site to air dry or wipe with dry sterile gauze or cotton | | | |
| 7. Position the puncture site, holding the skin taut with one hand and holding the lancet in the other hand | | | |
| 8. Perform the capillary puncture, using a quick, firm stab | | | |
| 9. Wipe the first drop of blood away with sterile gauze or cotton | | | |
| 10. Massage the finger gently to produce the second drop of blood | | | |
| 11. Fill a capillary tube two thirds to three-quarters full using the second drop of blood (fill to the line if using pre-calibrated capillary tubes) | | | |
| 12. Fill a second tube in the same manner | | | |
| 13. Place the clean end of the capillary tubes into the sealing clay | | | |
| 14. Apply pressure to the puncture site by pressing with dry sterile gauze or cotton | | | |
| 15. Place used lancet and used capillary tubes in a biohazard container | | | |
| 16. Dispose of used gauze or cotton properly | | | |
| 17. Clean and return equipment to proper storage | | | |
| 18. Clean work area with surface disinfectant | | | |
| 19. Wash hands with hand disinfectant | | | |

Comments:

Student/Instructor:

Date: ______________________ Instructor: ______________________

# LESSON 2-2

## Microhematocrit

### LESSON OBJECTIVES

After studying this lesson, you should be able to:

- Prepare a microhematocrit sample.
- Centrifuge a microhematocrit sample.
- Determine the microhematocrit value.
- Explain what the microhematocrit measures.
- List the normal values for a microhematocrit.
- List conditions that affect the microhematocrit value.
- List precautions that should be observed in performing the microhematocrit.
- Define the glossary terms.

### GLOSSARY

**buffy coat** / a light-colored layer of leukocytes and platelets which forms on the top of the red cell layer when a sample of blood is centrifuged or allowed to stand

**EDTA** / ethylene diamine tetraacetic acid; commonly used anticoagulant for hematological studies

**hematocrit** / the volume of erythrocytes packed by centrifugation in a given volume of blood and expressed as a percentage; abbreviated "crit" or Hct

**microhematocrit** / a hematocrit performed on a small sample of blood

**microhematocrit centrifuge** / a machine which spins capillary tubes at a high speed to cause rapid separation of liquid from solid components

**plasma** / the liquid part of the blood in which the cellular elements are suspended

## INTRODUCTION

The **microhematocrit** is a commonly performed test. It may be ordered separately or as part of a complete blood count (CBC). It is a simple procedure requiring only two to three drops of blood, which makes it an ideal test to follow the progress of anemic or bleeding patients.

The microhematocrit is a variation of a test called the **hematocrit.** The hematocrit is a test that is performed using one milliliter of blood in a Wintrobe tube (named for the person who developed the test). The test is based on the principle of separating the cellular elements of the blood from the liquid part, the **plasma.** In both hematocrit and microhematocrit procedures, the separation process is speeded up by centrifugation. After centrifugation, the red cells will be at the bottom of the tube, the white cells and platelets in the center, and the plasma at the top. The layer containing the white cells and platelets has a whitish-tan appearance and is commonly referred to as the **buffy coat** (Figure 2–4). From this separation the hematocrit or microhematocrit is determined by comparing the concentration of red cells to the volume of the whole blood sample. Laboratory personnel often refer to a hematocrit as a "crit" or abbreviate it with the letters Hct.

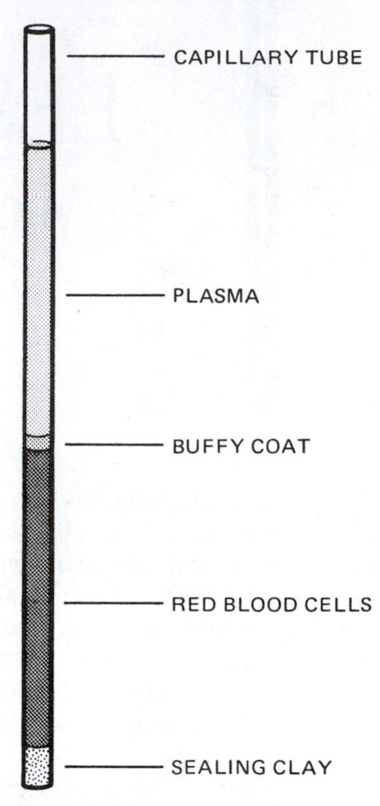


**Figure 2-4.** Diagram of packed cell column

### Preparing the Sample

The blood sample may be obtained from a capillary puncture or from a tube of venous blood which has had the anticoagulant **EDTA** added. The blood is drawn by capillary action into capillary tubes of very small diameter (Figure 2–5) which are sealed (Figure 2–6). To do this, the clean end of the tube is placed in sealing clay. This makes a tight seal and prevents contamination with blood. The tube is then placed in a special **microhematocrit centrifuge** (Figures 2–7, 2–8). The sealed ends of the tubes are placed against the rubber gasket and the open ends toward the center. After being centrifuged for the prescribed time (usually 3–5 minutes), the hematocrit (percentage) is read by placing the tube on a special microhematocrit reader (Figure 2–9). Some centrifuges, such as the Clay Adams Readacrit, have a built-in reading scale (Figure 2–7). Special precalibrated capillary tubes must be used with this type of centrifuge. Microhematocrits should be performed in duplicate. The average of the two results is reported. The two values should not vary by more than ± 2 percent.

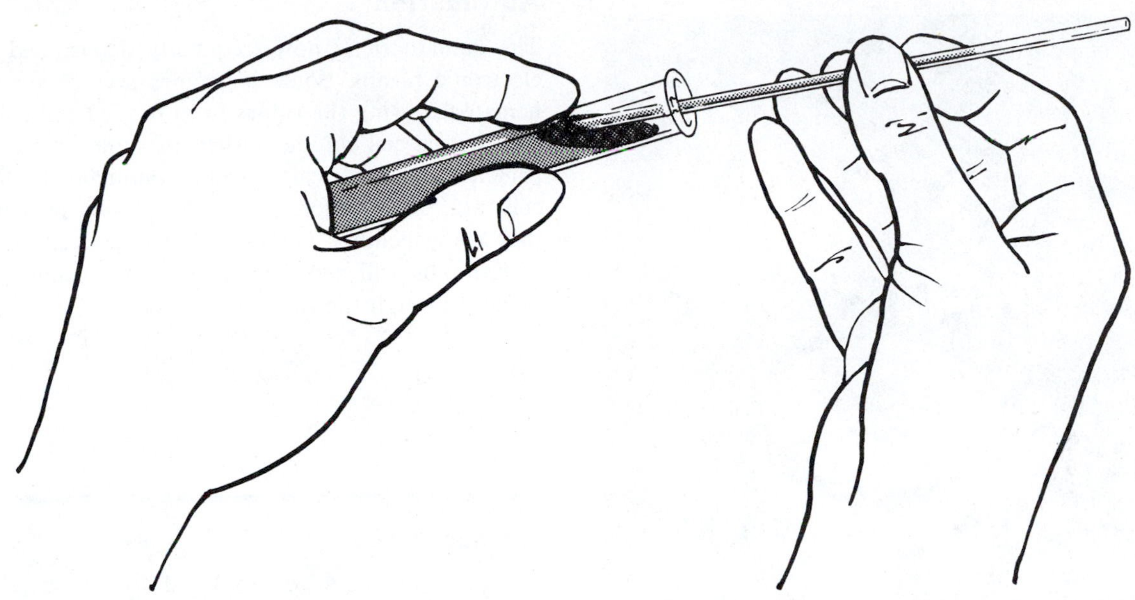

**Figure 2-5.** Filling the capillary tube from a tube of blood

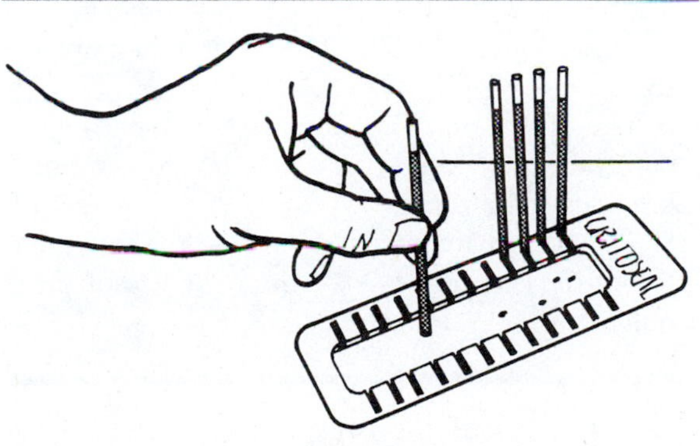

**Figure 2-6.** Sealing the capillary tube with sealing clay

## Normal Values

The normal microhematocrit value varies with the sex and age of the patient (Table 2–1). As you can see from the table, the values range from a low of 32% for a one-year-old to a high of 60% for a newborn.

**Table 2-1.** Normal Microhematocrit Values

| Age | Microhematocrit Values (%) Average | Range |
|---|---|---|
| Adult males | 47 | 42–52 |
| Adult females | 42 | 36–48 |
| Children (both sexes): | | |
| Newborn | 56 | 51–60 |
| One year | 35 | 32–38 |
| Six years | 38 | 34–42 |

## Factors that Influence Microhematocrit Values

The values obtained for microhematocrits can be influenced by physiological or pathological factors and by the handling of the specimen during the test procedure. Improper blood collection or the use of inadequately mixed blood can cause unreliable results.

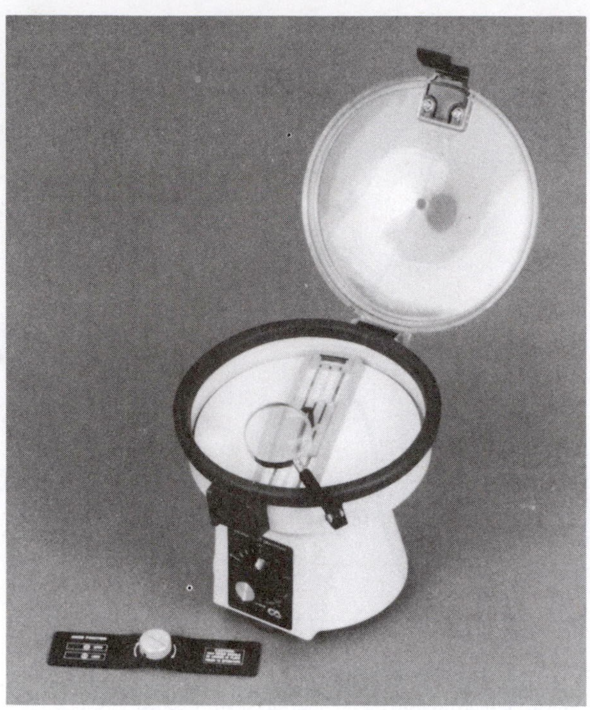

**Figure 2-7.** Microhematocrit centrifuge with built–in reader (*Photo courtesy of Clay Adams Division of Becton Dickinson & Co.*)

A low microhematocrit value can indicate an anemia or the presence of bleeding in a patient. An increased value may be caused by dehydration in the patient or by a condition such as polycythemia.

## Automation

The hematocrit is now frequently determined by electronic means. Some instruments calculate the hematocrit using the values from the red cell count and the red cell volume. Other instruments use the principle of electrical current conductance. Red cells are less conductive than the plasma in which they are suspended. Therefore, a high concentration of red cells will result in less current being conducted through the sample of blood.

### *Precautions*

- The recommended speed and time of centrifugation must be strictly followed.
- The clay seal must be tight or the contents of the tube may leak out.
- The sealed end of the capillary tube must be placed against the rubber gasket in the centrifuge.
- The inner centrifuge lid must be closed securely before closing the outer lid, to prevent breaking glass tubes.
- The microhematocrit should be read at the top of the red cell layer—not at the top of the buffy coat.

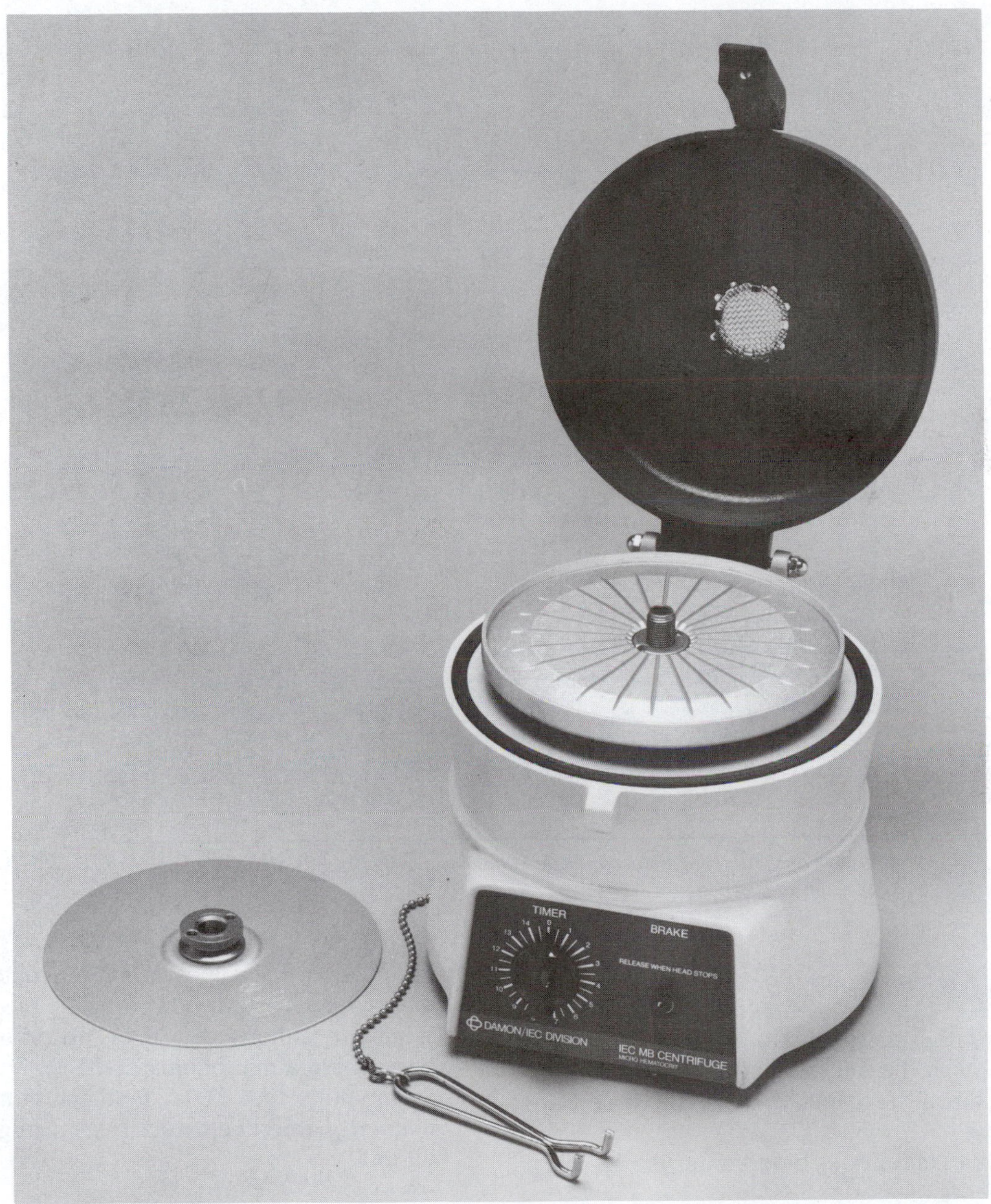


**Figure 2-8.** Microhematocrit centrifuge without reader (*Photo courtesy of International Equipment, Division of Damon*)

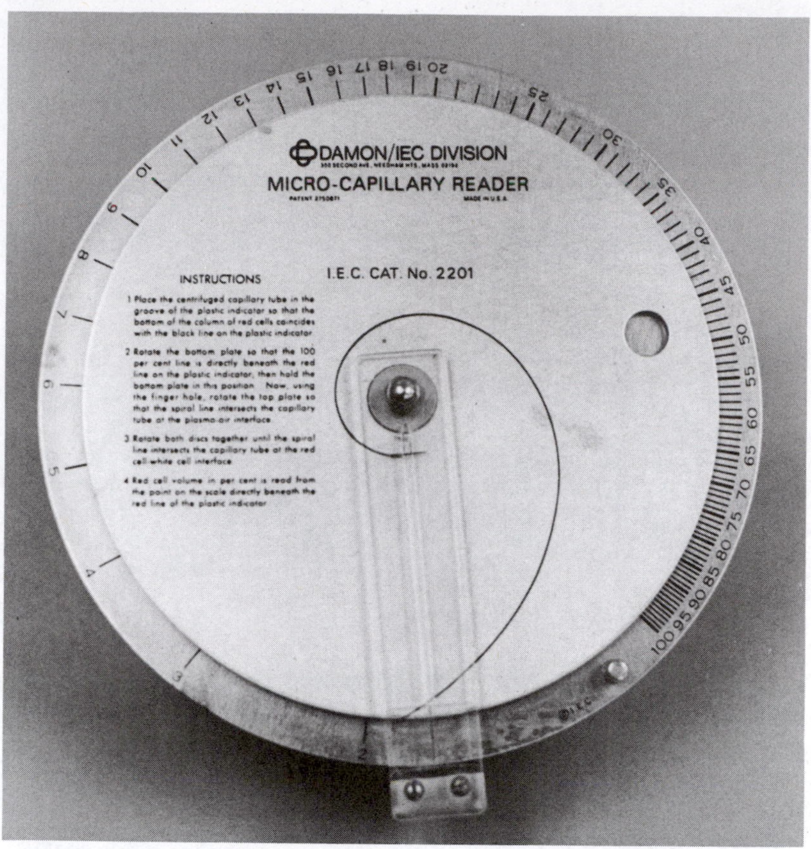


**Figure 2-9.** Microhematocrit reader (*Photo courtesy of International Equipment, Division of Damon*)

## *LESSON REVIEW*

1. Explain the microhematocrit procedure.
2. What does the microhematocrit measure?
3. Why must the capillary tube be sealed securely?
4. By what action does blood enter the capillary tube?
5. What is the usual length of time for centrifugation?
6. Name a condition which could cause a decreased microhematocrit value.
7. Give the normal values of microhematocrit for males, females, and newborns.
8. What precautions should be observed when performing a microhematocrit?
9. Define buffy coat, EDTA, hematocrit, microhematocrit, microhematocrit centrifuge, and plasma.

## *STUDENT ACTIVITIES*

1. Re-read the information on microhematocrit.
2. Review the glossary terms.
3. Practice performing a microhematocrit test on several blood samples as outlined on the Student Performance Guide.
4. Repeat the microhematocrit procedure on a blood sample, lengthening or shortening the centrifugation time. Record the results and give the reason for the different values obtained in the previous microhematocrit.
5. Demonstrate the importance of using well-mixed blood: perform a microhematocrit on a well-mixed sample; allow the sample tube to stand upright two minutes and perform another microhematocrit without re-mixing the blood. Compare the results and explain the difference.

# Student Performance Guide

NAME ______________________________

DATE ______________________________

## LESSON 2–2 MICROHEMATOCRIT

### Instructions

1. Practice the microhematocrit procedure.
2. Demonstrate the microhematocrit procedure satisfactorily for the instructor. All steps must be completed as listed on the instructor's Performance Check Sheet.
3. Complete a written examination successfully.

### Materials and Equipment

- hand disinfectant
- capillary tubes, plain and with heparin
- pre-calibrated capillary tubes (optional)
- sealing clay or vinyl putty
- microhematocrit centrifuge and reader
- tube of anticoagulated venous blood
- paper towels or soft laboratory tissue
- 70% alcohol
- gauze or cotton balls, sterile
- blood lancets, sterile, disposable
- surface disinfectant
- biohazard container

*Note:* Consult the instruction manual for the centrifuge being used. Refer to the specific procedure being performed.

## Procedure

S = Satisfactory
U = Unsatisfactory

| You must: | S | U | Comments |
|---|---|---|---|
| 1. Wash hands with hand disinfectant | | | |
| 2. Assemble equipment and materials | | | |
| 3. Fill two capillary tubes using a tube of EDTA anticoagulated blood: | | | |
| a. Mix the tube of blood thoroughly by rocking tube from end to end gently 20 to 30 times | | | |
| b. Remove cap from tube, avoiding contamination of hands with blood | | | |
| c. Tilt the tube so that blood is very near the top edge of the tube | | | |
| d. Insert a plain capillary tube beneath the surface of the blood and fill to two thirds by capillary action (if using pre-calibrated tubes, fill to the line) Note: Wipe the outside of the filled capillary tube with tissue, if necessary, to remove excess blood | | | |
| e. Seal the tube by placing the clean end into the tray of sealing clay | | | |
| f. Fill a second tube in the same manner | | | |
| 4. Fill two capillary tubes from a capillary puncture: | | | |
| a. Wash hands | | | |
| b. Assemble equipment and materials | | | |
| c. Perform a capillary puncture | | | |
| d. Wipe away the first drop of blood | | | |
| e. Place one end of a heparinized capillary tube into the second drop of blood | | | |
| f. Allow the tube to fill two thirds by capillary action. A slight downward angle of the tube may be necessary (if using pre-calibrated tubes, fill to the line) | | | |
| g. Fill a second tube in the same manner | | | |
| h. Wipe the outside of the filled capillary tube with soft tissue, if necessary, to remove excess blood | | | |
| i. Seal the capillary tube by placing one end into the tray of sealing clay (the sealing clay will stay cleaner if dry/clean end of the capillary tube is sealed) | | | |
| 5. Check to see if the interior sealing clay edge appears level in tubes | | | |

| You must: | S | U | Comments |
|---|---|---|---|
| 6. Place tubes into the microhematocrit centrifuge with sealed ends securely against the gasket (balance the centrifuge by placing the tubes opposite each other) | | | |
| 7. Fasten the lids securely | | | |
| 8. Set the timer and adjust the speed if necessary | | | |
| 9. Centrifuge for the prescribed time | | | |
| 10. Allow centrifuge to come to a complete stop and unlock lid | | | |
| 11. Determine the microhematocrit values using one of the following methods:<br>A. A centrifuge which requires calibrated tubes and has a built-in scale: | | | |
| (1) Position the tubes as directed by the manufacturer's instructions to obtain the microhematocrit value | | | |
| B. A centrifuge which can accept any microhematocrit tubes:<br>(1) Remove capillary tubes from centrifuge carefully | | | |
| (2) Place tube on the microhematocrit reader provided | | | |
| (3) Follow instructions on the reader to obtain the hematocrit value | | | |
| 12. Average the values from the two tubes and record the hematocrit | | | |
| 13. Dispose of the capillary tubes in a biohazard container | | | |
| 14. Clean and return equipment to proper storage | | | |
| 15. Clean the work area with surface disinfectant | | | |
| 16. Wash hands with hand disinfectant | | | |

Comments:

Student/Instructor:

Date: ______________________ Instructor: ______________________

# LESSON 2-3

## Blood Diluting Pipets

## LESSON OBJECTIVES

After studying this lesson, you should be able to:

- Identify the parts of a blood diluting pipet.
- Explain the function of a blood diluting pipet.
- Dilute a blood sample using the white blood cell diluting pipet.
- Dilute a blood sample using the red blood cell diluting pipet.
- Dispense drops one at a time from a filled blood diluting pipet.
- Clean a blood diluting pipet.
- Calculate the dilutions made with red and white blood cell diluting pipets.
- Explain the proper care of a blood diluting pipet.
- List the precautions to be observed when using blood diluting pipets.
- Define the glossary terms.

## GLOSSARY

**aspiration** / act of drawing in by suction

**capillary action** / the action by which a fluid will enter a tube or pipet because of the attraction between the glass and liquid

**diluting fluid** / diluting solution which will not damage the cells being counted

**erythrocyte** / red blood cell; RBC; transports oxygen to the tissue and carbon dioxide ($CO_2$) to the lungs

**leukocyte** / white blood cell; WBC; protects from disease

**micropipet** / pipet which holds a very small volume

**red cell diluting pipet** / pipet used to dilute blood for a red cell count; RBC pipet

**white cell diluting pipet** / pipet used to dilute blood for white cell count; WBC pipet

## INTRODUCTION

Before blood cells may be counted microscopically, blood must be diluted. This is because cellular elements in the blood are so concentrated. Blood diluting pipets are valuable pieces of equipment which are used to dilute blood and other body fluids. To use the reusable Thoma-style pipets, blood (or other sample) and **diluting fluid** are mixed within the pipet. A count is then performed using the diluted sample, a counting chamber, and a microscope. The Thoma-style pipets are used mostly for **erythrocyte, leukocyte,** and platelet counts. However, they may also be used for sperm counts, counting cells in spinal fluid, synovial fluids, or other body fluids. Red and white cell pipets are shown in Figure 2-10.

## PARTS OF A BLOOD DILUTING PIPET

Blood diluting pipets have three basic parts: (1) a long calibrated stem into which the sample and diluting fluid are aspirated, (2) the bulb in which the contents are mixed, and (3) the short stem to which rubber tubing and the mouthpiece are attached (Figure 2-10). Blood diluting pipets may differ in the markings on the stems and the size of the mixing bulb. Only pipets manufactured according to specifications of the National Bureau of Standards (NBS) and certified by the NBS to have a ± 1% accuracy should be used for clinical work.

### The Red Cell Diluting Pipet

The **red cell diluting pipet** is used to dilute blood for an erythrocyte count (Figure 2-11). The 0.5 mark on the long stem is the mark to which blood is drawn. The 101 mark on the short stem is the mark to which diluting fluid (mixed with sample) is drawn. The red bead identifies the pipet as an RBC pipet and also mixes the contents. The bulb is the area where sample and diluting fluid are combined in exact proportions and mixed.

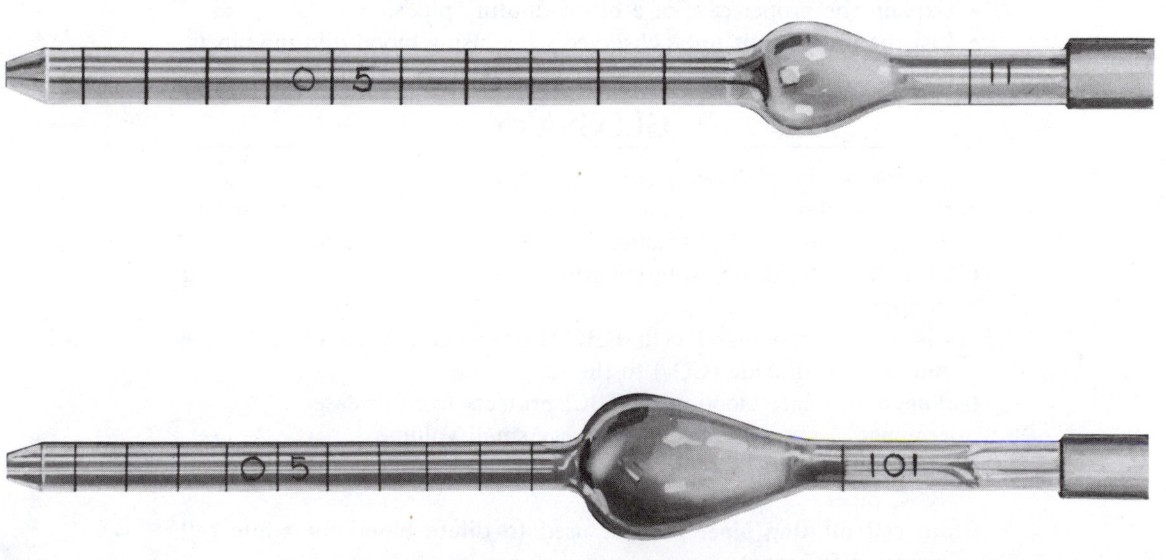


**Figure 2-10.** Red (bottom) and white (top) cell diluting pipets (*Photo courtesy of Reichert Scientific Instruments*)

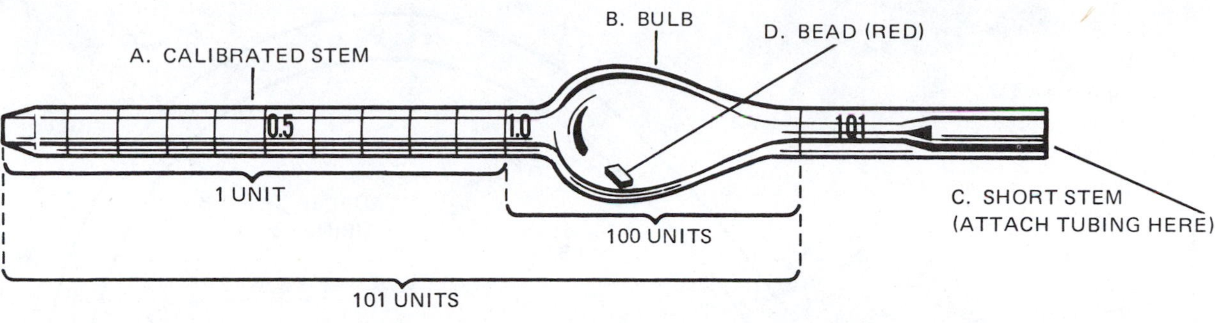


**Figure 2-11.** Parts of a red cell diluting pipet

## The White Cell Diluting Pipet

The **white cell diluting pipet,** shown in Figure 2–12, is used to dilute blood for a leukocyte count. The pipet is designed like the RBC pipet except that it holds a smaller volume and, therefore, makes a lower dilution. The 0.5 mark on the long stem is the mark to which blood is drawn. The 11 mark is the mark to which diluting fluid (mixed with blood) is drawn. In the bulb the blood and diluting fluid are combined in exact proportions and mixed. The white or clear bead aids in mixing the contents and in identifying the WBC pipet.

# USING A BLOOD DILUTING PIPET

Blood diluting pipets are all used similarly. The important steps in using a pipet are: filling the pipet, mixing the contents, and dispensing the diluted sample. Pipets must be clean and dry when used in order to make accurate dilutions. When a pipet is completely dry, the mixing bead will roll freely in the bulb.

Cell counts provide valuable information to the physician. It is important that the cell counts be as accurate as possible. Therefore, it is important that blood dilutions be performed carefully and precisely. If anticoagulated venous blood is used, it must be mixed by gentle inversion 20–30 times before sampled. (Do not shake!)

## Filling the Pipet

Both sample and diluting fluid are aspirated into the pipet by using rubber tubing and mouthpiece (and safety filter if used) attached to the short stem (Figure 2–12). The tubing is attached to the pipet and the tip of the pipet is placed into the sample. The sample is then carefully and slowly drawn up to the 0.5 mark by **aspiration** or **capillary action** (Figure 2–13). The excess sample is then wiped from the outside of the pipet tip with soft tissue, taking care not to touch the tip of the pipet, thereby withdrawing some of the sample. Diluting fluid is then carefully aspirated to the 11 or 101 mark (Figure 2–14). The pipet should be slowly rotated while fluid is aspirated. It is important that the dilutions are accurate. Therefore, the sample must be drawn exactly to the 0.5 mark and the diluting fluid exactly to the 11 or 101 mark.

## Mixing Fluids

Once the pipet is filled, the index finger is placed over the pipet tip and the rubber tubing is carefully

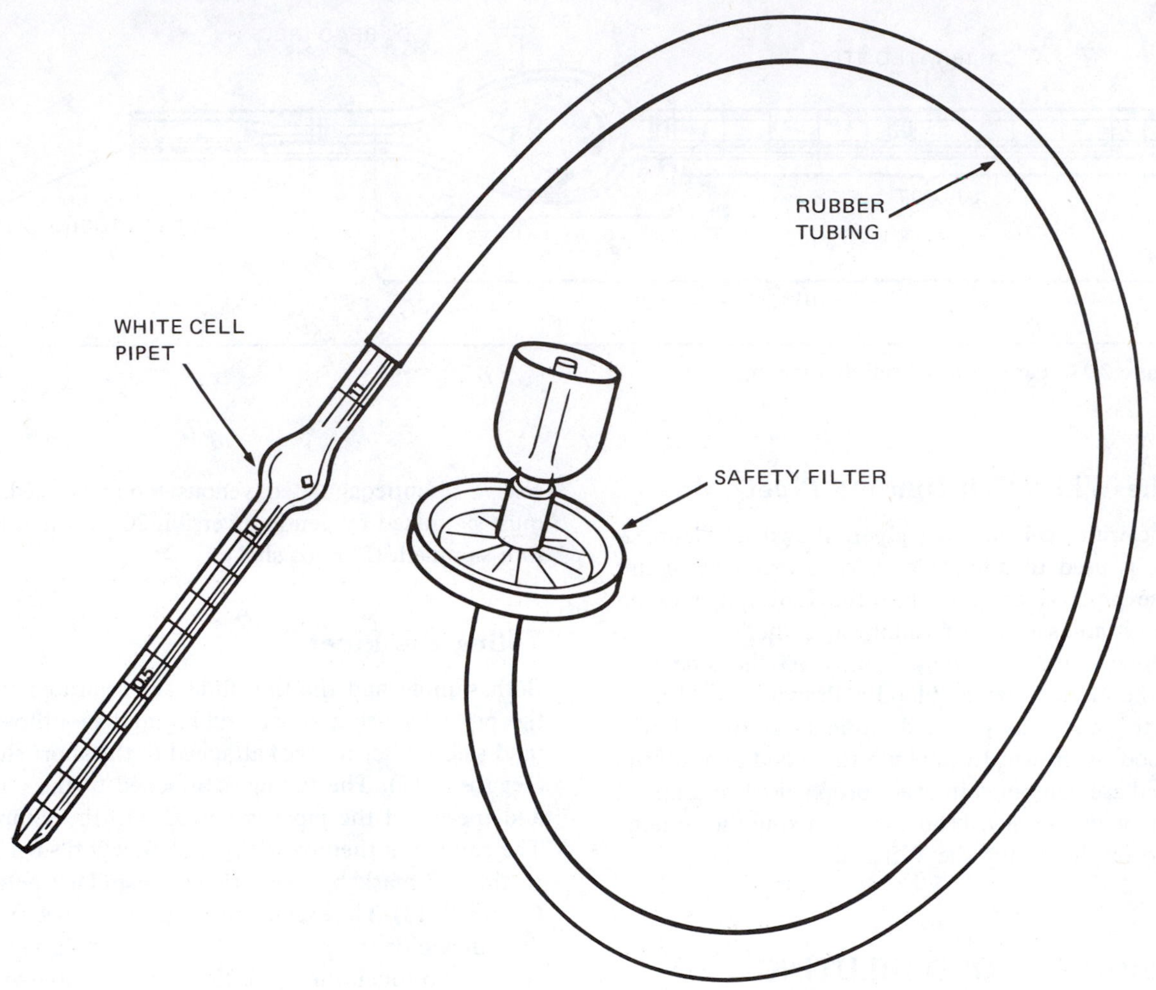


**Figure 2-12.** White cell diluting pipet with rubber tubing, safety filter and mouthpiece attached

removed while the pipet is held in a horizontal position. The contents of the pipet are then mixed by using hand rotation or a pipet shaker. For hand mixing, the pipet is held carefully so that the thumb covers one end of the pipet and the middle or index finger covers the other end (Figure 2–15). The pipet is then rotated in a figure-eight motion for two or three minutes. If an automatic shaker is used, the pipet should be carefully inserted into the shaker (Figure 2–16). The timer should be set for the proper shaking time (at least two minutes).

### Dispensing Fluids

Fluid should be dispensed from the pipet as soon as shaking is completed to avoid settling of the con-

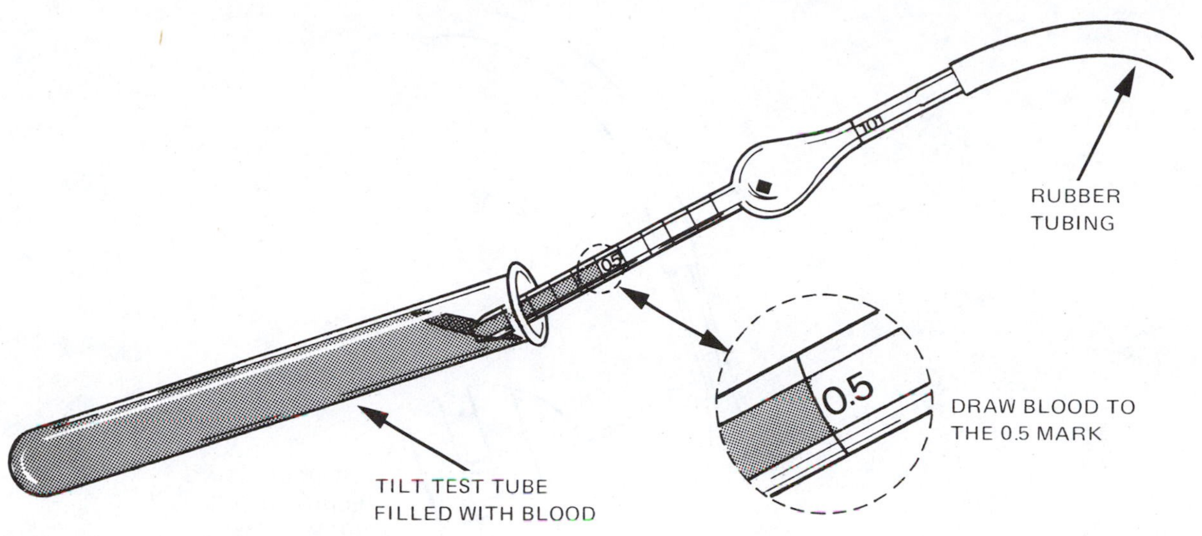


**Figure 2-13.** Aspirating a sample using the RBC pipet

tents. The pipet should be held as shown in Figure 2–17 with the index finger over the short stem of the pipet to control the flow of the fluid. Four to five drops of fluid should be expelled from the pipet onto gauze, cotton, or paper towel which should then be discarded. These first drops consist mostly of diluting fluid and do not contain the proper cell concentration. The next drop in the pipet may then be introduced into a counting chamber for the cell count.

## CALCULATING DILUTIONS FOR THE RBC PIPET

The long stem of most RBC pipets has ten divisions. Some types have a mark for each ten divisions; others have only a 0.5 and 1.0 mark. The 0.5 mark represents 0.5 unit and the 1.0 mark represents 1.0 unit. The bulb of the RBC pipet contains 100 units of volume; therefore, 101 units of volume are contained from the tip of the pipet to the 101 mark. When a sample is drawn into the pipet bulb and mixed, the dilution occurs only in the bulb. (The stem contains only diluting fluid and is not considered.) Therefore, the sample is diluted to a total volume of 100 units (Figure 2–11). Example: Draw 0.5 unit of blood into the pipet stem and dilute by drawing diluting fluid to the 101 mark. The mixing bulb now has 0.5 unit of blood in 100 units of the total diluted sample. The dilution factor may be determined by dividing 100 by 0.5. The dilution factor is 200, or a 1:200 dilution of the sample has been made. Many dilutions are possible if the pipet being used is marked in 0.1 unit divisions. The formula below is used to calculate the dilution factor for the blood diluting pipets:

$$\frac{\text{bulb units}}{\text{blood units}} = \text{dilution factor}$$

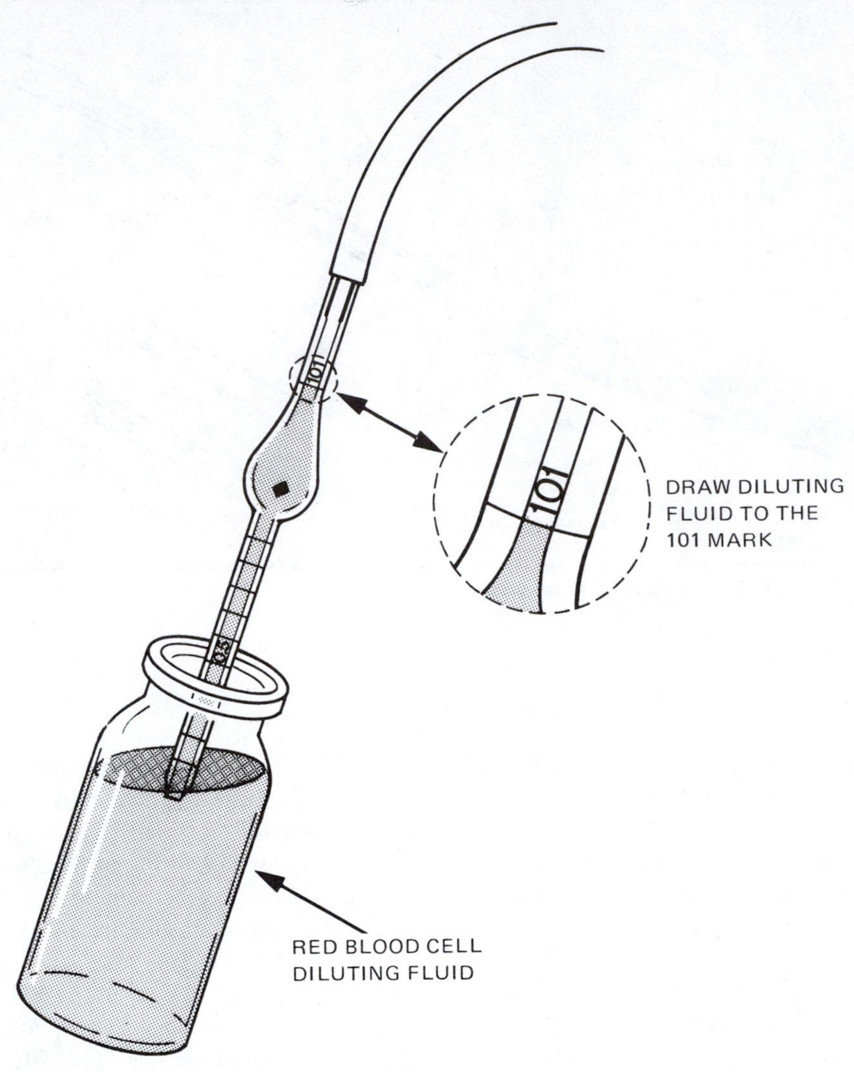


**Figure 2-14.** Diluting a sample using the RBC pipet

## CALCULATING DILUTIONS FOR THE WBC PIPET

The WBC pipet is similar to the RBC pipet except that the bulb contains 10 units of volume. Therefore, a sample drawn to the 0.5 mark and diluted to the 11 mark would contain 0.5 unit of sample in ten units of total diluted sample, a 1:20 dilution.

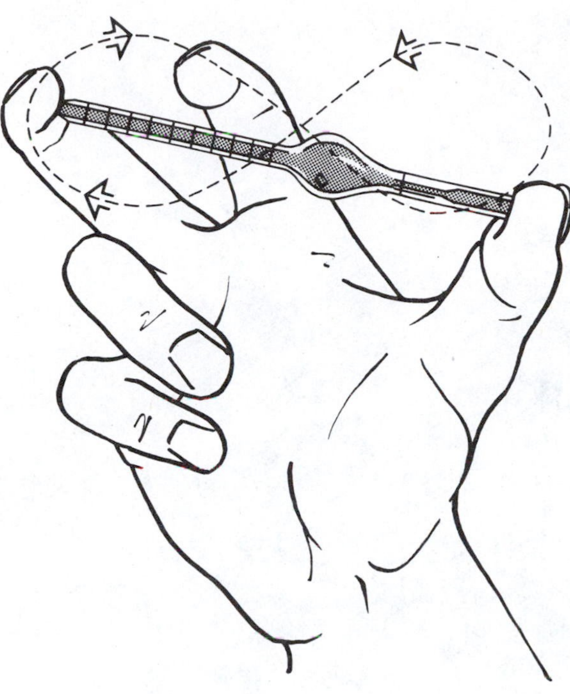

**Figure 2-15.** Manual rotation of blood diluting pipet using figure-eight motion

## CARE AND CLEANING OF BLOOD DILUTING PIPETS

Blood diluting pipets should be cleaned thoroughly immediately after each use. If immediate cleaning is not possible, the pipet should be placed in a detergent solution (or in water) to prevent drying.

The pipet may be cleaned using a suction apparatus (Figure 2–18). The pipet should be cleaned with laboratory detergent (do not use soap), rinsed with distilled water, and dried with acetone. Pipets should be handled gently; they break easily, particularly at the point where the bulb joins the stem.

Blood diluting pipets are delicate and special care should be taken when they are used. They should be transported carefully and stored so that the tips are protected and will not become chipped.

### *Precautions*

- Wipe blood from outside surface of pipet using a soft tissue, avoiding touching the tip of the pipet.
- Hold the pipet upright when filling and keep the tip of the pipet beneath the surface of the fluid to avoid entry of air bubbles into the pipet. Air bubbles will alter the dilution. If air bubbles occur, the filling procedure must be repeated using a clean, dry pipet.
- Do not draw blood sample past the 0.5 mark (or diluting fluid past the 11 or 101 mark) since this will affect the accuracy of the dilution. If this occurs, repeat the filling procedure using a clean, dry pipet.

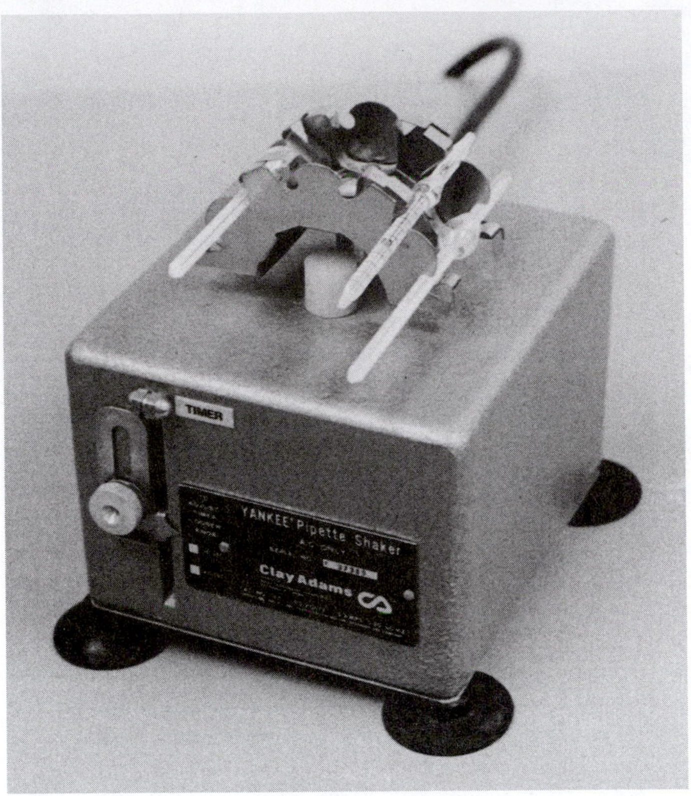


**Figure 2-16.** Automatic pipet shaker (*Photo courtesy of Clay Adams Division of Becton Dickinson & Co.*)

- Always use a clean, dry pipet to perform a dilution.
- Store used pipets in water or a cleaning solution until they can be cleaned. Do not allow sample to dry in the pipet.
- Do not use a pipet with a chipped tip.
- A safety filter may be used to prevent accidental aspiration of biological samples during pipetting.

## SELF-FILLING BLOOD DILUTING MICROPIPETS

Self-filling, self-measuring disposable systems are available for counting erythrocytes, leukocytes, and platelets. These disposable systems consist of the **micropipet,** pipet shield, and a sealed plastic reservoir containing a pre-measured volume of diluting fluid (Figure 2–19). The sample is collected in the micropipet, introduced into the reservoir, and the contents are mixed and dispensed from the reser-

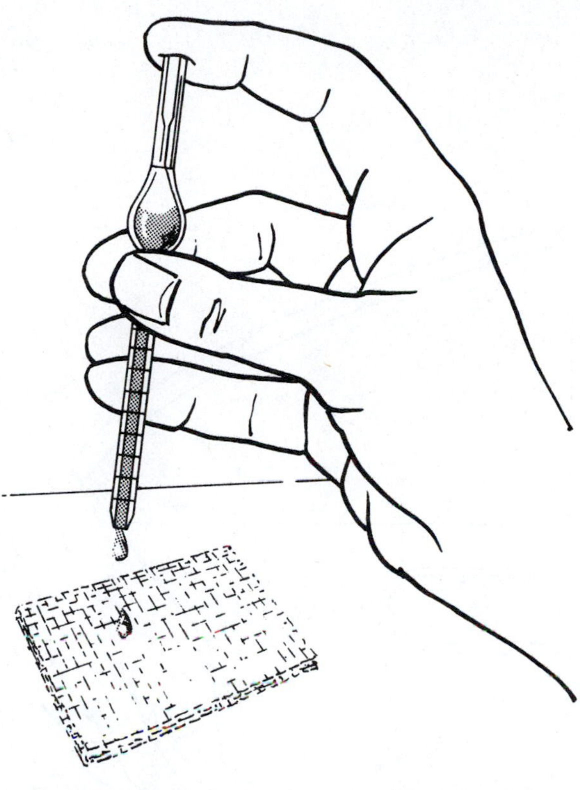

**Figure 2-17.** Dispensing four to five drops from blood diluting pipet onto a gauze pad

voir. Correct use of these self-filling, self-measuring systems usually provides a more accurate dilution than the blood diluting pipets, especially when used by inexperienced technicians. Using these systems eliminates the need for mouth-pipetting.

## *LESSON REVIEW*

1. What is the function of the WBC pipet?
2. What mark is above the bulb of the WBC pipet?
3. What is the function of the RBC pipet?
4. The sample is drawn to what mark on the RBC pipet?
5. What is the function of the bulb?
6. What are the functions of the bead?
7. Explain the proper care of blood diluting pipets.
8. What might affect the accuracy of dilutions made with blood diluting pipets?
9. What dilution is made when the blood sample is drawn to the 0.5 mark and diluting fluid to the 101 mark in the RBC pipet?
10. How should a blood diluting pipet be cleaned?

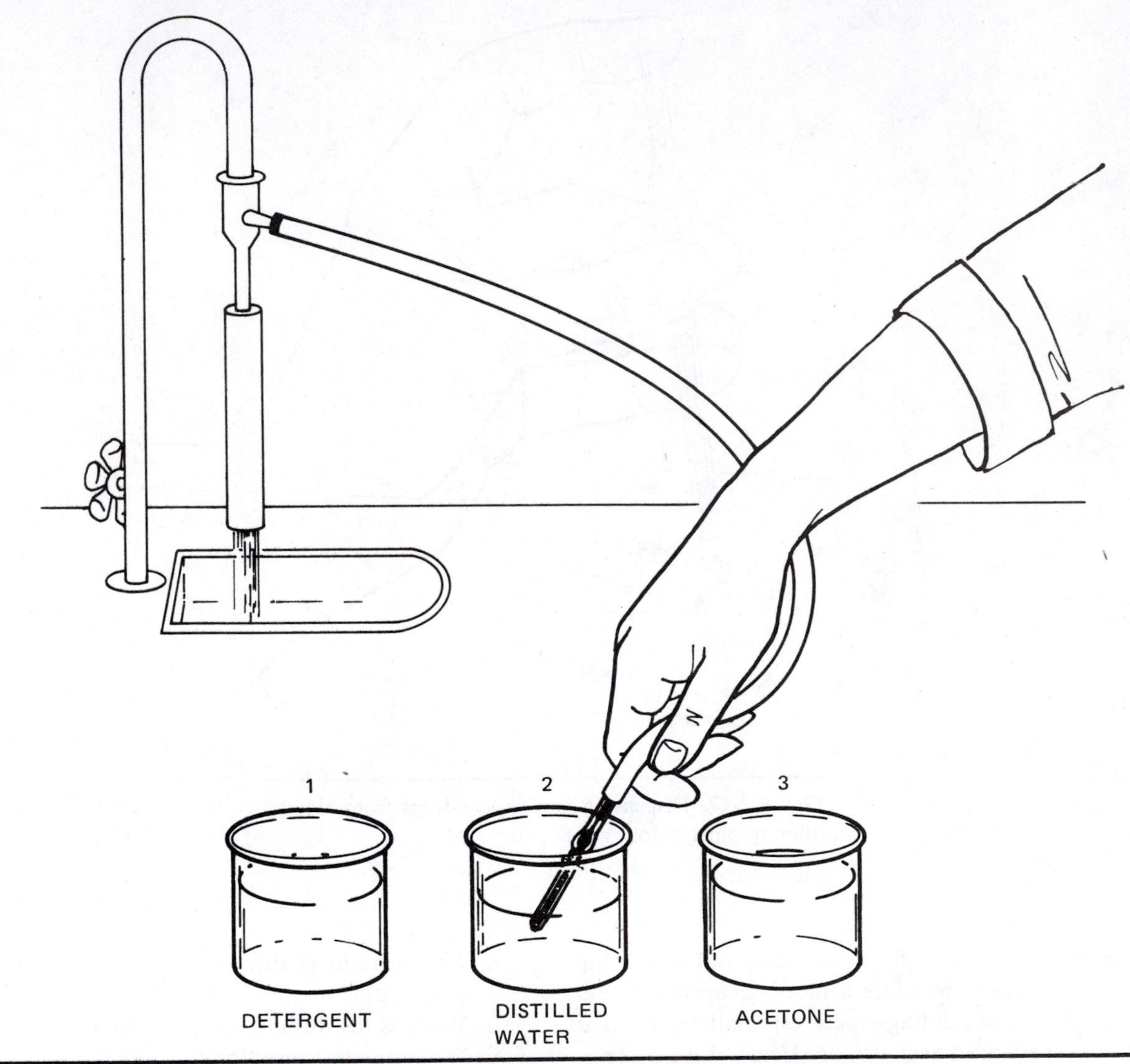


**Figure 2-18.** Cleaning a blood diluting pipet using suction apparatus

11. Draw and label the parts of the RBC pipet.
12. Draw and label the parts of the WBC pipet.
13. Define aspiration, capillary action, diluting fluid, erythrocyte, leukocyte, micropipet, red cell diluting pipet, and white cell diluting pipet.

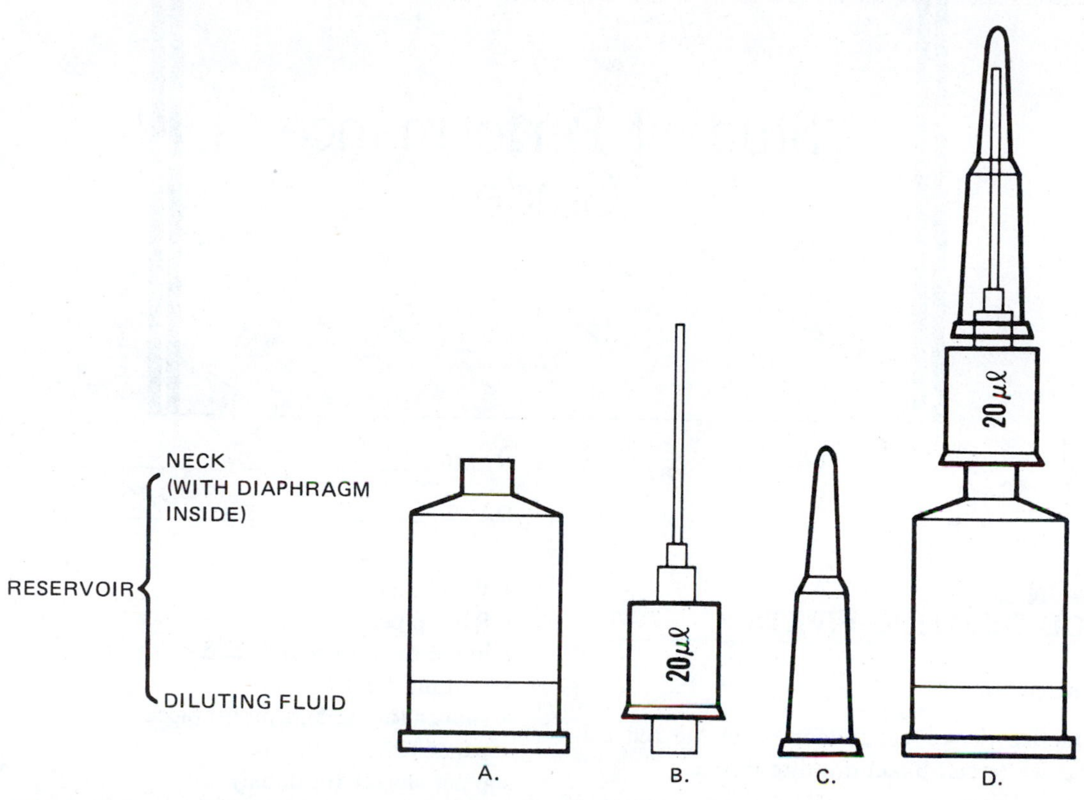


**Figure 2-19.** Parts of a disposable blood diluting unit such as Unopette®. A) Pre-filled reservoir containing pre-measured diluting fluid and sealed with diaphragm, B) capillary pipet with overflow chamber and capacity marking, C) pipet shield, and D) assembled unit

## *STUDENT ACTIVITIES*

1. Re-read the information on blood diluting pipets.
2. Review the glossary terms.
3. Practice the procedure for using the WBC and RBC blood diluting pipets as outlined on the Student Performance Guide.

# Student Performance Guide

NAME ______________________________

DATE ______________________________

## LESSON 2–3 BLOOD DILUTING PIPETS

### Instructions

1. Practice the procedure for using the red cell and white cell blood diluting pipets.
2. Demonstrate the red and white blood diluting pipet procedures satisfactorily for the instructor. All steps must be completed as listed on the Instructor's Performance Check Sheet.
3. Complete a written examination successfully.

### Materials and Equipment

- hand disinfectant
- WBC pipet
- RBC pipet
- blood or diluted red food coloring
- diluting fluid or water
- rubber tubing and mouthpiece
- paper towels or gauze
- pipet shaker (optional)
- suction apparatus for cleaning (optional)
- laboratory detergent
- distilled water
- acetone
- soft laboratory tissue
- surface disinfectant
- biohazard container
- safety filter

**Procedure** S = Satisfactory U = Unsatisfactory

| You must: | S | U | Comments |
|---|---|---|---|
| 1. Wash hands with hand disinfectant | | | |
| 2. Assemble equipment and materials | | | |

| You must: | S | U | Comments |
|---|---|---|---|
| 3. Connect mouthpiece to rubber tubing | | | |
| 4. Connect the rubber tubing to the end of the WBC pipet having the 11 mark | | | |
| 5. Hold the WBC pipet between the thumb and index finger (like holding a pencil) | | | |
| 6. Position the mouthpiece between the lips | | | |
| 7. Hold a tube of well-mixed blood or diluted red food coloring in the opposite hand and tilt the tube so that the sample is near the lip of the tube (Figure 2–13) | | | |
| 8. Place the tip of the pipet beneath the surface of the sample | | | |
| 9. Draw the sample slowly to the 0.5 mark, using the rubber tubing as a straw (by aspiration). Do not allow air bubbles to enter, or draw sample past the 0.5 mark | | | |
| 10. Wipe the outside of the pipet stem with a soft tissue to remove all sample (avoid touching pipet tip) | | | |
| 11. Select previously opened diluting fluid or water; tilt the container and insert the tip of the pipet beneath the surface of the fluid. Slowly rotate the pipet while aspirating the fluid exactly to the 11 mark. Hold pipet upright to prevent entry of air bubbles (Figure 2–14) | | | |
| 12. Place the index finger over the tip of the pipet and carefully remove the rubber tubing | | | |
| 13. Hold the pipet horizontally and mix by either method: (a) Place pipet on the automatic pipet shaker and turn the shaker on for at least two minutes or, | | | |
| (b) Mix contents for two to three minutes by rotating in a figure-eight motion while holding pipet with middle finger and thumb over ends | | | |
| 14. Hold the pipet in a horizontal position when mixing is completed | | | |
| 15. Place index finger firmly over the end of the pipet which has the 11 mark to control the flow of fluid | | | |

| You must: | S | U | Comments |
|---|---|---|---|
| 16. Discharge four to five free-falling drops of fluid, one drop at a time, on a gauze pad or paper towel while holding the pipet at a 45° angle or in a nearly vertical position (raise the index finger slightly from the pipet end to allow drops to flow) | | | |
| 17. Wash and dry the pipet using (1) detergent, (2) distilled water, and (3) acetone (for drying) | | | |
| 18. Return pipet and other materials to the proper storage area | | | |
| 19. Repeat procedure using the RBC pipet (draw diluting fluid to 101 mark in RBC pipet) | | | |
| 20. Clean equipment and return to proper storage | | | |
| 21. Clean work area with surface disinfectant | | | |
| 22. Wash hands with hand disinfectant | | | |
| Comments:<br><br>Student/Instructor: | | | |

Date: ______________________ Instructor: ______________________

# LESSON 2–4

## The Hemacytometer

### LESSON OBJECTIVES

After studying this lesson, you should be able to:

- Identify the parts of a hemacytometer.
- Identify the hemacytometer areas where red cells and white cells are counted, using the microscope.
- Fill the hemacytometer using a blood diluting pipet.
- Clean and dry the hemacytometer and coverglass.
- Write the general formula for calculating cell counts using a hemacytometer.
- List the precautions to observe when using the hemacytometer.
- Define the glossary terms.

### GLOSSARY

**hemacytometer** / a heavy glass slide made to precise specifications and used to count cells microscopically; a counting chamber

**hemacytometer coverglass** / a special coverglass of uniform thickness used with a hemacytometer

## INTRODUCTION

The **hemacytometer** is used to count erythrocytes, leukocytes, and platelets in the blood. It may also be used to count cells in other body fluids. The hemacytometer is a heavy glass slide manufactured to meet the specifications of the National Bureau of Standards (NBS). When viewed from the top, it has two raised platforms surrounded by depressions on three sides (Figure 2–20). Each raised surface contains a ruled counting area which is marked off by precise lines etched into the glass. The depressions surrounding these platforms are sometimes called "moats." The raised areas and the depressions form an "H."

### Coverglass

A special coverglass is used with the hemacytometer. Only a **hemacytometer coverglass** of uniform thickness which meets NBS specifications should

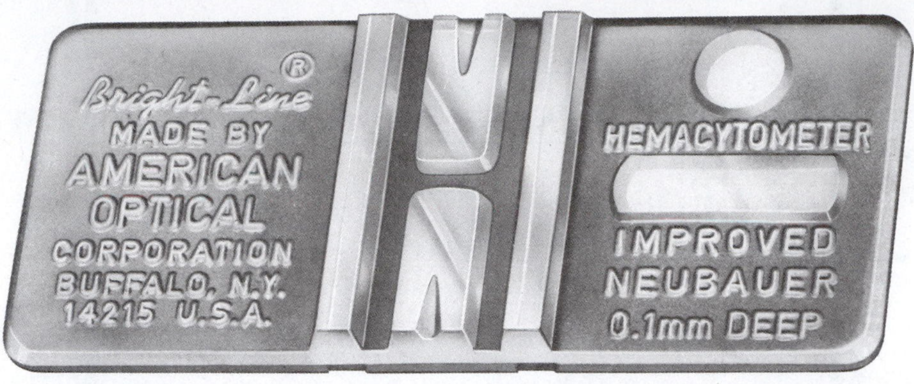


**Figure 2-20.** Hemacytometer (top view) (*Photo courtesy of Reichert Scientific Instruments*)

be used. The coverglass is positioned so that it covers both ruled areas of the hemacytometer (Figure 2–21). The coverglass confines the fluid in the chamber and regulates the depth of that fluid. The depth of the fluid in the Neubauer-type hemacytometer is 0.1 mm with the coverglass in place (Figure 2–22).

### Counting Areas

A hemacytometer has two ruled areas. These areas are composed of etched lines which define squares of specific dimensions. The most commonly used hemacytometer is the type with Neubauer ruling. In the Neubauer-type counting chamber, each ruled area consists of a large square, 3 mm × 3 mm. This area of 9 $mm^2$ is divided into nine equal squares, each of which is 1 $mm^2$ (Figure 2–23).

***WBC Counting Area.*** The WBC counting area consists of the four large corner squares labeled "W" in Figure 2–24. Each of these large corner squares is subdivided into sixteen smaller squares. All four large corner squares on both sides of the chamber are used to count WBC.

***RBC Counting Area.*** The center squares on both sides of the chamber are used to count the red blood cells. Each center square is subdivided into twenty-five smaller squares. Only the four corner squares and the center square within the large center square are used to count RBC (Figure 2–25).

## FILLING THE HEMACYTOMETER

A clean coverglass should be positioned so that it covers both ruled areas of a clean hemacytometer. Then the hemacytometer is filled or charged. This is done by touching the tip of a filled blood diluting pipet to the point where the coverglass and the raised platform on one side meet (Figure 2–26). The fluid from the pipet will flow by capillary action into one side of the hemacytometer, using one-half to one drop of fluid. The opposite side of the chamber is then filled in the same manner. (Some hemacytometers have a V-shaped trough on each raised platform to guide the placement of the pipet tip when filling.)

The fluid should flow into the chamber in a smooth, unbroken stream. It should not be allowed

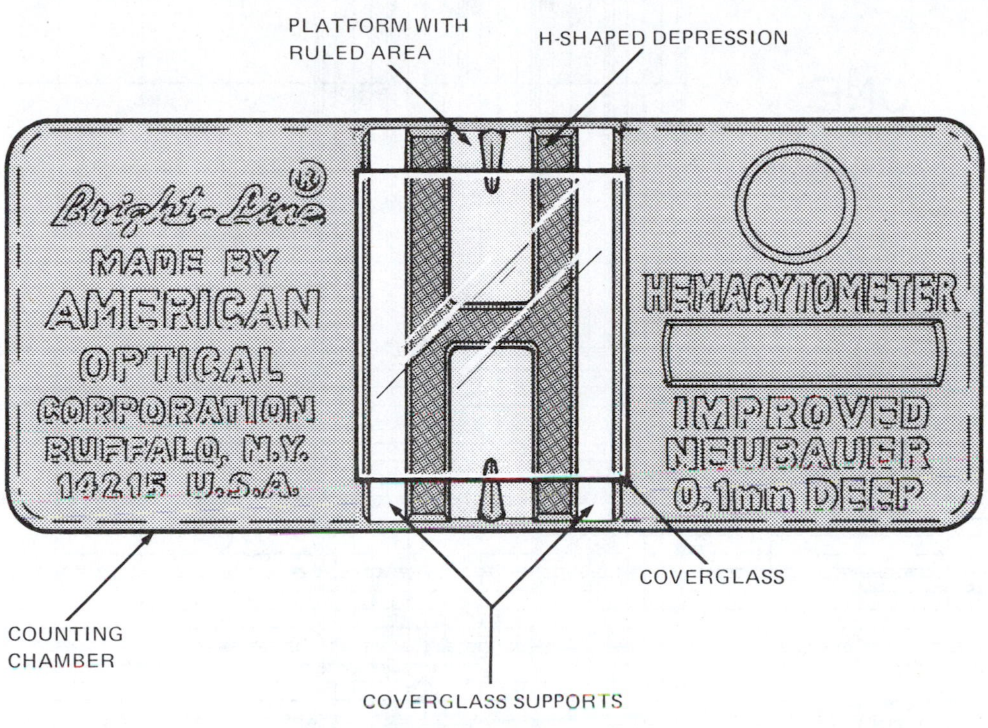


**Figure 2-21.** Hemacytometer with coverglass in place

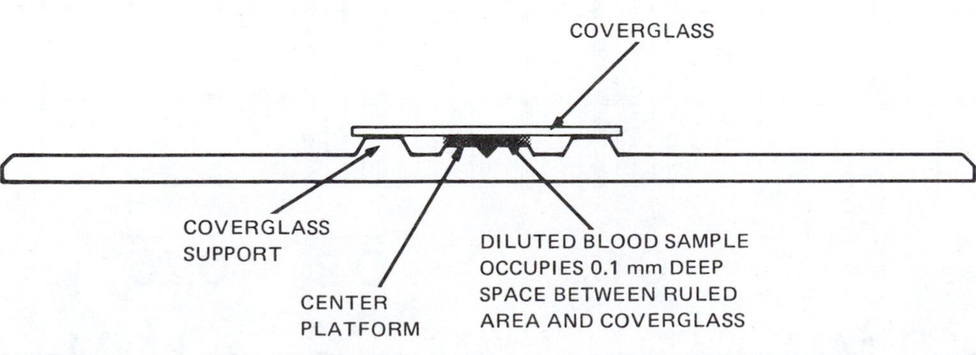


**Figure 2-22.** Side view of hemacytometer with coverglass in place

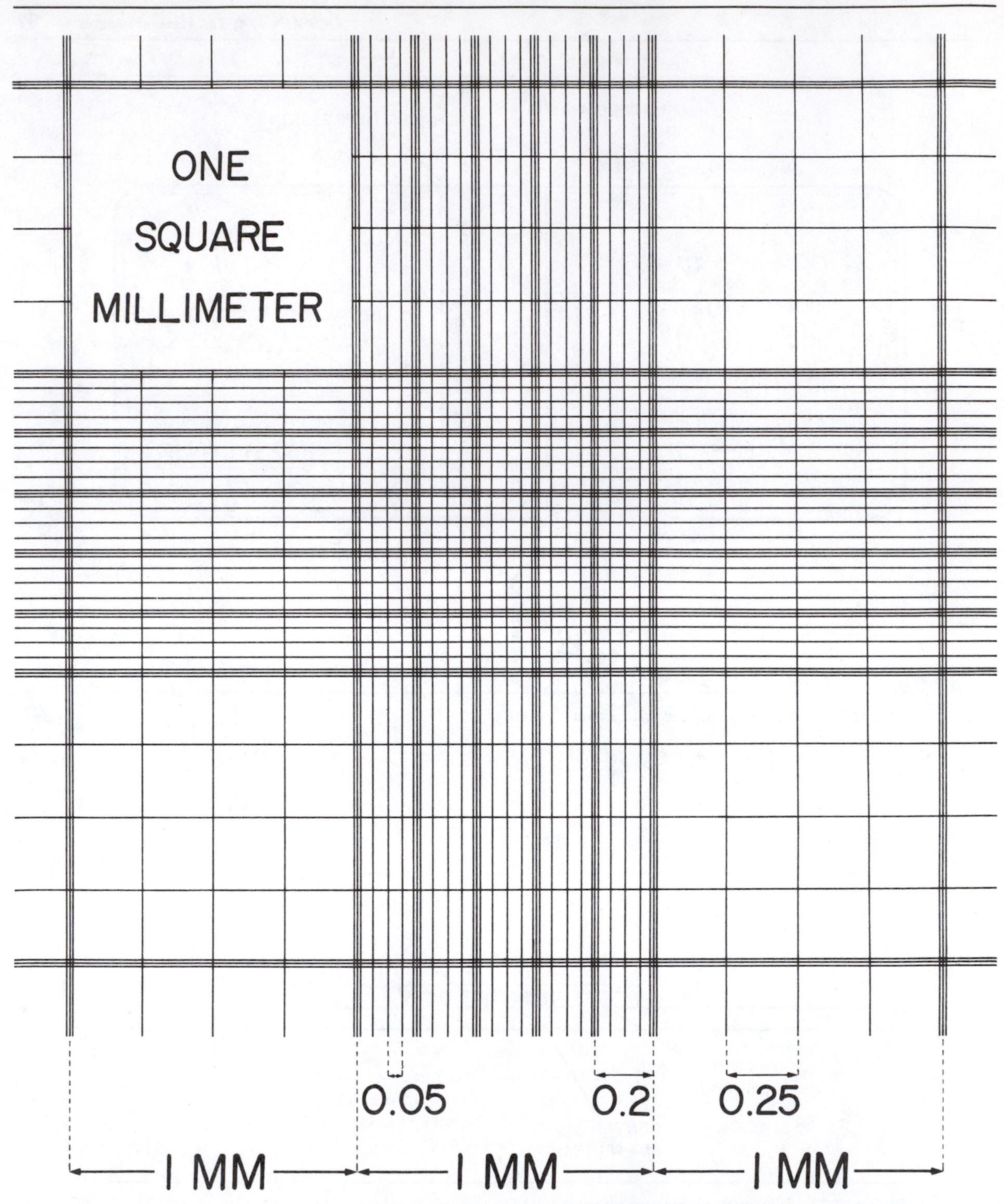


**Figure 2-23.** Ruled area of hemacytometer showing dimensions

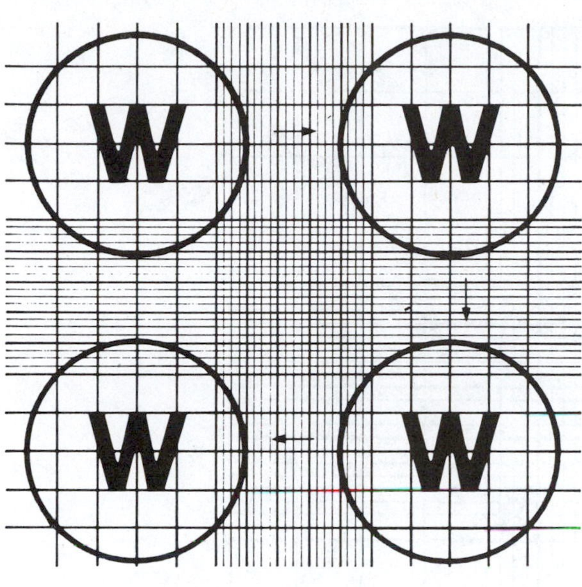


**Figure 2-24.** WBC counting area

to overflow into the depressions or moats. After the hemacytometer has been correctly filled, it should then stand two minutes to allow the cells to settle.

## Viewing the Ruled Areas

The hemacytometer should be placed on the microscope stage with the low power (10×) objective in place so that one of the ruled areas is located over the light source. The coarse adjustment knob should be used to carefully move the hemacytometer and objective closer together. This adjustment is continued until the objective is almost touching the coverglass. Looking into the eyepiece (ocular), the coarse adjustment knob is then used to increase the distance between the objective and the hemacytometer. This is continued until the etched lines come into view. The fine adjustment knob is then used to bring the etched lines into sharp focus. The etched lines are more easily viewed when the condenser or the light source of the microscope is lowered.

When the ruled area is in sharp focus, the white cell counting areas are located by moving the hemacytometer carefully (or moving the stage of the microscope if the microscope has a mechanical stage). After the white cell counting area has been observed, the central square used for the red cell counts should be located. The high power (40×) objective should then be carefully rotated into place. The five small squares used in a red cell count should be located. If the microscope is parfocal, the ruled area may be brought into focus with only a slight rotation of the fine adjustment.

Once all parts of the ruled area of one side have been located, the hemacytometer should be carefully moved so that the second ruled area can be viewed. When moving the hemacytometer from one side to the other, the low power objective should be in position. The oil immersion objective is never used with a hemacytometer.

## Counting Pattern

A counting pattern of left-to-right, right-to-left must be used to insure that cells are counted only one time. The count should begin in the upper left corner of a square and proceed in a serpentine manner (Figure 2–27).

Squares are divided by boundary lines which may be single, double, or triple. When triple lines are present, the center line is considered the boundary. When double lines are present, the outer line is considered the boundary. All cells within a square, cells which touch the left boundary of the square, and cells which touch the top boundary of the square are counted. Cells which touch the right boundary of a square and cells which touch the lower boundary (Figure 2–28) of a square should not be counted in that square even though they may lie within the square. The cells in the designated squares should be counted on both sides of the chamber. The results for each side should be re-

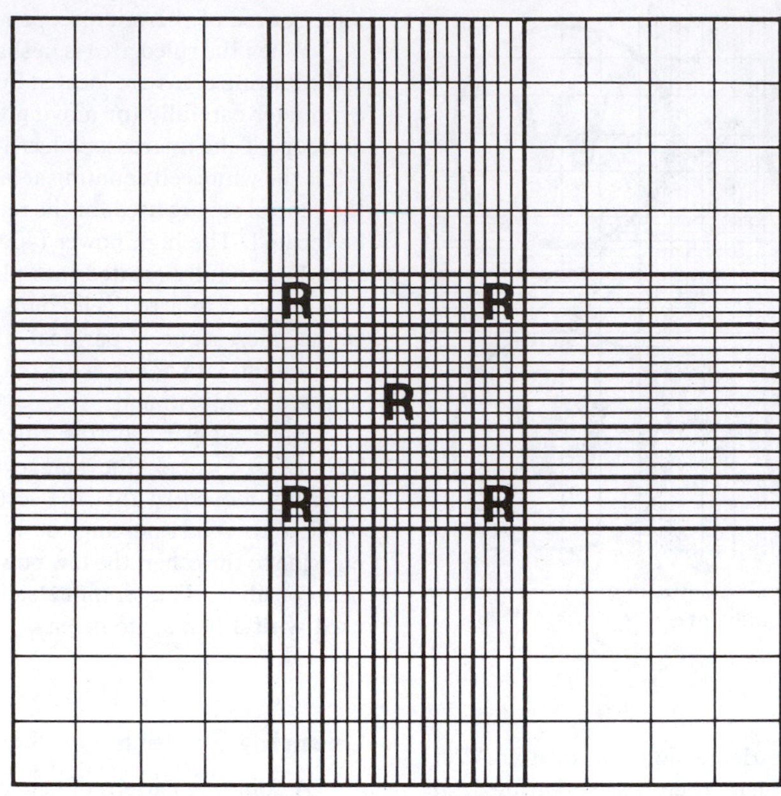


**Figure 2-25.** RBC counting area. The four corner squares and center square (labeled "R") within the large center square are used to count red blood cells.

corded. The counts for the two sides are then totaled and the average is calculated.

## Calculation of Cell Counts

The total number of cells per cubic millimeter ($mm^3$) of the sample can be calculated from the average number of cells which were counted. This is because the ruled areas of the hemacytometer contain an exact volume of diluted sample. Since only a small volume of diluted sample is counted, a general formula must be used to convert the count into the number of cells/$mm^3$:

$$C/mm^3 = \frac{Avg \times D\ (mm) \times DF}{A\ (mm^2)}$$

Where: $C/mm^3$ = Number of cells/$mm^3$
Avg = Average # of cells counted
D (mm) = Depth factor in mm
DF = Dilution factor
A ($mm^2$) = Area counted ($mm^2$)

The dilution factor used in the formula is determined by the dilution obtained with the blood diluting pipet. The depth factor used in the formula is always 10 (the counting chamber is 0.1 mm deep;

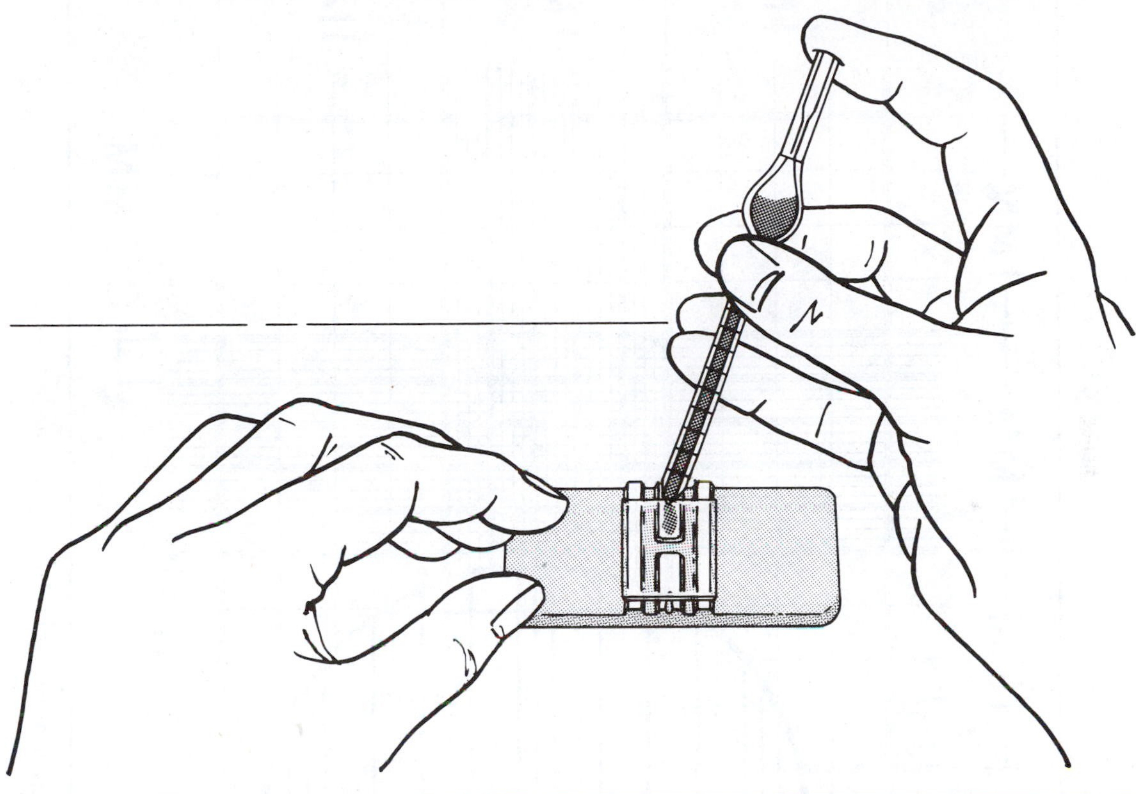

**Figure 2-26.** Filling the hemacytometer

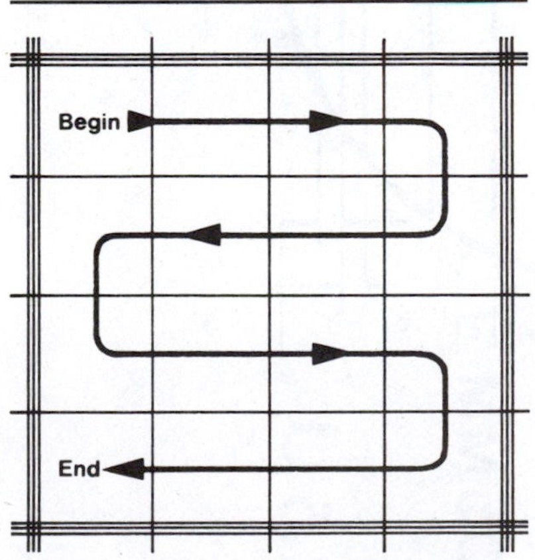


**Figure 2-27.** Left-to-right, right-to-left counting pattern (shown here in one of the large corner squares)

the depth is converted to 1 mm by multiplying by 10). The area counted will vary for each type of cell count and is calculated using the dimensions of the ruled area.

## Care of the Hemacytometer

The hemacytometer is an expensive piece of equipment which must be handled carefully. It should be held by the sides and bottom only, to avoid getting fingerprints on the raised ruled areas. Before and after each use, the raised surfaces should be wiped with lens paper dipped in 70% alcohol. The hemacytometer should then be immediately dried and polished with lens paper. The coverglass should be handled by the edges, and both sides cleaned

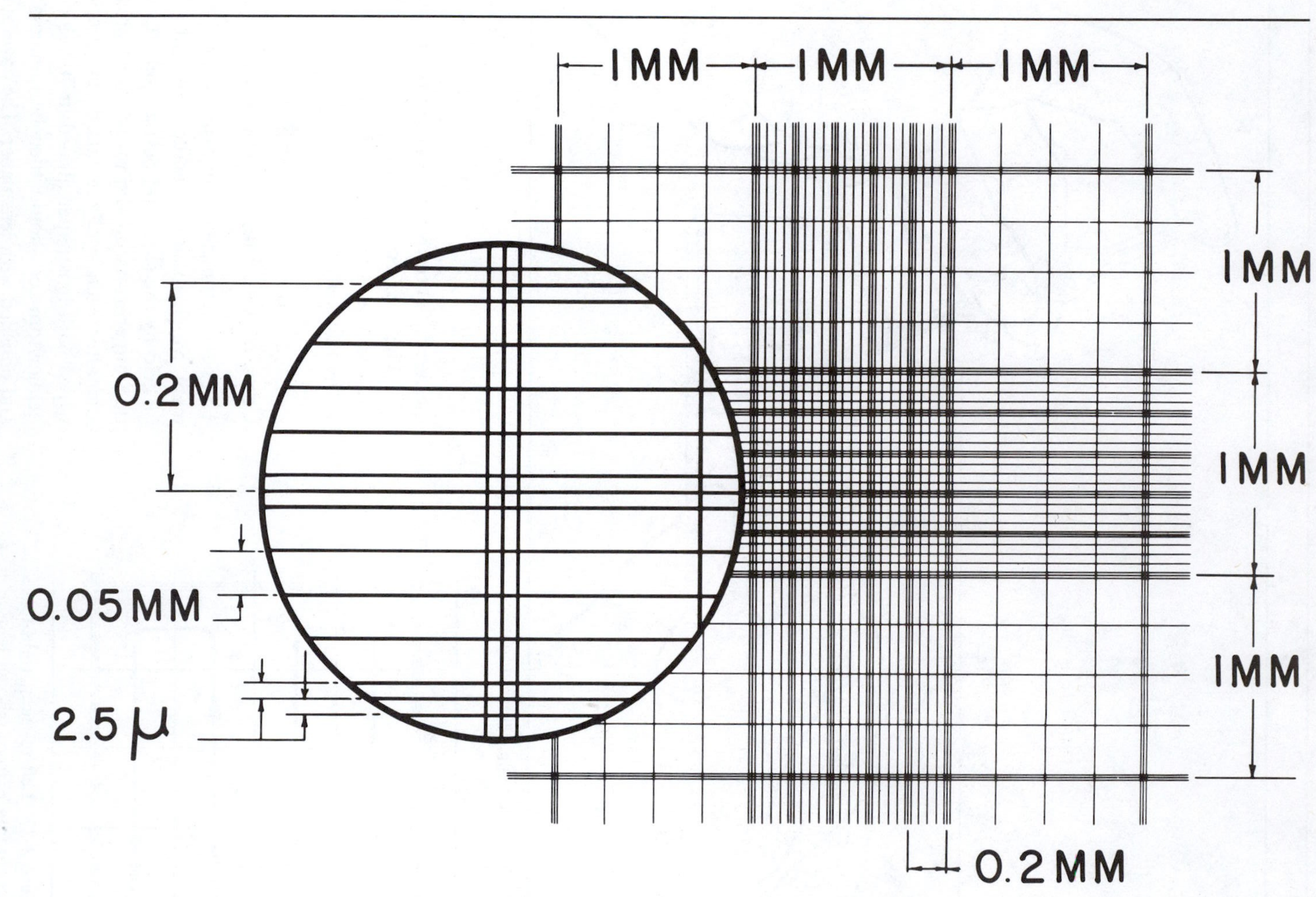


**Figure 2-28.** Boundaries and dimensions of ruled area (*Photo courtesy of Reichert Scientific Instruments*)

in the same manner as the hemacytometer. When not in use, the hemacytometer should be stored in a container to keep dirt and dust off the surface and to protect the ruled areas from scratches. When transporting the hemacytometer, it should be held carefully and placed on a secure surface.

### *Precautions*

■ Use care when focusing the microscope on the ruled areas.
■ Be certain that the hemacytometer and coverglass are free from dirt and oil before use.
■ Store and handle the hemacytometer and coverglass carefully to avoid scratches.

## *LESSON REVIEW*

1. What are the dimensions of the ruled areas of the hemacytometer?
2. What is the depth of the hemacytometer chamber with the coverglass in place?
3. What counting pattern is used to avoid counting cells more than once?
4. Which microscope objective is used to first locate the etched lines?
5. What is the proper procedure for cleaning the hemacytometer and coverglass?
6. Which squares are counted for a WBC count?
7. Which squares are counted for an RBC count?
8. What rule is used for counting cells that touch the boundaries of the squares?
9. What is the general formula used to calculate cell counts using the hemacytometer?
10. Define hemacytometer and hemacytometer coverglass.

## *STUDENT ACTIVITIES*

1. Re-read the information on the hemacytometer.
2. Review the glossary terms.
3. Practice filling the hemacytometer.
4. Practice locating the WBC counting areas as outlined on the Student Performance Guide.
5. Practice locating the RBC counting areas as outlined on the Student Performance Guide.

# Student Performance Guide

NAME ____________________

DATE ____________________

## LESSON 2–4 THE HEMACYTOMETER

### Instructions:

1. Practice the procedure for using the hemacytometer.
2. Demonstrate the procedure for using the hemacytometer satisfactorily for the instructor. All steps must be completed as listed on the instructor's Performance Check Sheet.
3. Complete a written examination successfully.

### Materials and Equipment

- hand disinfectant
- hemacytometer
- hemacytometer coverglass
- lens paper
- 70% ethyl or isopropyl alcohol
- blood (optional)
- blood diluting pipets
- rubber tubing with mouthpiece
- microscope
- RBC diluting fluid (optional)
- WBC diluting fluid (optional)
- suction apparatus for cleaning pipets (optional)
- paper towels or gauze
- laboratory detergent
- distilled water
- acetone
- pipet shaker (optional)
- soft tissue
- surface disinfectant
- biohazard container

**Procedure** S = Satisfactory U = Unsatisfactory

| You must: | S | U | Comments |
|---|---|---|---|
| 1. Wash hands with hand disinfectant | | | |
| 2. Assemble equipment and materials | | | |

| You must: | S | U | Comments |
|---|---|---|---|
| 3. Use lens paper and alcohol to carefully clean hemacytometer and coverglass | | | |
| 4. Place the coverglass carefully over the ruled areas (chamber) of the hemacytometer | | | |
| 5. Follow the procedure in the blood diluting pipet lesson and make a cell dilution (or fill pipet with distilled water) | | | |
| 6. Discharge four to five drops from the pipet onto a paper towel or gauze | | | |
| 7. Wipe excess fluid from the tip of the pipet using soft tissue | | | |
| 8. Hold the pipet at a 45° angle and touch the tip to the point where the coverglass and the hemacytometer meet, placing index finger on the short stem of pipet to regulate flow (do not move coverglass) | | | |
| 9. Allow fluid to flow into one side of the chamber by capillary action (the chamber should fill in one smooth flow without flooding over into the depressions) | | | |
| 10. Fill the other side of the chamber in the same manner | | | |
| 11. Position the low power (10×) objective in place | | | |
| 12. Place the hemacytomcter on the microscope stage securely with one ruled area over the light source | | | |
| 13. Look directly at the hemacytometer and turn the coarse adjustment knob to bring the microscope objective and the hemacytometer close together, continuing until the objective is almost touching the coverglass. Note: Use coarse adjustment with care | | | |
| 14. Look into the eyepiece and slowly turn the coarse adjustment knob in the opposite direction until the etched lines come into view | | | |
| 15. Rotate the fine adjustment knob until the lines are in clear focus | | | |
| 16. Find all nine large squares of one side of the chamber by moving the stage or the hemacytometer | | | |

| You must: | S | U | Comments |
|---|---|---|---|
| 17. Locate four large corner squares used for WBC count (Figure 2–24) | | | |
| 18. Scan squares using left-to-right, right-to-left counting pattern and observe boundaries | | | |
| 19. Locate the center square used for the RBC count (Figure 2–25) | | | |
| 20. Rotate the high power (40×) objective carefully into position and adjust focus using the fine adjustment knob until the etched lines appear distinct | | | |
| 21. Locate the four small corner squares and the center square used for the RBC count (Figure 2–25) | | | |
| 22. Scan counting area using left-to-right, right-to-left pattern and observe boundaries | | | |
| 23. View the second ruled area, repeating steps 16–22 | | | |
| 24. Rotate the low power objective into position | | | |
| 25. Remove the hemacytometer carefully from the microscope stage | | | |
| 26. Clean the hemacytometer and the coverglass carefully using alcohol and lens paper | | | |
| 27. Dry the hemacytometer and coverglass with lens paper | | | |
| 28. Clean and return all equipment to proper storage | | | |
| 29. Clean work area with surface disinfectant | | | |
| 30. Wash hands with hand disinfectant | | | |

Comments:

Student/Instructor:

Date: ______________________ Instructor: ______________________

# LESSON 2–5

## The Red Blood Cell Count

### LESSON OBJECTIVES

After studying this lesson, you should be able to:

- Explain the function of red blood cells.
- List the normal red cell counts for males and females.
- Name a condition or disease associated with an increased red cell count.
- Name two conditions or diseases associated with a decreased red cell count.
- State an important property of a red cell diluting fluid.
- Name three red cell diluting fluids.
- Perform a manual red cell count.
- Calculate the results of a red cell count.
- List two precautions to be observed when performing a red cell count.
- Define the glossary terms.

### GLOSSARY

**anemia** / decrease below normal in the red cell count or in the blood hemoglobin level

**erythrocytosis** / increase above normal in the number of red cells in circulation

**hemolysis** / the destruction of red blood cells resulting in the liberation of hemoglobin from the cells

**isotonic solution** / a solution which has the same concentration of dissolved particles as that solution with which it is compared

### INTRODUCTION

The blood is composed of three groups of cellular elements. These are (1) the red blood cells (RBC) or erythrocytes; (2) the white blood cells (WBC) or leukocytes; and (3) the platelets or thrombocytes. These cells are vital components of the blood. They are essential for proper functioning of body systems.

Each group of blood cells has a unique function. Leukocytes are important in preventing and fighting infection. Platelets help stop blood flow or hemorrhage by participating in the clotting mechanism. The red blood cells, the most numerous cells in the blood, transport oxygen to tissues. Red blood cells also carry carbon dioxide to the lungs.

**Table 2-2.** Normal RBC Counts in Adult Males and Adult Females

| Sex | Normal RBC Count |
|---|---|
| Adult male | $4.5–6.0 \times 10^6/mm^3$ |
| Adult female | $4.0–5.5 \times 10^6/mm^3$ |

## THE RED CELL COUNT

A red cell count is a commonly performed procedure. It is usually a part of a complete blood count (CBC). The red cell count approximates the number of circulating red cells. If the count falls below or above the normal range, an individual may experience a variety of symptoms. A red cell count helps the physician diagnose and treat many diseases.

### Normal Values

The normal values for red blood cell counts range from approximately 4 million per cubic millimeter of blood ($4.0 \times 10^6/mm^3$) to six million per cubic millimeter ($6.0 \times 10^6/mm^3$). Males usually have slightly higher RBC counts than females (Table 2–2).

Red cell counts may be reported as the number of cells per cubic millimeter ($mm^3$), microliter ($\mu l$), or liter (L) of blood. For example, a count of $5.6 \times 10^6$ RBC/$mm^3$ (or $\mu l$) would be reported as $5.6 \times 10^{12}$ RBC/L.

### Conditions Associated with Changes in Red Cell Counts

The condition in which the oxygen-carrying capacity of blood is below normal is called **anemia.** Usually when a person is anemic the red cell count is decreased. Examples of conditions with decreased red cell counts are iron deficiency anemia and sickle cell anemia. Anemias may also be due to deficiencies of vitamins such as $B_{12}$ or folic acid.

An increased red cell count is called **erythrocytosis.** People who live in high altitudes have erythrocytosis because of the lower oxygen content of the air. Polycythemia vera is a disease in which the red cell count is greatly increased.

## PERFORMING A MANUAL RED CELL COUNT

***Diluting Fluids.*** There are several fluids which may be used to dilute blood for an RBC count. The diluting fluid used for RBC counts must be an **isotonic solution.** This prevents **hemolysis,** or destruction of the red cells. Commonly used diluting fluids are Hayem's, Gower's, and Dacie's.

***Procedure.*** A capillary sample or a well-mixed anticoagulated blood sample is drawn into the RBC pipet to the 0.5 mark. Red cell diluting fluid is then drawn into the pipet to the 101 mark. A second pipet is filled in the same manner. The contents of the pipets are mixed thoroughly. The first 4 to 5 drops are discarded. A coverglass is positioned on the hemacytometer. The tip of the pipet is touched to the edge of the coverglass and one side of the chamber is allowed to fill by capillary action. Using the second pipet, the opposite side is then filled in the same manner. If the fluid overflows into the depression around the platforms, or if air bubbles occur, the chamber should be cleaned and refilled.

After allowing the cells to settle for two to three minutes, the hemacytometer is placed carefully on the microscope stage. The RBC ruled area is located using the low power (10×) objective. The high power (40×) objective is then rotated into place to perform the count.

The RBC count is performed using the center square of the ruled area as shown in Figure 2–29. Within the center square are twenty-five smaller squares. Of these twenty-five squares, the four corner squares and the center square (marked a, b, c, d, and e) are counted. Each of these five squares in turn contains four rows of squares. All cells within each of the five squares are counted using the left-to-right, right-to-left counting pattern. Be sure to include the cells touching the top and left boundary of the squares. The cells touching the right boundary and the cells touching the lower boundary of each square are not counted. Neither are the cells beyond these boundaries (Figure 2–30).

A hand counter is used to tabulate the red cells in the five designated squares. The numbers for each of the five squares are recorded and totaled. If the number of cells in a square varies from any other square on the same side by more than 25 cells, the count must be repeated. A count is then performed in the five squares of the second side of the chamber in the same manner. The two totals are then averaged.

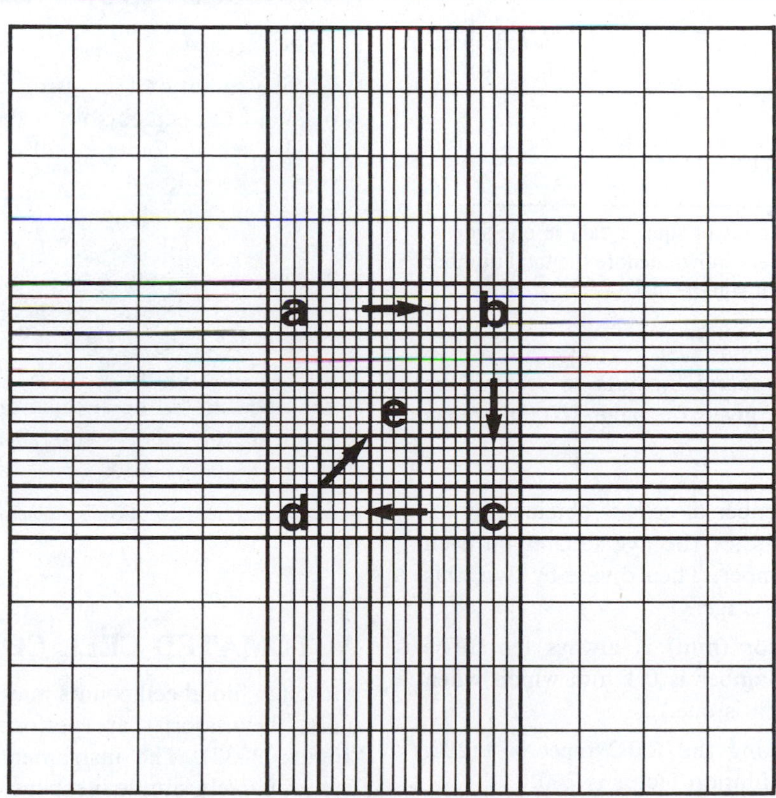


**Figure 2-29.** RBC counting area

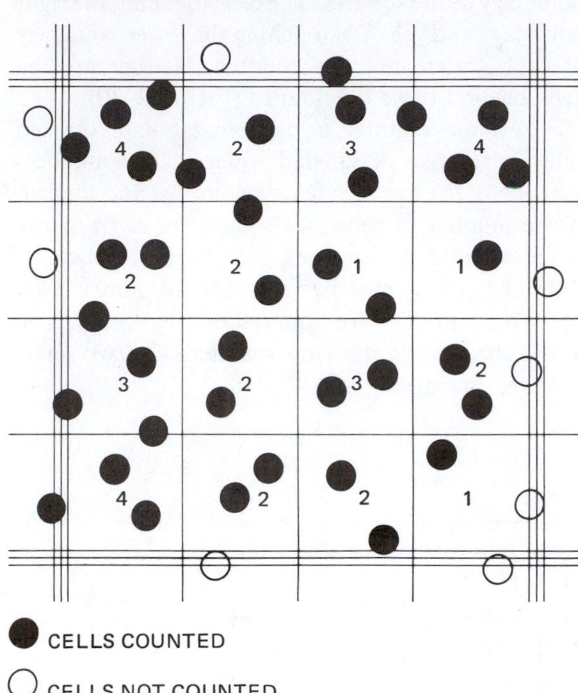


**Figure 2-30.** Sample count in square "a" on one side of chamber. The numbers shown denote the total number of cells counted in each square.

*Calculations.* The general formula to use for the hemacytometer was given on page 100. It breaks down as shown.

1. The average number of cells is obtained by totaling the counts for the five squares on each side of the chamber. Then divide by two; this gives you the average.
2. The depth factor (mm) is always ten. (The depth of the chamber is 0.1 mm which when multiplied by ten is one.)
3. The dilution using the RBC pipet is 1:200. Therefore, the dilution factor is 200.
4. The area counted is 0.20 mm². (Each square, a to e, has a length of 0.2 mm and a width of 0.2 mm. This gives each square an area of 0.04 mm². Since five squares are counted, the area is 5 × 0.04 mm² or 0.20 mm².) Substitute these numbers into the formula as shown below.

$$\text{C/mm}^3 = \frac{\text{Avg} \times 10 \times 200}{0.20}$$
$$= \text{average \# cells} \times 10{,}000$$

When an RBC count is performed this way, the count/mm³ may be calculated two ways: (1) simply adding four zeroes to the average number of cells counted or, (2) the average count may be multiplied by 10,000. A sample calculation is shown in Figure 2–31.

### *Precautions*

- All precautions for using blood-diluting pipets and the hemacytometer must be followed.
- The hemacytometer and coverglass must be free of dirt and oil.
- Proper counting methods should be carefully followed.
- The count from one small square (a to e) to another should not vary by more than twenty-five. Any greater variation indicates an uneven distribution of cells. In such cases, the chamber should be cleaned and refilled.
- Clean any spills with surface disinfectant.
- Wash hands after procedure is completed.

## AUTOMATED CELL COUNTS

Although blood cell counts may be performed manually, the majority are performed by automation (Figure 2–32). The instruments used may range from relatively simple inexpensive counters, to very elaborate and expensive equipment. Simple counters may be used in a physician's office or a small hospi-

1. Count the cells:

| Side 1 | | Side 2 | |
|---|---|---|---|
| Square | Cells counted | Square | Cells counted |
| a | 100 | a | 105 |
| b | 95 | b | 115 |
| c | 90 | c | 100 |
| d | 90 | d | 106 |
| e | 105 | e | 94 |
| Total | 480 | Total | 520 |

2. Compute the average:
   A. $480 + 520 = 1000$ cells
   B. $1000 \div 2 = 500$ average

3. Calculate the count:

$$\text{RBC/mm}^3 = \frac{\text{average \# cells counted} \times \text{depth factor (mm)} \times \text{dilution factor}}{\text{area counted (mm}^2\text{)}}$$

$$\text{RBC/mm}^3 = \frac{500 \times 10\ \text{(mm)} \times 200}{0.2\ \text{mm}^2}$$

$$\text{RBC/mm}^3 = 500 \times 10000\ \text{mm}^3$$

$$\text{RBC/mm}^3 = 5{,}000{,}000 \text{ or } 5.0 \times 10^6/\text{mm}^3$$

**Figure 2-31.** Sample calculation of an RBC count

tal. More elaborate equipment may be found in large hospitals and reference laboratories. Some instruments count only erythrocytes and leukocytes. Others count erythrocytes, leukocytes, and platelets.

Most automated cell counters operate on one of two principles. In some instruments, the cells to be counted are diluted in a fluid which conducts an electrical current. The cells are aspirated through a special narrow opening called an aperture. As the cells are aspirated, they interrupt the flow of the current across the opening. Each interruption is recorded and counted as a cell. In other instruments, the diluted blood sample is aspirated into a special channel which is so narrow that only one cell can pass through at a time. As the cells pass through the channel, they interrupt a laser beam. The interruptions of the beam are counted as cells. Most automated instruments complete a cell count in less than one minute.

Use of automated cell counters has improved the accuracy of cell counts and the efficiency of laboratories. Another advantage of using automated counters is that less skill or experience is required to operate the equipment than to perform a manual cell count.

Despite the widespread use of these instruments, every laboratory needs to maintain the equipment and trained personnel necessary to perform manual counts. Most spinal fluid and other body fluids must be examined manually. Many platelet counts are also performed manually. In some cases, the cell counts may be too low to use automated

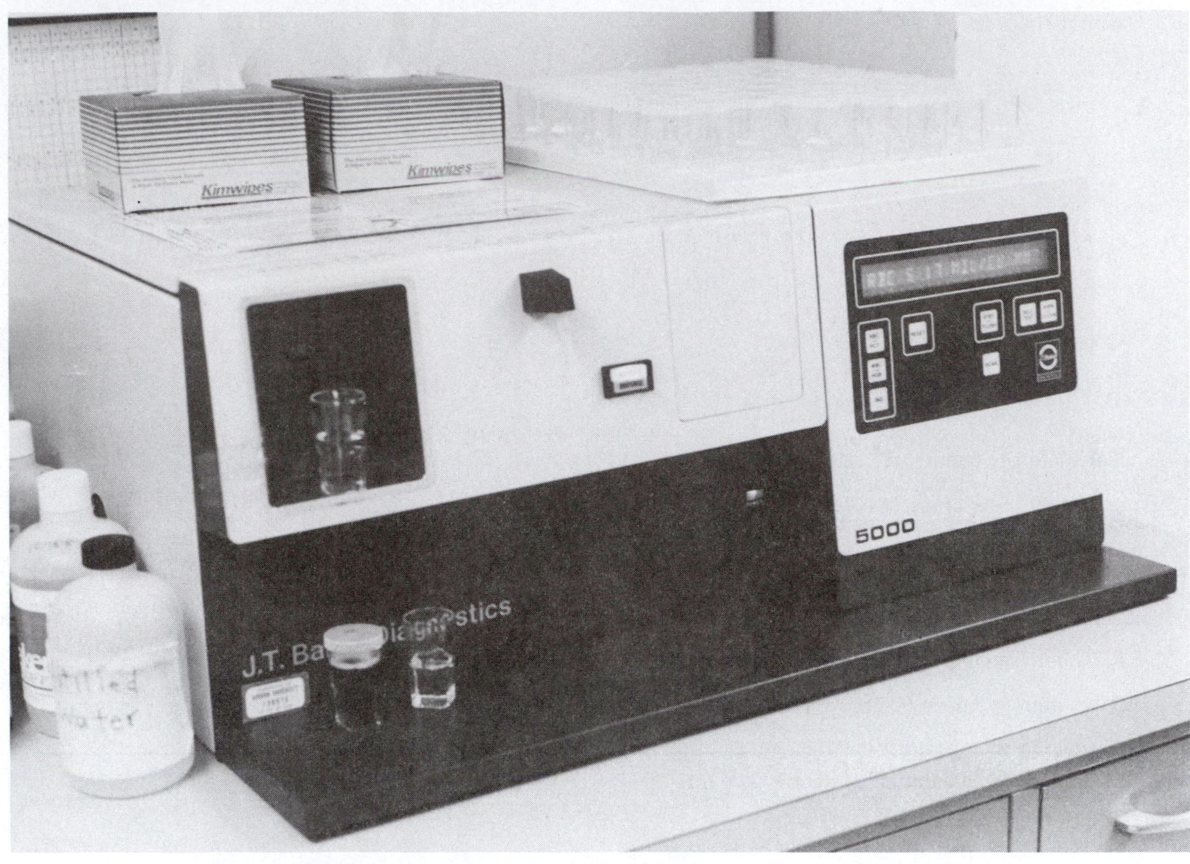


**Figure 2-32.** Automated cell counters (*Photos courtesy of Auburn University* [*above*], *and East Alabama Medical Center* [*page 113*], *photographer John Estridge*).

counters. The samples must then be counted manually. Such cases may be due to disease or drug treatments such as those for cancer.

## *LESSON REVIEW*

1. Name the three types of cellular elements found in the blood.
2. What is the function of the red cell?
3. What is the normal RBC count for a male—a female?
4. Name three diseases or conditions in which the red cell count is usually abnormal.
5. Which squares of the counting chamber are used in performing a red cell count?
6. Name three common red cell diluting fluids and state one requirement of a red cell diluting fluid.

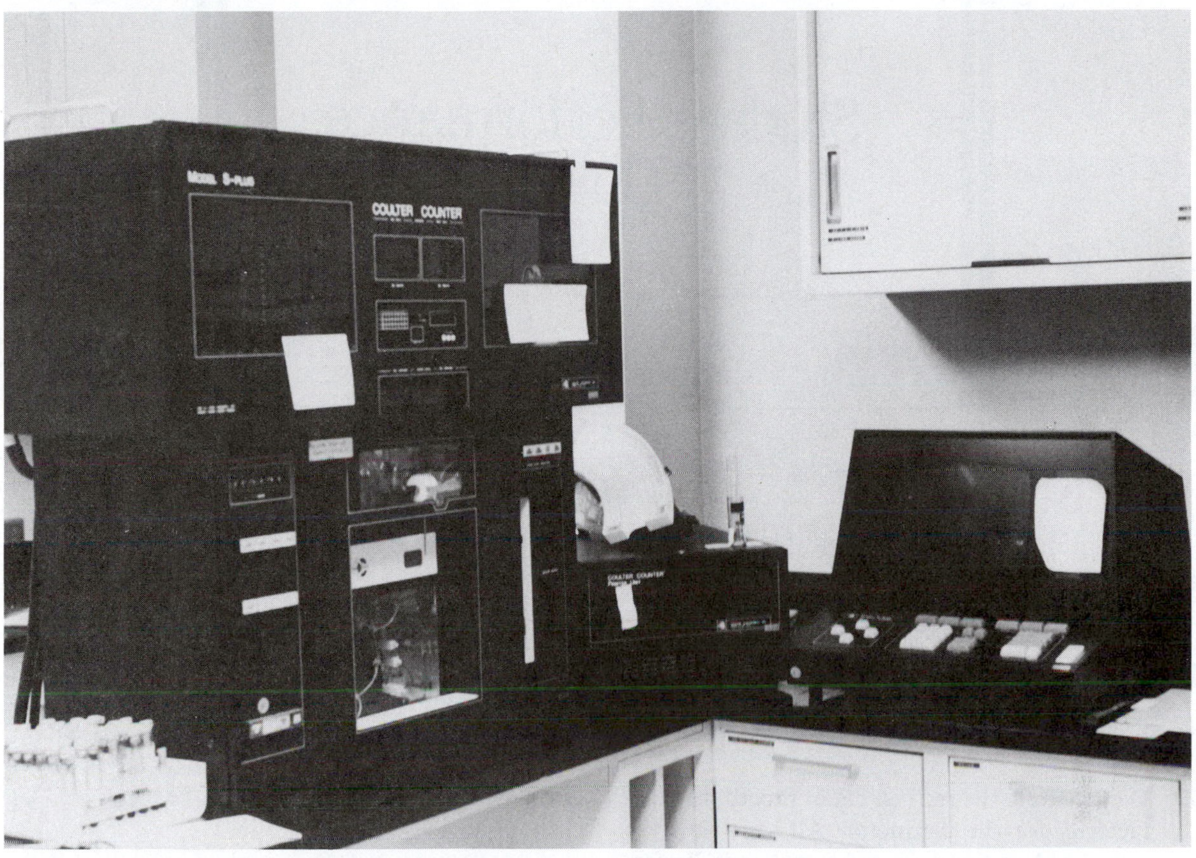


**Figure 2-32** (*cont*)

7. What is the usual dilution made when using an RBC pipet?
8. How is a red cell count calculated?
9. What precautions should be observed when performing a RBC count?
10. Define anemia, erythrocytosis, hemolysis, and isotonic solution.

## STUDENT ACTIVITIES

1. Re-read the information on red cell counts.
2. Review the glossary terms.
3. Practice making different dilutions with the RBC pipet by varying the mark to which the blood is drawn. Calculate the resulting dilutions.
4. Experiment to see what happens when red cells are exposed to 0.1N Hydrochloric acid (0.1N HCl) or to water.
5. Practice performing and calculating a red cell count as outlined in the Student Performance Guide, using the worksheet.

# Student Performance Guide

NAME ______________________

DATE ______________________

## LESSON 2–5
## THE RED BLOOD CELL COUNT

### Instructions

1. Practice performing and calculating a red cell count.
2. Demonstrate the red cell count procedure satisfactorily for the instructor. All steps must be completed as listed on the instructor's Performance Check Sheet.
3. Complete a written examination successfully.

### Materials and Equipment

- hand disinfectant
- RBC pipet
- rubber tubing with mouthpiece
- red blood cell diluting fluid
- hemacytometer with coverglass
- microscope
- hand counter
- pipet washer (optional)
- automatic pipet shaker (optional)
- gauze
- lens paper
- soft tissue
- detergent
- 70% ethyl or isopropyl alcohol
- capillary or EDTA anticoagulated blood specimen
- worksheet
- materials for capillary puncture
- surface disinfectant
- biohazard container
- safety filter

**Procedure**

S = Satisfactory
U = Unsatisfactory

| You must: | S | U | Comments |
|---|---|---|---|
| 1. Wash hands with hand disinfectant | | | |
| 2. Assemble equipment and materials | | | |

| You must: | S | U | Comments |
|---|---|---|---|
| 3. Attach rubber tubing and mouthpiece to RBC pipet | | | |
| 4. Hold pipet between thumb and index finger | | | |
| 5. Place mouthpiece between lips | | | |
| 6. Tilt well-mixed tube of blood and insert pipet tip (invert tube twenty to thirty times to mix) | | | |
| 7. Draw blood up to the 0.5 mark on the pipet. *Note:* Do not allow blood to pass the 0.5 mark | | | |
| 8. Wipe excess blood from pipet exterior with tissue to avoid the transfer of cells to the diluting fluid | | | |
| 9. Insert pipet tip into diluting fluid being careful not to allow cells to flow into diluting fluid | | | |
| 10. Draw the diluting fluid up to the 101 mark on the pipet. *Note:* Do not fill the pipet past the 101 mark | | | |
| 11. Place finger over the tip of pipet and remove the rubber tubing from stem | | | |
| 12. Fill a second pipet in the same manner | | | |
| 13. Mix contents of pipets manually or by automatic shaker:<br>A. Manual Method<br>(1) Hold pipet horizontally with thumb and middle finger over the ends of pipet | | | |
| (2) Mix for two to three minutes by rotating the pipet gently in a figure-eight motion | | | |
| B. Automatic Shaker<br>(1) Place pipets securely on automatic shaker and turn shaker on | | | |
| (2) Allow shaker to complete the cycle (usually two minutes) and come to a full stop | | | |
| (3) Remove pipets from shaker | | | |
| 14. Fill the hemacytometer:<br>a. Position a clean hemacytometer coverglass over the counting chamber | | | |
| b. Place the index finger over the tip of the short stem of pipet to control the flow of fluid | | | |
| c. Discard the first four to five drops of fluid from the long stem of the pipet | | | |

| You must: | S | U | Comments |
|---|---|---|---|
| d. Touch the tip of the pipet to the edge of the coverglass and counting chamber | | | |
| e. Allow the fluid to flow under the coverglass until one side of the counting chamber is completely full (usually one half to one drop). Do not overfill | | | |
| f. Fill the opposite side in the same manner using the second pipet | | | |
| g. Allow the cells to settle about two minutes | | | |
| 15. Place hemacytometer on the microscope stage and secure | | | |
| 16. Locate the central square of the ruled area using low power (10×) magnification | | | |
| 17. Switch to high power (40×) and focus with fine adjustment | | | |
| 18. Count the red cells:<br>a. Count the RBCs in the four corner squares and center square (a, b, c, d, and e) of the large central square using the left-to-right and right-to-left counting pattern | | | |
| b. Count the RBCs lying within each square, including the cells touching the top boundary, and the cells touching the left boundary. Do not count the cells touching the right or lower boundary | | | |
| 19. Record results from side 1 on the worksheet | | | |
| 20. Count side 2 in the same manner | | | |
| 21. Record results from side 2 on the worksheet | | | |
| 22. Average the counts from sides 1 and 2 | | | |
| 23. Use the formula to calculate the RBC count and either:<br>a. Multiply the average number of cells counted times the depth factor, times the dilution factor. Divide this by the area counted, or | | | |
| b. Multiply the average number of cells by 10,000 | | | |
| 24. Record RBC count on worksheet | | | |
| 25. Clean pipets carefully | | | |
| 26. Clean hemacytometer and coverglass carefully using 70% alcohol and lens paper | | | |

| You must: | S | U | Comments |
|---|---|---|---|
| 27. Dispose of specimen properly | | | |
| 28. Clean and return equipment to proper storage | | | |
| 29. Clean work area with surface disinfectant | | | |
| 30. Wash hands with hand disinfectant | | | |
| Comments: | | | |
| Student/Instructor: | | | |

Date: ______________________ Instructor: ______________________

# Worksheet

NAME ____________________ DATE __________

## LESSON 2–5 THE RED BLOOD CELL COUNT

| Side 1 | Number of cells counted |
|---|---|
| Square a | ______ |
| Square b | ______ |
| Square c | ______ |
| Square d | ______ |
| Square e | ______ |
| Total cells counted side 1 = | ______ |

| Side 2 | Number of cells counted |
|---|---|
| Square a | ______ |
| Square b | ______ |
| Square c | ______ |
| Square d | ______ |
| Square e | ______ |
| Total cells counted side 2 = | ______ |
| Total of sides 1 and 2 | ______ |
| Average of two sides (divide by two) | ______ |
| Multiply average number of cells × 10 × 200 and divide by 0.2 = | ______ = RBC/mm³ |
| or | |
| Add four zeroes to the average number of cells = | ______ = RBC/mm³ |

# LESSON 2–6

## The White Blood Cell Count

## LESSON OBJECTIVES

After studying this lesson, you should be able to:

- List the normal white cell count for adults, children, and newborn infants.
- Name a condition that causes leukocytosis and one that causes leukopenia.
- Perform a manual white blood cell count.
- Calculate the results of a white blood cell count.
- List the precautions to observe when performing a white blood cell count.
- List two white blood cell diluting fluids and state the function of each.
- Define the glossary terms.

## GLOSSARY

**immunity** / resistance to disease or infection

**leukocytosis** / increase above normal in the number of leukocytes in the blood

**leukopenia** / decrease below normal in the number of leukocytes in the blood

## INTRODUCTION

The white blood cell count or leukocyte count is a routine part of a complete blood count (CBC). The white blood cell count gives an approximation of the total number of leukocytes in circulating blood.

Five types of white blood cells (WBC) or leukocytes are present in the blood. These are neutrophils, eosinophils, basophils, monocytes, and lymphocytes. The white cells play an important role in providing **immunity** and fighting infections.

**Table 2-3.** Normal Leukocyte Counts

| Age | Leukocyte Count (cells/mm³) Average | Range |
|---|---|---|
| Newborn | 18,000 | 9,000–30,000 |
| One year | 11,000 | 6,000–14,000 |
| Six years | 8,000 | 4,500–12,000 |
| Adult | 7,400 | 4,500–11,000 |

### Normal Values

The normal white cell count varies with age (Table 2–3). Newborn infants usually have a WBC count of 9,000–30,000/mm$^3$. The count drops rapidly and children have a normal count ranging from 5,000–14,000/mm$^3$. By adulthood the normal WBC count is 4,500–11,000/mm$^3$.

### Factors that Influence White Cell Counts

Once adulthood is reached, the WBC count remains stable unless an individual experiences a physical, emotional, or pathological condition that influences the count. Many factors may affect the white cell count. The changes in WBC counts due to factors such as stress, exercise, and anesthesia are temporary while changes due to disease may last until the disease is under control. Most commonly, any increase or decrease in leukocytes is produced by a change in concentration of only one cell type.

An elevated white cell count, **leukocytosis,** may be related to physiologic conditions such as exercise, exposure to sunlight, obstetric labor, and anesthesia. Leukocytosis can also be due to pathologic conditions such as bacterial infections or leukemia.

A decrease below the normal number of leukocytes is called **leukopenia.** This condition may be caused by some viral infections or by exposure to ionizing radiation, some chemicals, and the drugs used in chemotherapy.

## PERFORMING A MANUAL WBC COUNT

### Diluting Fluids

A white cell count is performed similarly to a RBC count. The diluting fluids used for WBC counts should be solutions which will not damage the leukocytes but will destroy the erythrocytes in the sample. The red blood cells must be destroyed because they are present in such large numbers they will interfere with the count. Two common WBC diluting fluids are 2% acetic acid and 0.1 N Hydrochloric acid.

### Diluting the Sample

The sample is diluted by filling a WBC pipet to the 0.5 mark with blood. The WBC diluting fluid is then drawn into the pipet to the 11 mark. The contents of the pipet are mixed to assure even distribution of cells. Four to five drops of fluid are dis-

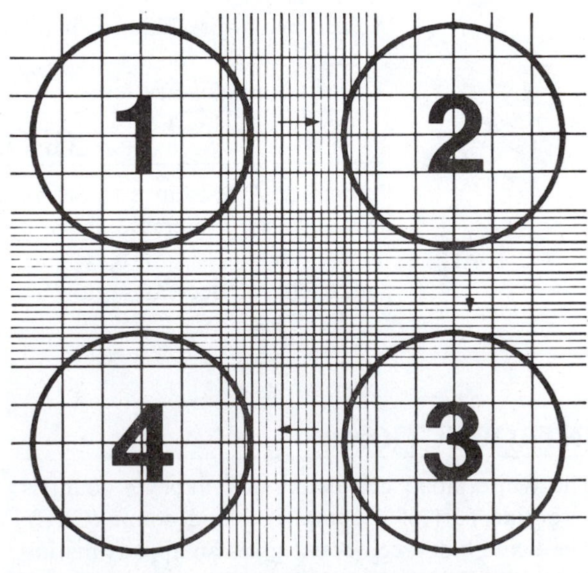


**Figure 2-33.** WBC counting area

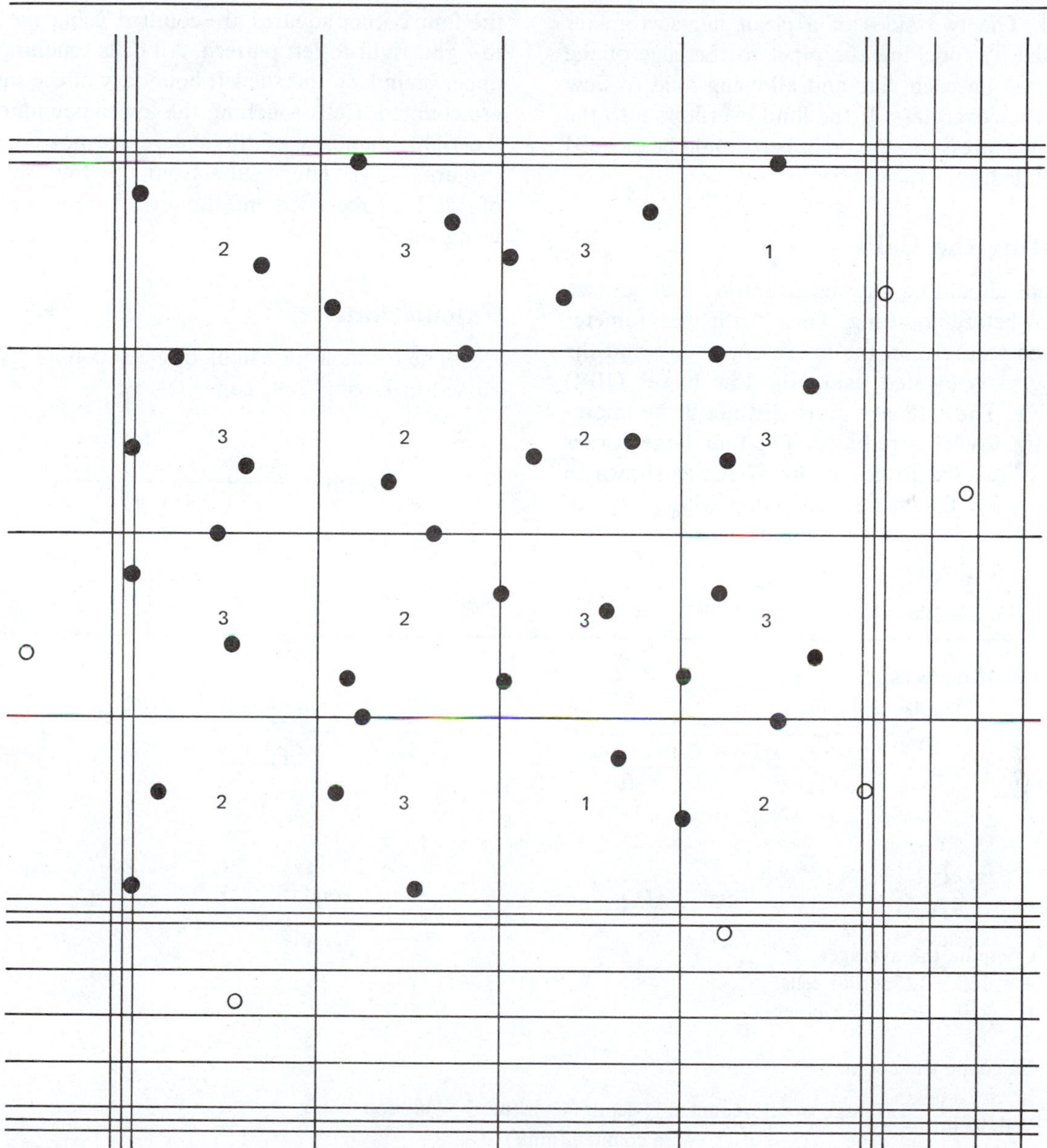


**Figure 2-34.** Sample count in square one (1) of WBC counting area. The numbers shown denote the total number of cells counted in each square.

carded. The two sides of a clean hemacytometer are filled by touching the pipet to the edge of the coverglass on each side and allowing fluid to flow under the coverglass. If the fluid overflows into the moat or depression, the chamber should be cleaned and refilled.

## Counting the Cells

The cells should be allowed to settle for about two minutes before counting. Then the hemacytometer is placed securely on the microscope stage and the ruled grid is located using the low power (10×) objective. The cells are more distinct if the microscope light level is reduced. The four large corner squares are used to count the WBC, as shown in Figure 2–33. The white cells lying within each of the four corner squares are counted using the left-to-right, right-to-left pattern. All cells touching the upper boundary and the left boundary of the square are counted. Cells touching the lower boundary or the right boundary of the square are not counted (Figure 2–34). The results from the four squares of side 1 are recorded and the procedure is repeated using side 2.

## Calculations

The formula for calculating cell counts (as discussed in Lesson 2–4, page 100) is:

$$C/mm^3 = \frac{Avg \times D\ (mm) \times DF}{A\ (mm^2)}$$

**Figure 2-35.** Sample calculation of a WBC count

1. Count the cells:

| Side 1 | | Side 2 | |
|---|---|---|---|
| Square | Cells counted | Square | Cells counted |
| 1 | 30 | 1 | 30 |
| 2 | 25 | 2 | 26 |
| 3 | 27 | 3 | 35 |
| 4 | 33 | 4 | 34 |
| Total | 115 | Total | 125 |

2. Compute the average:
   A. 115 + 125 = 240 cells
   B. 240 ÷ 2 = 120 average

3. Calculate the count:

$$WBC/mm^3 = \frac{\text{average \# cells counted} \times \text{depth factor (mm)} \times \text{dilution factor}}{\text{area counted (mm}^2\text{)}}$$

$$WBC/mm^3 = \frac{120 \times 10\ mm \times 20}{4\ mm^2}$$

$$WBC/mm^3 = 120 \times 50\ mm^3$$

$$WBC/mm^3 = 6{,}000\ (\text{or } 6.0 \times 10^3)/mm^3$$

For the WBC count, the dilution factor is 20 and the area counted is 4 $mm^2$. To calculate a WBC count, the number of cells counted on each side of the chamber is totaled. The average of the two sides is calculated. The numbers are then substituted into the formula.:

$$\text{WBC/mm}^3 = \frac{\text{Average \# cells} \times 10 \times 20}{4 \text{ mm}^2}$$
$$= \text{Average \# cells} \times 50$$

A sample calculation for a WBC count is shown in Figure 2–35.

### *Precautions*

- Observe all precautions for using blood diluting pipets and the hemacytometer.
- If the number of cells in a large square varies from any other square on the same side by more than ten cells, repeat the count after cleaning and refilling the chamber.
- For optimum safety, use a safety filter when pipeting to prevent accidental aspiration of sample.

## AUTOMATED WHITE CELL COUNTS

Most instruments that count RBC will also count WBC. Some of the instruments can even differentiate between types of leukocytes. Although automated cell counters aid in the efficiency of laboratories, manual counts are still performed in some circumstances. Therefore, laboratory personnel should be trained in performing manual WBC counts.

## *LESSON REVIEW*

1. Give the normal WBC count for newborns, children, and adults.
2. Name three factors that may cause leukocytosis.
3. Name three factors that may cause leukopenia.
4. Describe the procedure for performing a WBC count.
5. What areas of the hemacytometer are used for a WBC count?
6. What dilution is made?
7. Write a formula for calculating the WBC count.
8. Name two WBC diluting fluids.
9. What is the function of a WBC diluting fluid?
10. Define immunity, leukocytosis, and leukopenia.

## *STUDENT ACTIVITIES*

1. Re-read the information on the white blood cell count.
2. Review the glossary terms.
3. Practice performing WBC counts as outlined in the Student Performance Guide, using the worksheet.
4. Calculate the WBC counts when the average number of cells counted is 100; 125; and 175.

# Student Performance Guide

NAME ____________________

DATE ____________________

## LESSON 2–6
## THE WHITE BLOOD CELL COUNT

### Instructions

1. Practice performing and calculating a white cell count.
2. Demonstrate the white cell count satisfactorily for the instructor. All steps must be completed as listed on the instructor's Performance Check Sheet.
3. Complete a written examination successfully.

### Materials and Equipment

- surface disinfectant
- microscope
- WBC diluting fluid
- WBC diluting pipet
- rubber tubing with mouthpiece
- hemacytometer with coverglass
- hand counter
- 70% alcohol
- lens paper
- soft tissue
- EDTA anticoagulated blood sample
- automatic pipet shaker (optional)
- pipet washer (optional)
- WBC worksheet
- hand disinfectant
- biohazard container
- safety filter

### Procedure

S = Satisfactory
U = Unsatisfactory

| You must: | S | U | Comments |
|---|---|---|---|
| 1. Wash hands with hand disinfectant | | | |
| 2. Assemble equipment and materials | | | |

| You must: | S | U | Comments |
|---|---|---|---|
| 3. Place a clean hemacytometer coverglass over a clean hemacytometer | | | |
| 4. Attach rubber tubing and mouthpiece to WBC pipet | | | |
| 5. Hold pipet in hand between thumb and index finger | | | |
| 6. Place mouthpiece between lips | | | |
| 7. Tilt well-mixed tube of blood and insert pipet tip | | | |
| 8. Draw blood up to the 0.5 mark on the pipet. *Note:* Do not allow blood to pass the 0.5 mark | | | |
| 9. Wipe the excess blood from the outside of the pipet stem to avoid the transfer of cells to the diluting fluid (avoid touching the pipet tip with tissue) | | | |
| 10. Draw the WBC diluting fluid up to the 11 mark on the pipet. *Note:* Do not fill past the 11 mark | | | |
| 11. Place finger over the tip of pipet and remove the rubber tubing | | | |
| 12. Mix the contents of the pipet using the manual method or an automatic pipet shaker (see Lesson 2–3) | | | |
| 13. Place the index finger over the top of the pipet to control the flow of fluid | | | |
| 14. Discard the first 4 or 5 drops of fluid from the pipet | | | |
| 15. Touch the tip of the pipet to the edge of the coverglass and counting chamber | | | |
| 16. Allow the fluid to flow under the coverglass until one side of the chamber is completely full (usually one-half to one drop) | | | |
| 17. Fill the opposite side of the chamber in the same manner | | | |
| 18. Allow cells to settle for about two minutes | | | |
| 19. Place hemacytometer carefully on the microscope stage and secure | | | |
| 20. Locate the ruled area of the chamber using the low power (10×) objective | | | |

| You must: | S | U | Comments |
|---|---|---|---|
| 21. Locate the correct area for counting WBC (four large corner squares) | | | |
| 22. Count all the WBC lying within the four large corner squares (1, 2, 3, and 4) using the boundary rule | | | |
| 23. Record results from side 1 on worksheet | | | |
| 24. Repeat steps 21–22 using side 2 | | | |
| 25. Record results from side 2 on the worksheet | | | |
| 26. Average the total cells counted on the two sides of the chamber | | | |
| 27. Use the formula to calculate the WBC count and record on worksheet | | | |
| 28. Clean WBC pipet carefully | | | |
| 29. Clean hemacytometer and coverglass carefully | | | |
| 30. Clean and return equipment to proper storage | | | |
| 31. Dispose of specimen properly | | | |
| 32. Clean work area with surface disinfectant | | | |
| 33. Wash hands with hand disinfectant | | | |

Comments:

Student/Instructor:

Date: ______________________ Instructor: ______________________

# Worksheet

NAME ________________________________________ DATE ______________

## LESSON 2–6 THE WHITE BLOOD CELL COUNT

| Side 1 | Number of cells counted |
|---|---|
| Square 1 | ______________ |
| Square 2 | ______________ |
| Square 3 | ______________ |
| Square 4 | ______________ |
| Total cells counted side 1 = | ______________ |

| Side 2 | Number of cells counted |
|---|---|
| Square 1 | ______________ |
| Square 2 | ______________ |
| Square 3 | ______________ |
| Square 4 | ______________ |
| Total cells counted side 2 = | ______________ |
| Total of sides 1 and 2 | ______________ |
| Average of two sides (divide by 2) | ______________ |
| Multiply average number of cells × 10 × 20 and divide by 4 = | ______________ = WBC/mm³ |
| or | |
| Multiply average number of cells by 50 = | ______________ = WBC/mm³ |

# LESSON 2–7

## Preparation of a Blood Smear

### LESSON OBJECTIVES

After studying this lesson, you should be able to:

- Discuss the purpose and importance of the blood smear.
- List the components that may normally be observed in a blood smear.
- Prepare a blood smear.
- Preserve a blood smear.
- List the precautions to observe when preparing a blood smear.
- Define the glossary terms.

### GLOSSARY

**CBC** / complete blood count; a commonly performed group of hematological tests

**fixative** / preservative; chemical which prevents deterioration of cells or tissues

**morphology** / study of form and structure of cells, tissues, organs

## INTRODUCTION

A blood smear enables the technologist to view the cellular components of blood in as natural a state as possible. The **morphology,** or structure, of the cellular components can then be studied. The erythrocytes, leukocytes, and platelets are viewed to evaluate relative numbers, size, structure, and maturity. It is important that the cell morphology and relative distribution of cells are altered as little as possible while preparing the smear.

Examining a stained blood smear is a routine part of the **CBC.** A blood smear is prepared by spreading blood on a microscope slide. The smear is dried and stained. The blood components may then be viewed microscopically, identified, and evaluated, as in the white cell differential count. Careful examination of a well-prepared blood smear can provide valuable information to the physician in the diagnosis and treatment of many diseases such as leukemia, sickle cell anemia, and malaria.

## PREPARING A BLOOD SMEAR

It is a waste of time to stain smears that are poorly prepared. The results of the microscopic evaluation of a poorly prepared smear may be misleading and unreliable. Thus, each step involved in preparing a smear should be followed correctly.

## Specimen

The best specimen for a blood smear is capillary blood which has had no anticoagulant added. However, a satisfactory smear may be made from venous blood which has the anticoagulant EDTA added to it, provided the smear is made within two hours of collection. Other anticoagulants should not be used since they change the morphology of the cells.

## Cleaning the Slides

The slides that are used to make a blood smear must be entirely free of grease and dust. Slides may be purchased pre-cleaned. Or, slides may be washed with soap and water, rinsed thoroughly in hot water, and then distilled water, dipped in 95% ethyl alcohol, and polished with a clean, lint-free cloth. Clean slides may be stored in 95% ethyl alcohol and should be handled by the edges only.

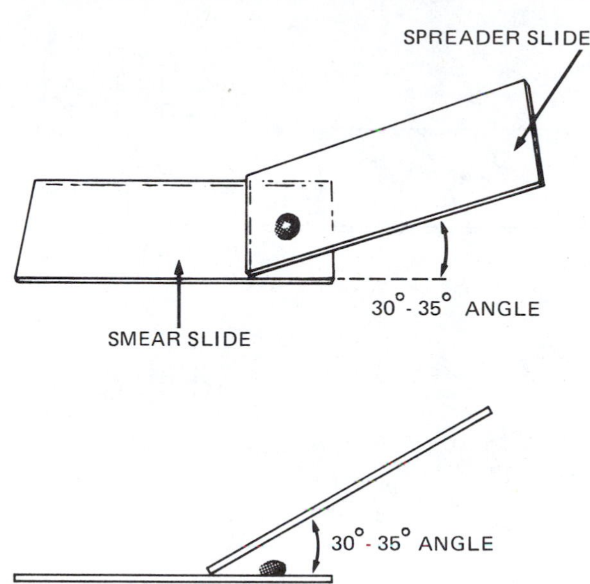


**Figure 2-36.** Position the spreader slide in front of the drop of blood.

# MAKING THE SMEAR: TWO-SLIDE METHOD

There are several methods of spreading the blood on a slide which result in good smears. Each individual needs to find the technique that is least awkward and that provides good results. The blood smear can be prepared by placing one-half drop of blood about one-half to three-fourths inch from the right end (left end for left-handed) of a pre-cleaned slide which has been placed on a flat surface. The end of a second "spreader" slide is brought to rest at a 30–35° angle in front of the drop of blood (Figure 2–36).

The spreader is then brought back into the drop of blood until the drop spreads along 3/4 of the edge of the spreader slide. This should be performed in a smooth, quick sliding motion. As soon as the blood spreads along the edge of the spreader, the spreader is pushed to the left (right for left-handed) with a quick, steady motion (avoiding pressure on the slide) to spread the blood (Figure 2–37). Each end of the spreader slide should be used only one time unless the slide is cleaned and kept unchipped. The smear is allowed to air dry as quickly as possible. It is then ready for staining or preserving. Smears may be labeled with pencil in the thick area of the blood.

## Preserving and Staining

Dried smears should be stained immediately. If this is not possible, however, the slide may be immersed in methanol in a Coplin jar for thirty to sixty seconds and allowed to air dry. It may then be stained at a later date. The methanol is a **fixative** or preservative that prevents changes or deterioration of cellular components.

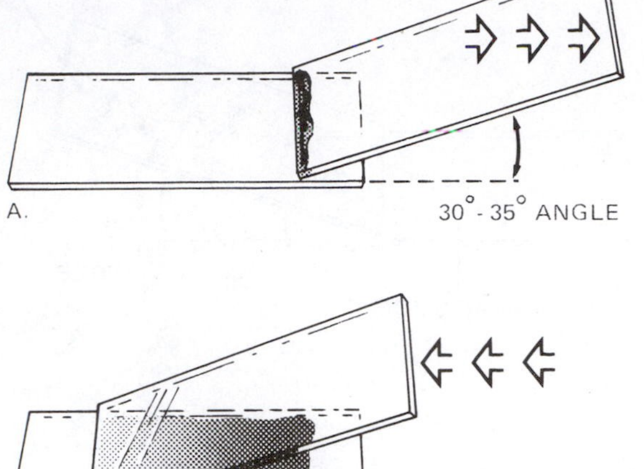


Figure 2-37. Spreading the blood with a spreader slide

## Features of a Good Smear

A well-prepared smear is illustrated in Figure 2–38. The smear should cover about one-half to three-fourths of the slide and should show a gradual transition from thick to thin. It should have a smooth appearance with no holes or ridges and should have a feathered edge (about 1.5 cm long) at the thin end. When the smear is examined microscopically, the cells should be distributed evenly.

## Factors Affecting the Smear

The length and thickness of the smear are affected by the size of the drop of blood and the angle at which the spreader slide is held. Thick smears occur when the angle of the spreader is too high or the drop of blood is too large. Thin smears occur when the drop is too small or the angle is too low. Thin, uneven smears may also occur when too much pressure is applied to the spreader. The faster the spreading procedure the thinner the smear.

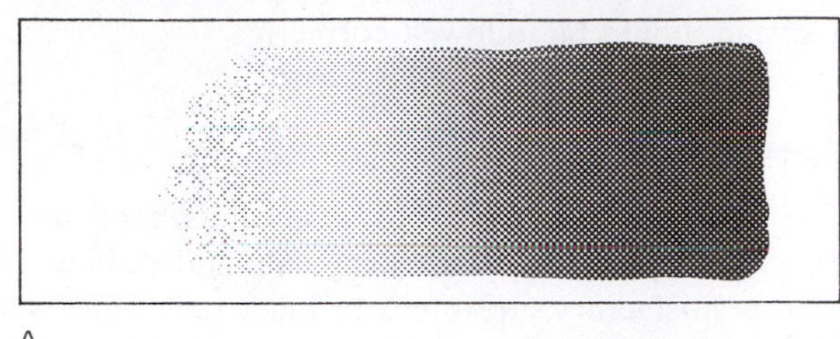


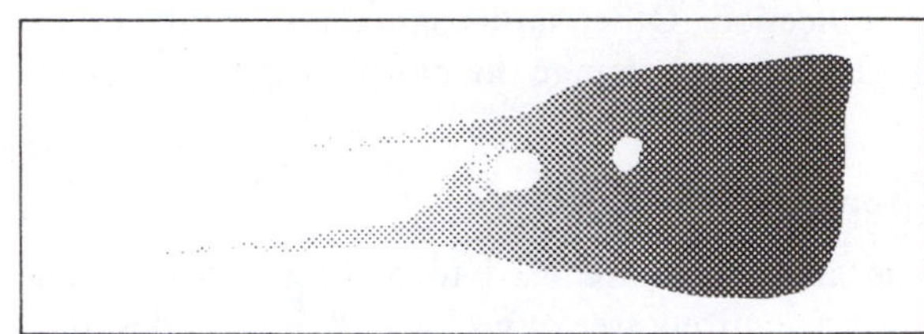


C.

**Figure 2-38.** Properly prepared smear A) vs improper smears B) and C)

Drying time may affect the appearance of the cellular elements. If high humidity causes slow drying, the cells may appear abnormal. For example, the red blood cells may appear moth-eaten.

### *Precautions*

- Methanol is poisonous; do not inhale fumes; wash hands thoroughly.
- The spreader slide should have a clean, pol-

ished end to prevent holes and streaks in the smear.

- The drop of blood should not be too small or too large.
- Delay between applying the drop and spreading the drop may cause uneven cell distribution.
- Hesitation or jerky motion when spreading the blood will cause uneven cell distribution.
- Smears should be stained within one to two hours after preparation or should be preserved.
- Smears should be dried as quickly as possible (do not blow on slides to dry them).
- To prevent clotting of the blood, capillary blood must be spread immediately.

## *LESSON REVIEW*

1. What is the purpose of a blood smear?
2. What components in the blood can be viewed on a smear?
3. What specimen(s) may be used for blood smears?
4. Explain the two-slide method for making a blood smear.
5. What are some of the errors to avoid when making a blood smear?
6. Describe and diagram the appearance of a properly prepared blood smear.
7. How may unstained blood smears be preserved?
8. Define CBC, fixative, and morphology.

## *STUDENT ACTIVITIES*

1. Re-read the information on preparing a blood smear.
2. Review the glossary terms.
3. Practice preparing blood smears by the two-slide method as outlined on the Student Performance Guide.

# Student Performance Guide

NAME ______________________

DATE ______________________

## LESSON 2–7 PREPARATION OF A BLOOD SMEAR

### Instructions

1. Practice preparing a blood smear.
2. Demonstrate the procedure for preparation of a blood smear satisfactorily for the instructor. All steps must be completed as listed on the instructor's Performance Check Sheet.
3. Complete a written examination successfully.

### Materials and Equipment

- hand disinfectant
- microscope slides
- 95% ethyl alcohol
- lint-free polishing cloth
- capillary tubes (plain and heparinized)
- slide rack
- hot water
- detergent
- distilled water
- methanol in covered staining (Coplin) jar
- EDTA anticoagulated blood specimen (fresh)
- materials for capillary puncture
- surface disinfectant
- biohazard container

**Procedure**

S = Satisfactory
U = Unsatisfactory

| You must: | S | U | Comments |
|---|---|---|---|
| 1. Wash hands with hand disinfectant | | | |
| 2. Assemble equipment and materials | | | |

| You must: | S | U | Comments |
|---|---|---|---|
| 3. Prepare several clean slides:<br>A. Use pre-cleaned slides, or<br>B. Clean slides with soap, rinse with hot water followed by distilled water, dip in 95% ethyl alcohol, and polish dry with clean lint-free cloth | | | |
| 4. Place a clean slide on a flat surface (be sure to touch only the edges of the slide with the fingers) | | | |
| 5. Obtain an anticoagulated blood sample (from the instructor) | | | |
| 6. Mix blood well and fill a plain capillary tube with blood | | | |
| 7. Dispense a small drop of blood from the capillary tube onto the slide about one-half to three-fourths inch from the right end (if left-handed, reverse instructions) | | | |
| 8. Place the end of a clean, polished unchipped spreader slide in front of the drop of blood at a 30–35° angle. Spreader should be lightly balanced with fingertips | | | |
| 9. Pull the spreader slide back into the drop of blood by sliding gently along the slide until the blood spreads along three-fourths of the width of the spreader | | | |
| 10. Push the spreader slide forward with a quick steady motion (use other hand to keep slide from moving while spreader is pushed) | | | |
| 11. Examine the smear to see if it is satisfactory | | | |
| 12. Repeat the procedure until two satisfactory smears are obtained | | | |
| 13. Allow the smear to air dry quickly (slide may be waved gently to accelerate drying) and label the slide | | | |
| 14. Place the dried smear in absolute methanol for thirty to sixty seconds to preserve the smear | | | |
| 15. Remove the slide from methanol and allow to air dry | | | |
| 16. Store slide for staining | | | |
| 17. Perform a capillary puncture, wipe away the first drop | | | |

| You must: | S | U | Comments |
|---|---|---|---|
| of blood, and fill one or two heparinized capillary tubes | | | |
| 18. Prepare two blood smears from capillary blood, repeating steps 7–16 | | | |
| 19. Dispose of blood specimens properly | | | |
| 20. Clean equipment and return to proper storage | | | |
| 21. Clean work area with surface disinfectant | | | |
| 22. Wash hands with hand disinfectant | | | |

Comments:

Student/Instructor:

Date: ______________________ Instructor: ______________________

# LESSON 2-8

## Staining a Blood Smear

### LESSON OBJECTIVES

After studying this lesson, you should be able to:

- Discuss the purpose of staining blood smears.
- Explain what information may be obtained from a stained blood smear.
- Stain a blood smear.
- List precautions to be observed for proper staining of a blood smear.
- Define the glossary terms.

### GLOSSARY

**anhydrous** / containing no water
**buffer** / a substance which prevents changes in the pH of solutions when additional acid or base is added
**cytoplasm** / the fluid portion of the cell outside the nucleus
**eosin** / a dye that produces a red stain
**methylene blue** / a dye that produces a blue stain
**nucleus, nuclei** / the central structure of a cell which contains DNA and controls cell growth and function
**polychromatic** / multicolored

## INTRODUCTION

Stains are applied to blood smears so that the formed elements may be more easily viewed and evaluated. A stained blood smear can provide important information regarding a patient's health. The evaluation of a blood smear often leads to the diagnosis or verification of disease.

A stained smear is evaluated in a procedure called the leukocyte differential count. Observations of erythrocyte, leukocyte, and platelet morphology, relative numbers of the types of leukocytes, and cellular maturity are made while examining the blood smear. Also, stained smears may be examined to identify blood parasites such as those that cause malaria. Bone marrow smears may be examined to evaluate blood cell production.

## DIFFERENTIAL OR POLYCHROMATIC STAINS

The stains commonly used for the routine microscopic examination of blood are called **polychromatic.** These stains are thus named because they contain dyes that will stain various components of cells different colors. Most polychromatic blood stains contain combinations of **methylene blue,** a blue stain; **eosin,** a red-orange stain; and methyl alcohol, a fixative. The different dyes are attracted to the different cell structures. The cells and structures are thus more easily visualized and differentiated (hence the name differential count). The two most commonly used differential blood stains are Wright's and Giemsa's.

## SPECIAL STAINS

Information gained during routine blood smear evaluation may cause a physician to order special blood stains for further study. These special stains may be used to stain specific components of cells such as iron granules or nucleic acids.

## STAINING PROCEDURES

Blood smears should be stained as soon as they have been thoroughly air-dried. If more than one or two hours will pass before staining, the smears should be preserved. Smears may be stained by a two-step method, quick-stain method, or by an automatic stainer. A quick-stain is adequate for most routine work, but the two-step method (or automatic stainer) should be used to evaluate cell abnormalities and bone marrow cells.

### Two-Step Method

In a two-step method, a stain such as Wright's stain is applied to the slide for approximately 1-3 minutes (Figure 2–39). Fixation occurs in this step because of the methyl alcohol in the stain. A **buffer** is then added to the stain until the buffer volume is about equal to the stain (Figure 2–40). Buffers are substances which prevent changes in the pH of solutions when additional acid or base is added. The stain is gently blown until a green metallic sheen appears (this occurs when the solutions mix), usually two

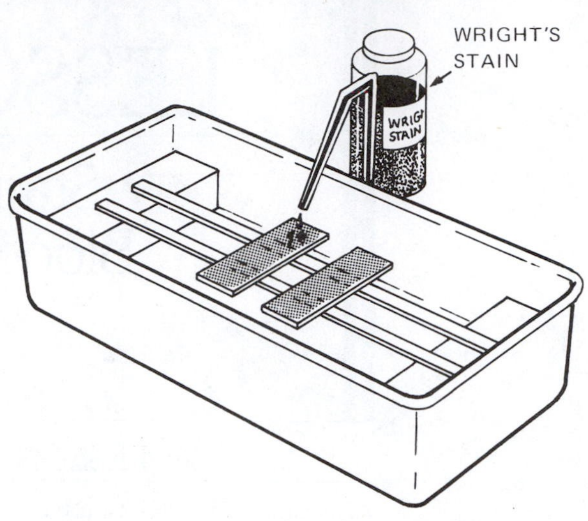


**Figure 2-39.** Apply Wright's stain to a blood smear.

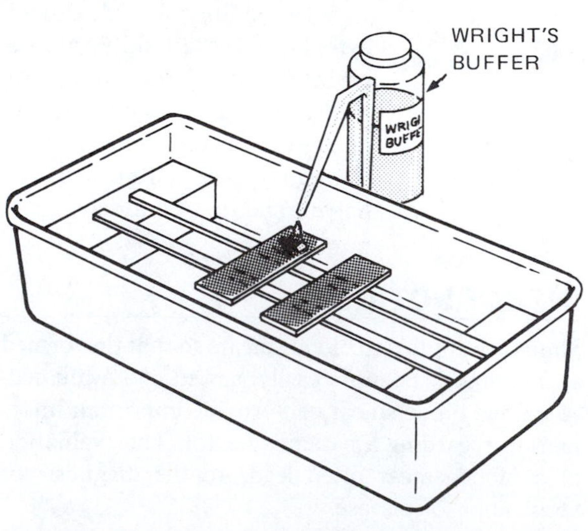


**Figure 2-40.** Apply buffer to Wright's stain.

to four minutes (Figure 2–41). Times may vary according to the stain and buffer used. The slide is rinsed gently, allowed to air dry, and can then be examined using the microscope.

### Quick Stains

Quick stains are variations of the polychromatic stains. In these quick stains, the slide is dipped into two or three solutions quickly, then rinsed and dried. The entire quick-staining method takes less than a minute whereas the two-step method requires 4-6 minutes. It may be easier for the inexperienced technician to obtain an adequate stain with quick methods, but experienced technicians can achieve superior results using the two-step method.

## APPEARANCE OF STAINED SMEAR AND CELLS

A properly stained smear should appear pinkish to the naked eye. When viewed microscopically, the red cells should appear pinkish-tan. The leuko-

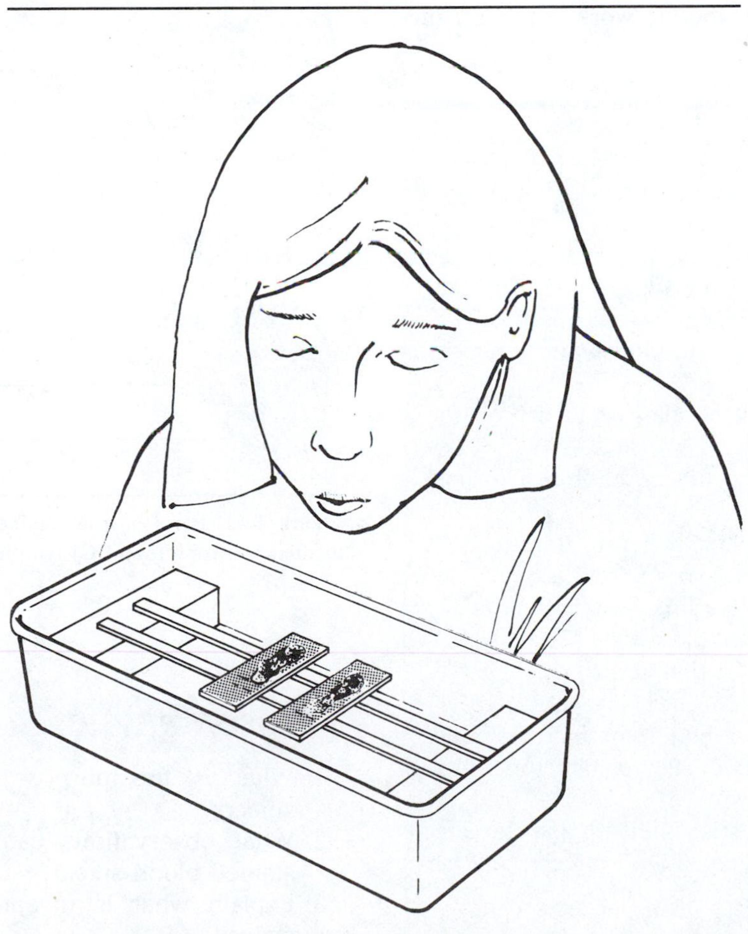

**Figure 2-41.** Mix buffer and stain.

cyte **nuclei** should appear purple. The leukocyte **cytoplasm** may vary from pink to blue or blue-gray, depending on the cell type (Figure 2–42). Variations in color intensities may be due to pH, timing, or characteristics of the stain and/or buffer. Colors are best evaluated using the oil immersion objective.

## STORAGE OF STAINED SMEARS

Stained smears should be stored in the dark in a covered dust-free slide box or container. If protected from light when not in use, the stains will last for years with little fading. Surfaces may be protected from scratches by mounting a permanent coverglass over the smear. For routine work, however, this is not necessary.

### *Precautions*

- Handle methyl alcohol with care; it is poisonous.
- Store stains tightly capped; methanol in the staining solution is **anhydrous** and the stain must be discarded if moisture is absorbed.
- Stains may precipitate and should be filtered often.
- Stain should not be allowed to dry on the slide before rinsing.
- Slides should be rinsed thoroughly after staining.
- Proper staining and buffering times should be observed for best staining results.
- Slides that are too pink may be due to (1) pH of stain or buffer too acidic, (2) wash time too long, or (3) stain time too short.
- Slides that are too blue may be due to (1) overstaining, (2) wash time or buffering time too short, or (3) pH of stain or buffer too alkaline.
- To avoid getting stain on hands and clothing, slides should be handled with forceps, and lab aprons or coats should be worn.

A. ERYTHROCYTE

CENTER AREA OF PALLOR (NO NUCLEUS)

SIDE VIEW SHOWING BICONCAVITY

B. NEUTROPHIL

NUCLEUS (LOBED)

CYTOPLASM

CYTOPLASMIC GRANULES

C. LYMPHOCYTE

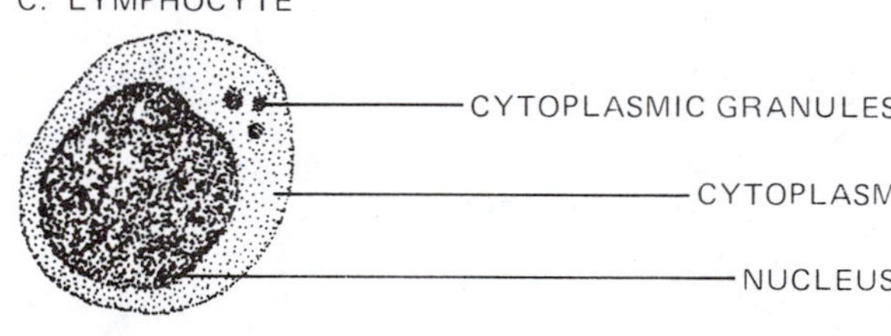


**Figure 2-42.** Parts of a A) stained erythrocyte, B) segmented neutrophil, and C) lymphocyte

## *LESSON REVIEW*

1. What is the purpose of staining blood smears?
2. What observations can be made from a stained blood smear?
3. Explain what is meant by polychromatic stains.

4. What two dyes are usually components of polychromatic blood stains?
5. Name two types of commonly used blood stains.
6. Which provides the most satisfactory stain, the two-step method or the quick stains?
7. How should a properly stained smear appear?
8. What is the proper method of storing slides?
9. Name four precautions that must be observed to achieve good staining results.
10. Define anhydrous, buffer, cytoplasm, eosin, methylene blue, nucleus, and polychromatic.

## *STUDENT ACTIVITIES*

1. Re-read the information on staining a blood smear.
2. Review the glossary terms.
3. Practice staining blood smears by the two-step method as outlined on the Student Performance Guide.
4. Practice staining blood smears by a quick method.
5. Compare smears stained by the two-step and quick methods. Observe the most desired effect.
6. Experiment with variations in the staining and buffering times using the two-step method. Explain the results.

# Student Performance Guide

NAME ______________________

DATE ______________________

## LESSON 2–8 STAINING A BLOOD SMEAR

### Instructions

1. Practice staining a blood smear.
2. Demonstrate the procedure for staining a blood smear satisfactorily for the instructor. All steps must be completed as listed on the instructor's Performance Check Sheet.
3. Complete a written examination successfully.

### Materials and Equipment

- hand disinfectant
- blood smears, freshly prepared or preserved
- Wright's stain and buffer
- staining rack
- immersion oil
- microscope
- lens paper
- forceps
- laboratory tissue
- lab apron or lab coat
- quick stain (optional)
- staining jars (optional)
- surface disinfectant
- biohazard container

*Note:* Stain characteristics may vary from lot to lot. Follow manufacturer's instructions for best results.

| **Procedure** | | | S = Satisfactory<br>U = Unsatisfactory |
|---|---|---|---|
| **You must:** | **S** | **U** | **Comments** |
| 1. Wash hands with hand disinfectant | | | |
| 2. Assemble equipment and materials | | | |

| You must: | S | U | Comments |
|---|---|---|---|
| 3. Obtain a dried blood smear | | | |
| 4. Stain a blood smear by one of the following methods:<br>A. Two-step method<br>(1) Place the smear on the staining rack or on a flat surface, blood side up | | | |
| (2) Flood the smear with Wright's stain but do not let stain overflow the sides of the slide | | | |
| (3) Leave stain on slide 1–3 minutes (get exact time from instructor) | | | |
| (4) Add buffer, dropwise, to the stain until the buffer volume is about equal to the stain | | | |
| (5) Blow gently on the surface of the fluid to mix the solutions. A green metallic sheen should appear on the surface | | | |
| (6) Allow buffer to remain on slide for 2–4 minutes (do not allow mixture to run off slide); get exact time from instructor | | | |
| (7) Rinse thoroughly and continuously with a gentle stream of tap or distilled water | | | |
| (8) Drain water from slide | | | |
| (9) Wipe the back of the slide with a wet gauze to remove excess stain | | | |
| (10) Stand smear on end to dry<br>or | | | |
| B. Quick stain<br>(1) Dip dried slide into solutions as directed by manufacturer's instructions (do not allow slide to dry between solutions) | | | |
| (2) Rinse slide (if instructed to do so) | | | |
| (3) Remove excess stain from the back of the slide with wet gauze | | | |
| (4) Allow slide to air dry by standing on end | | | |
| 5. Place thoroughly-dried slide on microscope stage, stain side up | | | |
| 6. Focus with low power (10X) objective | | | |
| 7. Scan slide to find area where cells are barely touching each other (in feathered edge of smear) | | | |
| 8. Place a drop of immersion oil on the slide | | | |

| You must: | S | U | Comments |
|---|---|---|---|
| 9. Rotate oil immersion lens carefully into position | | | |
| 10. Focus with fine adjustment knob only | | | |
| 11. Observe erythrocytes; color should be pinkish-tan | | | |
| 12. Observe leukocytes; nuclei should be purple | | | |
| 13. Observe platelets; they should appear purple and granular | | | |
| 14. Rotate 10X objective into position | | | |
| 15. Remove slide from microscope stage | | | |
| 16. Clean oil objective thoroughly with lens paper | | | |
| 17. Wipe oil from slide gently with soft tissue | | | |
| 18. Clean equipment and return to proper storage | | | |
| 19. Clean work area with surface disinfectant | | | |
| 20. Wash hands with hand disinfectant | | | |
| Comments: | | | |
| Student/Instructor: | | | |

Date: ______________________ Instructor: ______________________________

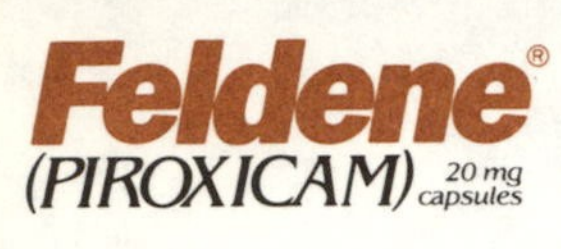
Feldene®
(PIROXICAM) 20 mg capsules

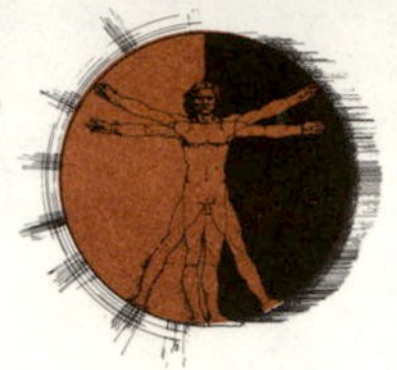

# LESSON 2–9

## Identification of Normal Blood Cells

### LESSON OBJECTIVES

After studying this lesson, you should be able to:

- State the importance of blood cell identification.
- List three features of cells which are evaluated in blood cell identification.
- Identify microscopically five types of leukocytes in normal blood.
- Identify platelets microscopically.
- Identify erythrocytes microscopically.
- List precautions to be observed in identifying cellular components of blood.
- Define the glossary terms.

### GLOSSARY

**band cell** / an immature neutrophil with a non-segmented nucleus; a stab cell

**basophil** / a leukocyte containing basophilic-staining granules

**basophilic** / blue in color; having affinity for the basic stain

**eosinophil** / an acid-staining leukocyte; numbers may increase in allergic reactions

**eosinophilic** / having affinity for the acid stain; reddish in color

**lymphocyte** / a small basophilic staining leukocyte having a round or oval nucleus and which is important in the immune process

**megakaryocyte** / a large bone marrow cell which releases platelets into the blood stream

**monocyte** / the largest of the leukocytes, usually has a convoluted nucleus

**neutrophil** / most numerous leukocyte, neutral staining; first line of defense against infection

**platelet** / thrombocyte; a small, disc-shaped fragment of cytoplasm from a megakaryocyte which plays an important role in blood coagulation

**vacuole** / a clear space in cytoplasm filled with fluid or air

## INTRODUCTION

Useful information can be gained from the microscopic identification and evaluation of blood cells from a stained smear. Many situations arise in medical practice in which the physician needs to know more concerning the blood cells than is provided by the cell counts alone. By microscopically viewing a blood smear, the technologist or physician can identify blood cells and evaluate any abnormalities present. Many hematologists say that more information is gained from a blood smear than from any other laboratory test.

The features of blood cells which must be observed and evaluated are: (1) cell size, (2) nuclear characteristics, and (3) cytoplasmic characteristics. The size of cells can be estimated by comparing them with red cells. The nucleus must be observed for shape, size, structure, and color. The cytoplasm is evaluated by noting the color, amount, and type of inclusions. When the information from these three observations is combined, the identification of most cells is possible. Beginners will find it necessary to consciously consider each of the properties of the cells. As experience is gained, the process becomes almost automatic for normal cells. Much practice is required to be able to recognize and classify the cells that may be seen in various disease states.

## BLOOD CELLS IN A NORMAL BLOOD SMEAR

The cells usually seen in a normal blood smear are described below. The descriptions are for cells as they would appear in Wright's stained smears. A leukocyte identification guide with abbreviated descriptions is given in Table 2–4, and Color Plates 1–10 depict typical appearances of stained cells.

### Erythrocytes

Red cells are the most numerous blood cells. Normal mature red cells stain pink-tan, have no nuclei, and are 6–8 micrometers in diameter. The pink-tan color is due to the staining of hemoglobin within the cells. Red cells are shaped like biconcave discs. Because they are thin in the center, the central area of the cell is paler than the margins.

### Platelets

**Platelets,** or thrombocytes, are the smallest of the stained blood elements. They are usually two to three micrometers in diameter, or one-third the diameter of a red cell. No nucleus is present because the platelet is simply a fragment of cytoplasm from a large bone marrow cell called a **megakaryocyte.** The cytoplasm stains bluish and usually contains small reddish-purple granules. Platelets may be round, oval, or have spiny projections.

### Leukocytes

The leukocytes are the largest of the normal blood components. Their sizes range from slightly larger than a red cell to more than twice the diameter of a red cell. Each of the five types of leukocytes has a characteristic appearance. The granular leukocytes—neutrophil, eosinophil, and basophil—contain many distinctive cytoplasmic granules, and may have segmented nuclei. The lymphocyte and monocyte have few, if any, easily visible cytoplasmic granules and have nonsegmented nuclei.

***Segmented neutrophil.*** Other names for the **neutrophil** are PMN (polymorphonuclear neutrophil)

**Table 2-4.** Leukocyte Identification Guide

| | Segmented Neutrophil | Neutrophilic Band (Stab) | Eosinophil | Basophil | Lymphocyte | Monocyte |
|---|---|---|---|---|---|---|
| | 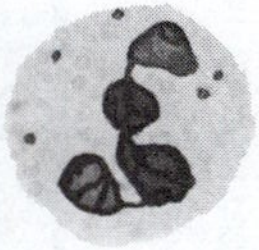 | 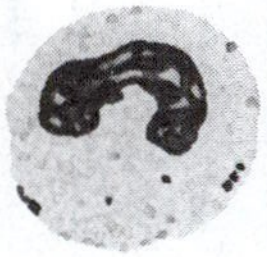 | 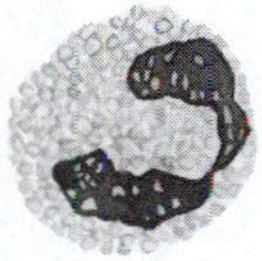 | 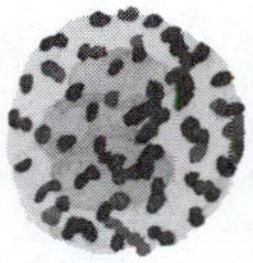 | 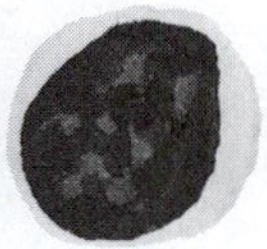 | 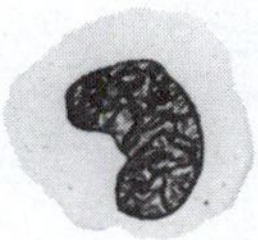 |
| **Cell Size** ($\mu$m) | 10–15 | 10–15 | 10–15 | 10–15 | 8–15 | 12–20 |
| **Nucleus** | | | | | | |
| *shape* | 2–5 lobes | sausage or U-shaped | bilobed | segmented | round, oval | horseshoe |
| *structure* | coarse | coarse | coarse | difficult to see | smudged (smoothly stained) | folded, convoluted |
| **Cytoplasm** | | | | | | |
| *amount* | abundant | abundant | abundant | abundant | scant | abundant |
| *color* | pink-tan | pink-tan | pink-tan | pink-tan | clear blue | opaque, blue-gray |
| *inclusions* | small, lilac granules | small, lilac granules | coarse, orange-red granules | coarse, blue-black granules | occasional red-purple granules | ground-glass appearance |

"poly," or "seg." The neutrophil nucleus is segmented into lobes, usually two to five, which are connected by a strand or filament. The nucleus stains a dark purple and has a coarse appearance. The cytoplasm is pale pink to tan and contains fine pink or lilac granules. The neutrophil is about twice the diameter of an erythrocyte and is the most numerous of the white cells in normal adult blood.

***Band or stab.*** The **band cell** is a younger (more immature) stage of the neutrophil. The staining characteristics are like the neutrophil, but the nucleus is not segmented.

***Eosinophil.*** The nucleus of the **eosinophil** is usually divided into two or three lobes and stains purple. The color of the cytoplasm is pink-tan but may be difficult to see because the cytoplasm is filled with large round or oval **eosinophilic** (red-orange) granules. Eosinophils are approximately the size of neutrophils but are much less numerous.

***Basophil.*** The nucleus of the **basophil** is segmented and stains light purple. However, the nuclear shape is often difficult to see. This is because numerous coarse blue-black granules often obscure the nucleus and cytoplasm. Basophils are seen only occasionally in normal smears.

***Lymphocyte.*** The smallest of the leukocytes are **lymphocytes.** Most lymphocytes are only slightly larger than an RBC. The nucleus is usually rather smooth, has a round or oval shape, and stains purple. The cytoplasm is **basophilic** or sky-blue and varies in amount. Occasionally, a few red-purple granules may be present in the cytoplasm.

***Monocyte.*** The **monocyte** is the largest circulating leukocyte. The nucleus may be oval, indented, or horseshoe-shaped and may have brain-like convolutions or folds. The cytoplasm is a dull gray-blue and may have an irregular outline. Very fine granules are distributed throughout the cytoplasm, giving the cytoplasm a ground-glass appearance. **Vacuoles** may be present. These appear as a clear space in the cytoplasm which is filled with fluid or air.

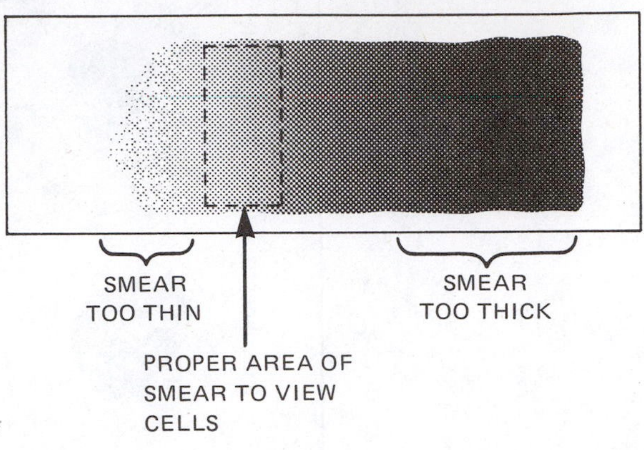


**Figure 2-43.** Proper area of slide to view

## METHOD OF OBSERVING A STAINED SMEAR

A well-prepared Wright's stained blood smear is used to learn cell identification. The smear should always be examined using immersion oil on the slide and the oil immersion objective. The light should be bright so that colors and small structures may be readily seen. The slide should be examined near the feathered edge of the smear. This is where the red cells are barely touching and do not overlap (Figure 2–43). In this area of the slide, the cells are easiest to identify because of their slightly flattened shape and large appearance.

### *Precautions*

- Oil immersion objective must be used for cell identification. If the field appears hazy, clean the objective and add an additional drop of oil to slide.

■ Cell identification may be difficult, inaccurate, or impossible with an improperly stained smear.

■ Much practice is required before cells can be identified with confidence.

## *LESSON REVIEW*

1. List three features of cells which must be considered before cell identification can be made.
2. Describe the appearance of a stained red blood cell.
3. What is the largest circulating leukocyte?
4. What is the stab or band cell?
5. Describe the appearance of a stained platelet.
6. What color granules are present in neutrophils—eosinophils—basophils?
7. What is the smallest leukocyte?
8. State the importance of blood cell identification.
9. What are the precautions to observe in identification of blood cells?
10. Define band cell, basophil, basophilic, eosinophil, eosinophilic, lymphocyte, megakaryocyte, monocyte, neutrophil, platelet, and vacuole.

## *STUDENT ACTIVITIES*

1. Re-read the information on blood cell identification.
2. Review the glossary terms.
3. Practice cell identification as outlined on the Student Performance Guide.
4. Practice identifying cells on additional stained smears or from unlabeled colored illustrations of cells.
5. Make simple drawings of each type of cell and label the parts.

# Student Performance Guide

NAME ______________________

DATE ______________________

## LESSON 2–9 IDENTIFICATION OF NORMAL BLOOD CELLS

### Instructions

1. Practice identifying erythrocytes, leukocytes, and platelets from a stained blood smear.
2. Identify erythrocytes, the five classes of leukocytes, and platelets satisfactorily for the instructor. All steps must be completed as listed on the instructor's Performance Check Sheet.
3. Complete a written examination successfully.

### Materials and Equipment

- hand disinfectant
- stained normal blood smear
- microscope
- lens paper
- immersion oil
- drawings (or photographs) and descriptions of stained blood cells
- soft laboratory tissue
- surface disinfectant

### Procedure

S = Satisfactory
U = Unsatisfactory

| You must: | S | U | Comments |
|---|---|---|---|
| 1. Wash hands with hand disinfectant | | | |
| 2. Assemble equipment and materials | | | |
| 3. Place stained smear on microscope stage and secure it with clips | | | |
| 4. Bring cells into focus using low power (10X) objective and coarse adjustment knob | | | |

| You must: | S | U | Comments |
|---|---|---|---|
| 5. Scan slide to find area of slide where cells are barely touching each other | | | |
| 6. Place one drop of immersion oil on slide | | | |
| 7. Rotate oil immersion objective carefully into position | | | |
| 8. Focus with fine adjustment knob until cells can be seen clearly | | | |
| 9. Raise the condenser and open the diaphragm to allow maximum light into objective | | | |
| 10. Scan slide to observe leukocytes | | | |
| 11. Study the smear until all five types of leukocytes have been identified correctly | | | |
| 12. Scan the slide to observe erythrocytes | | | |
| 13. Scan the slide to observe platelets | | | |
| 14. Rotate low power objective into position | | | |
| 15. Remove slide from microscope stage | | | |
| 16. Clean oil from objective thoroughly | | | |
| 17. Clean oil from slide gently | | | |
| 18. Repeat steps 3–17 with another stained smear | | | |
| 19. Wipe any oil from the microscope stage with soft laboratory tissue | | | |
| 20. Return equipment to proper storage | | | |
| 21. Clean work area with surface disinfectant | | | |
| 22. Wash hands with hand disinfectant | | | |

Comments:

Student/Instructor:

Date: ______________________ Instructor: ______________________

# LESSON 2–10

## Differential Leukocyte Count

### LESSON OBJECTIVES

After studying this lesson, you should be able to:

- List the normal values for a differential leukocyte count.
- Perform a differential leukocyte count.
- Report the results of a differential leukocyte count.
- Evaluate and report the morphology of the red cells.
- Evaluate platelets and estimate their numbers.
- List the precautions that should be observed when performing a differential leukocyte count.
- Define the glossary terms.

### GLOSSARY

**anisocytosis** / marked variation in the size of erythrocytes
**hypochromic** / having reduced color or hemoglobin content
**macrocytic** / having a larger than normal cell size
**microcytic** / having a smaller than normal cell size
**normochromic** / having normal color
**normocytic** / having a normal cell size and shape
**poikilocytosis** / significant variation in the shape of erythrocytes

### INTRODUCTION

The differential leukocyte count is part of a complete blood count. It is often referred to simply as a "diff." The purpose of the count is to obtain the percentage of each of the five types of leukocytes. The procedure involves counting either 100 or 200 white cells from a stained smear and recording each type observed. Afterwards, more information can be obtained from the same smear concerning the erythrocytes and platelets. The red cells can be evaluated for their morphology and hemoglobin content. The platelets can be evaluated for their morphology and an estimation can be made of the amount of platelets in circulation. Leukemias, anemias, and other diseases can often be diagnosed and monitored by the differential leukocyte count. For example, infectious mononucleosis produces a characteristic white cell differential and iron deficiency anemia produces small red cells with little hemoglobin.

## AREA OF THE SMEAR TO BE STUDIED

A specific area of the stained smear must be examined when doing the differential count and observing the red cells and platelets (Figure 2–44). The best area for observation is where the red cells are just touching but not overlapping when viewed microscopically. After a good observation area has been located using the low power objective (10X), the slide is scanned using the oil immersion objective (97X).

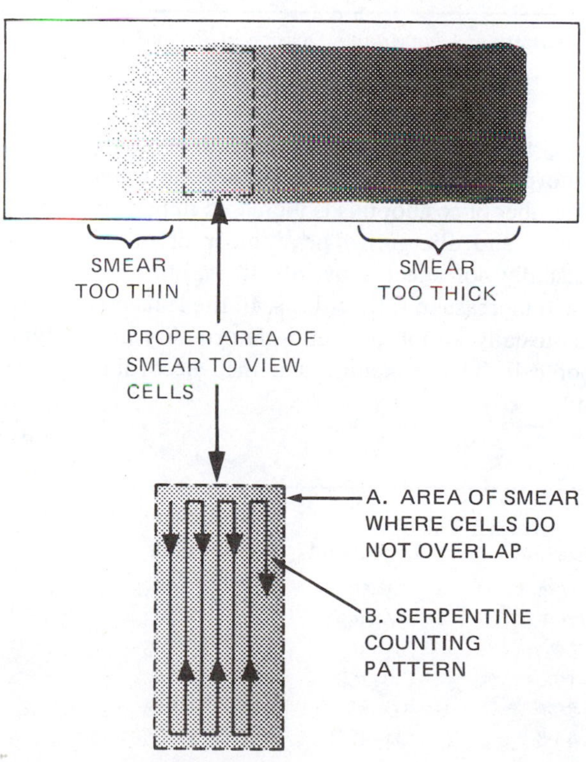


**Figure 2-44.** Proper area of slide to be viewed for differential count: A) closeup of proper area and B) counting pattern

## PERFORMING THE COUNT

When an area of the slide has been located in which the stain appears satisfactory and the cells are not crowded or distorted, 100 leukocytes are counted. A definite pattern, such as the one shown in Figure 2–44, must be followed to avoid counting the same cells twice. As the count is performed, a tally is kept of each type of white cell seen using a differential counter (Figure 2–45) or a tally counter. Any abnormalities of the cells are also noted.

After the leukocyte differential has been completed, the stained red cells and platelets are observed and evaluated. With some experience, the red cell size may be estimated as **normocytic** (normal size), **microcytic** (small), or **macrocytic** (large). The condition in which markedly different sized cells (red) are present in a smear is called **anisocytosis.** The hemoglobin content of the red cells can also be estimated. A red cell with the normal amount of hemoglobin is called **normochromic.** It stains evenly with only a small pale area in the center of the cell. A **hypochromic** red cell is one which has less than the normal amount of hemoglobin. It has only a ring of hemoglobin around the outer edge of the cell and a large pale area in the center. Normal red cells are round or slightly oval. The condition in which there is a significant variation in the shape of erythrocytes is called **poikilocytosis.** The platelets are also observed for any abnormalities in their morphology. At the same time, the average number of platelets seen in each oil immersion field is noted while examining ten to fifteen fields.

## NORMAL VALUES

The normal values of the differential count will vary with age. Normal values for adults and children are listed in Table 2–5. Children normally have a higher percentage of lymphocytes than adults.

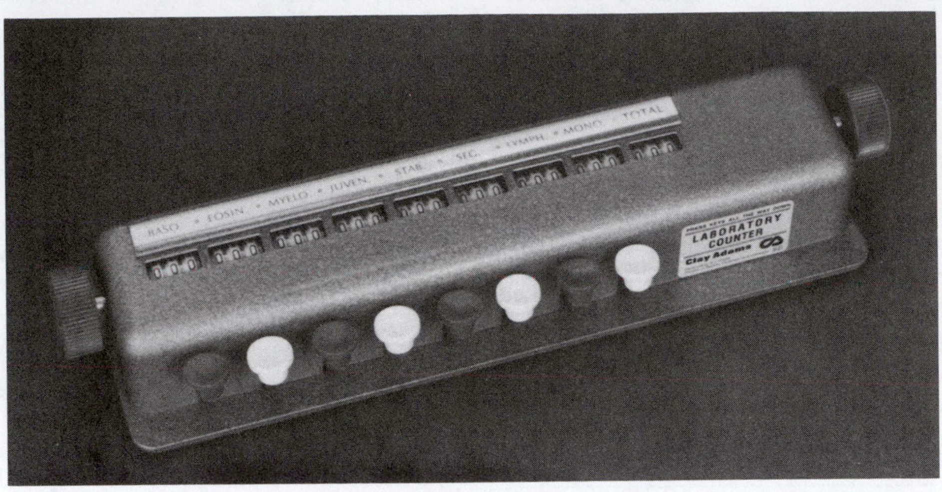


**Figure 2-45.** Differential counter (*Photo courtesy of Clay Adams Division of Becton Dickinson & Co.*)

## FACTORS AFFECTING THE DIFFERENTIAL LEUKOCYTE RATIOS

Many disease states can change the ratios of the different types of leukocytes. Bacterial infections usually cause an increase in the bands and segmented neutrophils. Viral infections can increase the number of lymphocytes and/or change their morphology, causing them to appear atypical. The number of eosinophils is increased in parasitic infections and allergies. The number of monocytes is usually not affected by infections, but occasionally will increase in tuberculosis. In the leukemias, there is usually an increase and abnormality in one type of cell. The leukemia is named according to the

**Table 2-5.** Normal Values for Differential Count

| Type of cell White cell | Normal Values | | | |
|---|---|---|---|---|
| | **1 month** | **six-year-old** | **12-year-old** | **adult** |
| neutrophil (seg) | 15–35% | 45–50% | 45–50% | 50–65% |
| neutrophil (band) | 7–13% | 0–7% | 6–8% | 0–7% |
| eosinophil | 1–3% | 1–3% | 1–3% | 1–3% |
| basophil | 0–1% | 0–1% | 0–1% | 0–1% |
| monocyte | 5–8% | 4–8% | 3–8% | 3–9% |
| lymphocyte | 40–70% | 40–45% | 35–40% | 25–40% |
| **Platelets** | An average of 5–15 platelets per oil immersion field is considered normal | | | |

predominant cell present. For example, an increased ratio of lymphocytes is found in the lymphocytic leukemias.

## FACTORS AFFECTING THE RED CELLS

Various diseases can affect the appearance of the stained red cells. Iron-deficiency anemia causes the red cells to be microcytic and hypochromic. Deficiencies of vitamins such as $B_{12}$ and folic acid cause the cells to be macrocytic.

## FACTORS AFFECTING THE PLATELETS

The platelets in the blood can be affected by several factors. In some leukemias, the number of platelets is below normal. Exposure to chemicals, radiation, or drugs used in cancer therapy can also cause a reduction of platelets. On the stained smear, the number may appear reduced if the platelets are clumped or have been pushed to the end of the smear.

## AUTOMATION

Automated instruments for differential leukocyte counts are used in many medical laboratories, especially those in larger hospitals. The instrument may operate on the principle of either enzyme staining characteristics or pattern recognition. In the enzyme staining method, 10,000 white cells are counted and differentiated in each sample. The pattern recognition method compares the morphology pattern of 100 to 200 white cells in the sample with hundreds of normal morphology patterns which are stored in the computer. Whichever method is used, a technologist must check all cells which have been designated as abnormal by the instrument.

### *Precautions*

- The condenser of the microscope should be raised until it is almost touching the bottom surface of the slide.
- The diaphragm of the microscope must be fully opened to allow maximum light.
- The differential count must be performed in a good area of the slide, following a definite pattern.
- The oil immersion objective should be rotated carefully into place to avoid touching the slide.
- The area being counted should be checked occasionally to insure that it is not near the edge of the smear where cells may be distorted.
- A more experienced technologist or a pathologist should be consulted if there is any difficulty in identifying cells.

## *LESSON REVIEW*

1. What is the purpose of the differential leukocyte count?
2. A differential is performed as a part of what hematological procedure?
3. What red cell information can be obtained from the smear?
4. Name some diseases which can be diagnosed or monitored by examining the smear.
5. What area of the smear should be used to perform the differential?
6. What method is used to avoid counting the same cells twice?
7. Which microscope objective is used to perform the differential?
8. What is the normal percentage of segmented neutrophils for an adult—for a child?
9. State the normal adult values for eosinophils, basophils, lymphocytes, and monocytes.

10. Bacterial infections usually increase the percentage of which cells?
11. What precautions should be observed when performing a differential leukocyte count?
12. Define anisocytosis, hypochromic, macrocytic, microcytic, normochromic, normocytic, and poikilocytosis.

## *STUDENT ACTIVITIES*

1. Re-read the information on the differential leukocyte count.
2. Review the glossary terms.
3. Practice performing a differential count as outlined on the Student Performance Guide, using the worksheet.
4. Perform differential counts on additional smears provided by the instructor.

# Student Performance Guide

NAME ______________________

DATE ______________________

## LESSON 2–10 DIFFERENTIAL LEUKOCYTE COUNT

### Instructions

1. Practice the procedure for performing the leukocyte differential count.
2. Demonstrate the procedure for performing the leukocyte differential count satisfactorily for the instructor. All steps must be completed as listed on the instructor's Performance Check Sheet.
3. Complete a written examination successfully.

### Materials and Equipment

- hand disinfectant
- microscope with oil immersion lens
- immersion oil
- lens paper
- soft tissue or soft paper towels
- stained blood smears
- differential report form
- blood atlas
- tally counter or differential counter
- worksheet
- surface disinfectant

**Procedure**

S = Satisfactory
U = Unsatisfactory

| You must: | S | U | Comments |
|---|---|---|---|
| 1. Wash hands with hand disinfectant | | | |
| 2. Assemble equipment and materials | | | |
| 3. Place stained blood smear on microscope stage and secure it with clips | | | |

| You must: | S | U | Comments |
|---|---|---|---|
| 4. Locate an area of the smear which is not near the edges and in which the red cells just touch, using the 10X objective | | | |
| 5. Place a drop of immersion oil on the area of the smear to be viewed | | | |
| 6. Rotate the oil immersion objective (97X) carefully into place | | | |
| 7. Insure that the area is one in which the stain is correct and the red cells just touch | | | |
| 8. Count 100 consecutive leukocytes moving the slide or mechanical stage so that consecutive microscopic fields are viewed. Use the counting pattern illustrated in Figure 2–44 | | | |
| 9. Record on worksheet how many of each type of leukocyte are seen and note any abnormalities | | | |
| 10. Observe the red cells in at least ten fields:<br>a. Note the hemoglobin content; record as normochromic or hypochromic | | | |
| b. Note the red cell size; record as normocytic, microcytic, or macrocytic. An approximation of the number of cells affected may be recorded using a plus system (1+ to 4+) or using terms such as small, moderate, large | | | |
| 11. Observe platelets in at least ten fields:<br>a. Note morphology | | | |
| b. Estimate the number per oil immersion field; record as normal, decreased, or increased | | | |
| 12. Rotate low power (10X) objective into position | | | |
| 13. Remove slide from microscope stage | | | |
| 14. Clean oil immersion objective thoroughly | | | |
| 15. Check microscope stage and condenser for oil and clean if necessary | | | |
| 16. Blot smear gently with lens paper or soft tissue | | | |

| You must: | S | U | Comments |
|---|---|---|---|
| 17. Clean equipment and return to proper storage | | | |
| 18. Wash hands with hand disinfectant | | | |
| Comments:<br><br>Student/Instructor: | | | |

Date: ______________________ Instructor: ______________________

# Worksheet

NAME ______________________________ DATE ____________

SPECIMEN NO. ____________

## LESSON 2–10
## DIFFERENTIAL LEUKOCYTE COUNT

| | | Normal Values (Adult) |
|---|---|---|
| Segmented Neutrophils | _____% | 50–65% |
| Lymphocytes | _____% | 25–40% |
| Monocytes | _____% | 3–9% |
| Eosinophils | _____% | 1–3% |
| Basophils | _____% | 0–1% |
| Bands | _____% | 0–7% |

Other ____________________

Platelet Estimate:

- □ appear adequate 5–15/oil immersion field
- □ appear decreased <4/oil immersion field
- □ appear increased >16/oil immersion field

RBC Morphology:

| | | Normal |
|---|---|---|
| Cell size: | □ normocytic<br>□ microcytic<br>□ macrocytic | normocytic (6–8 micrometers) |
| Cell color: | □ normochromic<br>□ hypochromic | normochromic |

Comments: ______________________________

______________________________

# UNIT 3
# Advanced Hematology

## UNIT OBJECTIVES

After studying this unit, you should be able to:

- Perform a venipuncture.
- Perform an erythrocyte sedimentation rate test.
- Perform a reticulocyte count.
- Perform a platelet count.
- Use a spectrophotometer.
- Measure the hemoglobin concentration of a blood sample.
- Calculate erythrocyte indices.
- Perform a capillary coagulation test.
- Perform a bleeding time test.

## OVERVIEW

The hematology procedures in this unit are ones which, for the most part, are not considered routine. These procedures give the physician additional information beyond that provided by the procedures in Unit 2. The lessons in this unit are generally ones which take more technical skill. They also require the worker to use judgement and to make use of principles learned earlier.

Venipuncture is presented as another method of obtaining a blood sample. This method is used routinely when the blood sample required is too large to be obtained by capillary puncture. Venipuncture also takes more skill than a capillary puncture. Since veins are used to administer drugs or other treatment, care must be taken not to damage the veins. An improperly performed venipuncture could have serious consequences for the patient. However, a properly performed venipuncture is a safe, convenient means of obtaining a blood sample.

The erythrocyte sedimentation rate (sed rate) is not considered a part of routine hematology. The results of the procedure can be used with other laboratory results to aid the physician in diagnosis. The sed rate is also used to follow the progress of some inflammatory disease processes.

The reticulocyte count tells the physician if the patient is producing a sufficient number of new red blood cells; the test is not routinely ordered. The results can be used to evaluate the treatment and progress of anemia patients.

The platelet count is frequently requested. It is included in advanced hematology because of technical difficulties in counting platelets. Since platelets are very small, any dirt or debris present in the sample could be confused with platelets. For this reason, all equipment and reagents must be very clean.

The measurement of hemoglobin by the cyanmethemoglobin method is considered a routine procedure. It is the method recommended and approved for clinical laboratories. The procedure requires a spectrophotometer. The two lessons are included in this unit because a spectrophotometer may not be available in all classrooms.

The calculation of the erythrocyte indices uses the red blood cell count, the hemoglobin value and the hematocrit. The physician can use these indices values to classify anemias and to evaluate anemia treatment.

The bleeding time test and the capillary coagulation test are not routinely done either. Both are screening procedures which can detect blood clotting disorders but are not specific for any certain one. They are presented as an introduction to the principles involved in hemostasis, the blood clotting process.

With the completion of units 2 and 3 many of the hematology procedures performed in medical laboratories will have been covered. However, these are actually only a few of a large number of tests available and are meant as illustrations of some basic laboratory principles.

The spectrophotometer, the hemoglobin, and the indices lessons should be studied in the order in which they appear. The remainder of the lessons in the unit are independent of each other.

# LESSON 3-1

## Venipuncture

## LESSON OBJECTIVES

After studying the lesson, you should be able to:

- Explain the venipuncture procedure to a patient.
- Select the equipment necessary to perform a venipuncture.
- Apply a tourniquet.
- Select a proper venipuncture site.
- Prepare a venipuncture site.
- Perform a venipuncture.
- Care for a puncture site after venipuncture.
- List the precautions to be observed when performing a venipuncture.
- Explain the use of vacuum tubes.
- Name three common anticoagulants and state when they are used.
- Define the glossary terms.

## GLOSSARY

**artery** / a blood vessel that carries oxygenated blood from the heart to the tissues

**gauge** / a measure of the diameter of a needle

**hematoma** / the swelling of tissue around a vessel due to leakage of the blood into the tissue

**hypodermic needle** / a hollow needle used for injections or for obtaining fluid specimens

**lumen** / the open space within a tubular organ or tissue

**median cephalic vein** / a vein located in the bend of the elbow and frequently used for venipuncture

**phlebotomy** / venipuncture; entry of a vein with a needle

**syringe** / a hollow, tube-like container with a plunger, used for injecting or withdrawing fluids

**tourniquet** / a band used to constrict the blood flow in the vein from which blood is to be drawn

**vein** / a blood vessel that carries deoxygenated blood to the heart
**venipuncture** / entry of a vein with a needle; a phlebotomy

## INTRODUCTION

The most common method of obtaining blood for laboratory examination is by venipuncture. In a **venipuncture,** sometimes called a **phlebotomy,** the blood is taken directly from a superficial **vein.** The vein is punctured with a needle and blood is collected in a syringe or tube. The venipuncture is a quick way to obtain a large sample of blood from which many different analyses can be made.

The venipuncture is a safe procedure when performed correctly by a skilled worker. The procedure should be performed with care. Every effort should be made to preserve the condition of the vein. Much observation and practice is required to become skilled and self-confident in the art of venipuncture.

## VENIPUNCTURE BY SYRINGE METHOD

Performing a venipuncture with a syringe involves several important steps. It is necessary that these steps be thoroughly understood before the procedure is attempted. The steps are (1) selecting proper

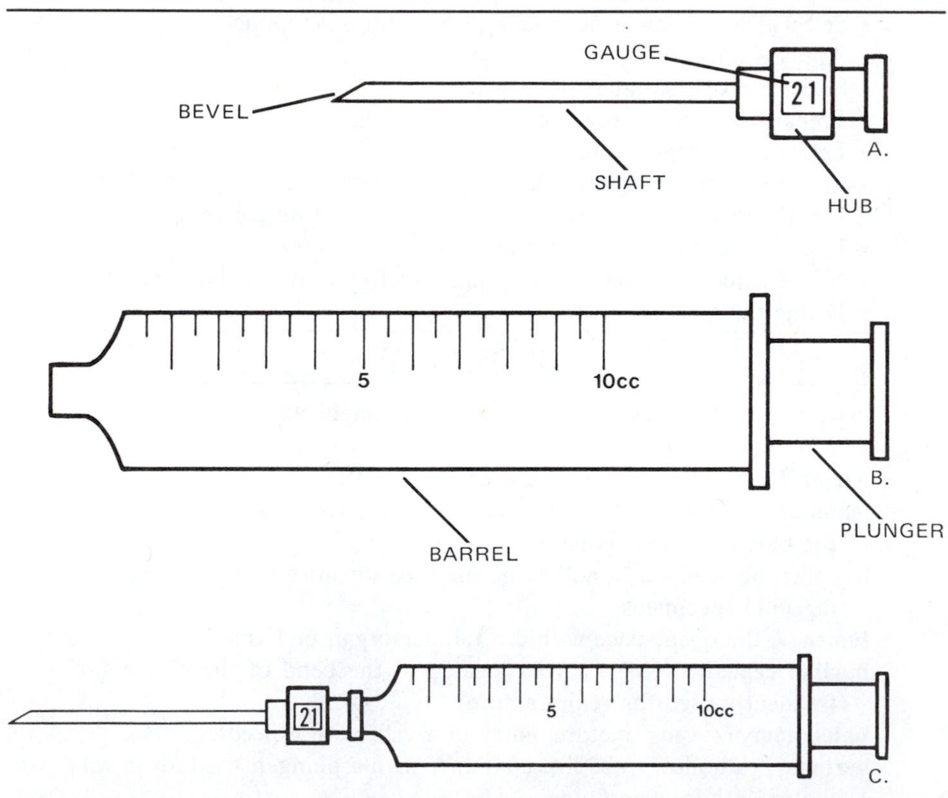


**Figure 3-1.** Materials for venipuncture: A) Hypodermic needle, B) syringe, and C) syringe and needle assembled

equipment, (2) preparing the patient for venipuncture, (3) applying the tourniquet, (4) preparing the puncture site, (5) obtaining the blood, and (6) care of the puncture site. When performing a venipuncture, the student must be supervised by a qualified instructor.

## Selecting the Equipment

The equipment required for venipuncture by syringe includes a sterile **syringe** and **hypodermic needle** (Figure 3–1), 70% alcohol, sterile gauze, tourniquet, and a blood collecting tube. Most laboratories use disposable syringes and needles. To maintain sterility, the syringe and needle should be assembled carefully. The tip of the syringe or the needle must not be touched. The needle should remain capped until ready to use. Needles of 20 to 22 **gauge** are usually used for venipuncture. (The higher the gauge, the smaller the needle.) The plunger of the syringe should be pushed up and down to see that it moves freely. It should then be left pushed completely into the barrel so that no air remains in the syringe. The needle should be positioned firmly on the syringe so that the bevel and the graduations of the syringe face in the same direction. The needle should be inspected carefully to see that the point is sharp and smooth. The needle should then be capped until used. All materials should be placed within easy reach of the venipuncturist.

## Preparation of Patient

The venipuncturist should always identify the patient by name and by checking the laboratory request form. If the patient is hospitalized, patient identification wristband should be checked. The procedure should be explained to the patient to minimize apprehension. The patient should be lying down or seated in a chair—not standing or sitting on a high stool. The venipuncturist should always be prepared for the occasional patient who may faint and should be trained to administer current first aid techniques should this occur. The patient's arm needs to be fully extended and firmly supported during the venipuncture procedure.

## Application of Tourniquet

A **tourniquet** is applied to the arm to slow the blood flow and make the veins more prominent. A small piece of rubber tubing may be used for this purpose. The tourniquet must be applied correctly. To do so, the tourniquet is placed under the arm above the elbow and the two ends are stretched and crossed over the top of the arm. While maintaining tension on the ends, one side should be looped and pulled halfway through in a slipknot (Figure 3–2). If the tourniquet is tied in this manner, it will release easily with a gentle pull on one end (Figure 3–3). The tourniquet should be applied to select the puncture site. It should then be released while the site is cleansed, and retied before the puncture is performed. *The tourniquet is always released before the needle is withdrawn from the vein* after the puncture has been completed. A tourniquet should never be tied tight enough to restrict blood flow in the **artery.** Neither should the tourniquet be left in place more than two minutes.

## Selection of Puncture Site

The puncture site should be carefully selected after inspecting both arms to locate the best vein. The vein most frequently used is the **median cephalic vein** of the forearm (Figure 3–4). The fingertips should be used to gently press on the veins to determine the direction of the vein and to estimate the size and depth of the vein (Figure 3–5). The vein will feel like an elastic tube.

## Preparation of the Puncture Site

The area around the puncture site should be cleansed thoroughly with 70% alcohol and a sterile gauze. The site may then be dried using dry sterile gauze, or it may be allowed to air dry. Once the site is cleansed, it should not be touched again except to enter the vein with the needle.

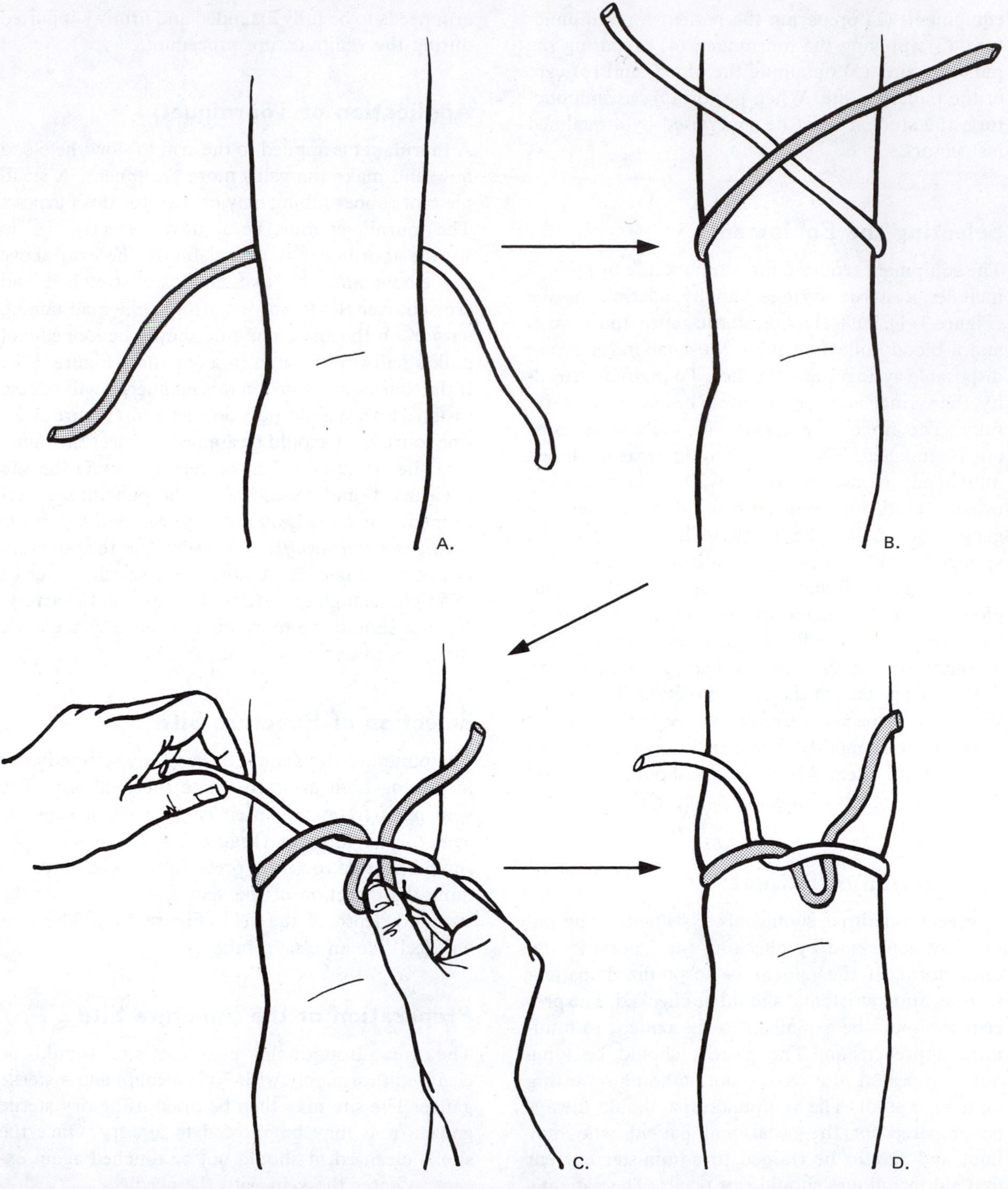


**Figure 3-2.** Tying a tourniquet

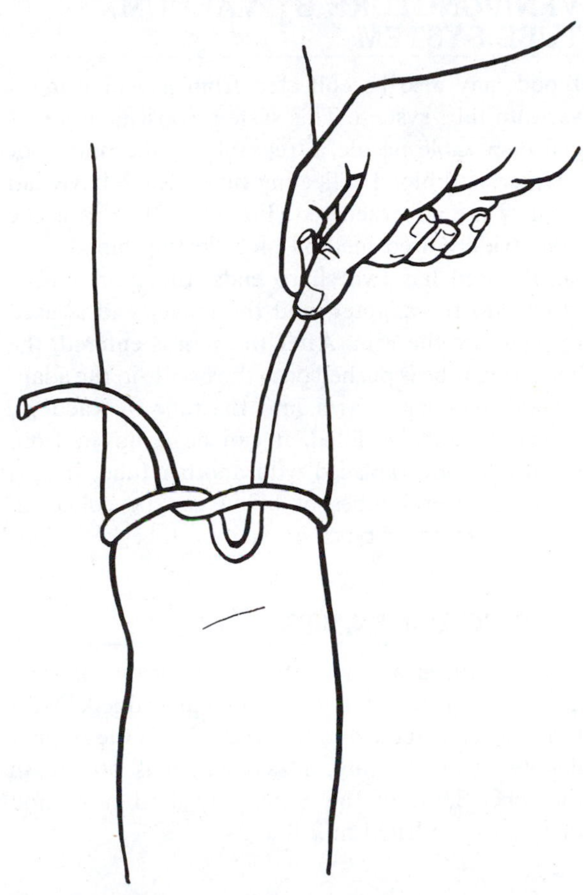

**Figure 3-3.** Releasing the tourniquet

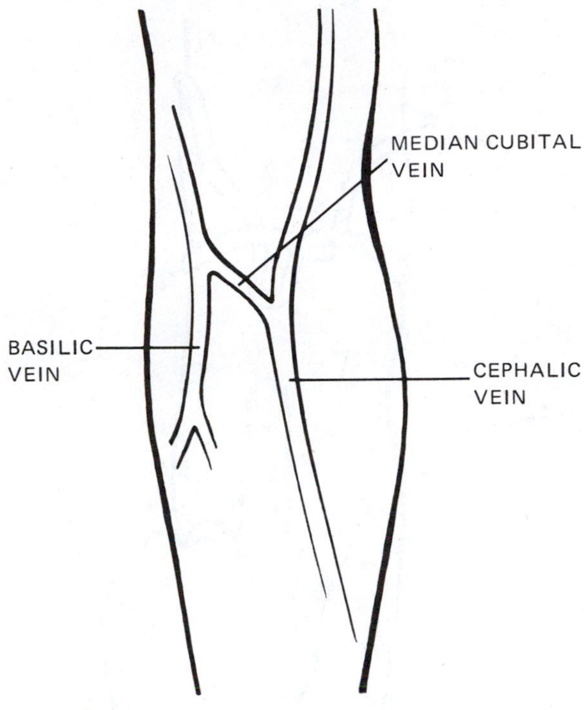


**Figure 3-4.** Veins most commonly used for venipuncture (left arm)

## Performing the Puncture

When the puncture site has been cleansed, the tourniquet should be reapplied to the arm, being careful not to touch the cleansed area. The syringe should be held in one hand at a 15–30° angle to the arm. The bevel should be up, and the needle should point in the same direction as the vein. Penetrating the vein at the proper angle will prevent penetrating both blood vessel walls. (The thumb may be placed about one inch below the point of entry, and the skin pressed and pulled toward the venipuncturist, to anchor the vein and lessen the pull of the needle on the skin.) The skin and vein should be entered in one smooth motion until the needle is in the **lumen** of the vein (Figure 3–6). The syringe and needle should then be held motionless while the plunger is gently pulled back with the other hand to draw blood into the syringe. The needle should be observed while the syringe is filling to be sure it is not pulled out of the vein. When the proper amount of blood has been obtained, the tourniquet should be released. The needle can then be withdrawn from the vein while gauze is placed over the puncture site (Figure 3–7). The needle should be capped, carefully removed from the syringe, and properly discarded. The blood should then be transferred to the appropriate blood collecting tube. The

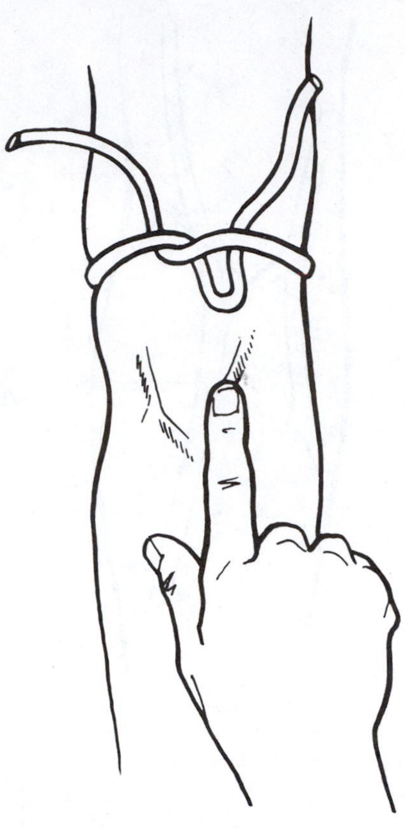

**Figure 3-5.** Palpating a vein with fingertip

tube should be labeled with the patient's name, identification number, date, time of collection, and initials of the venipuncturist.

### Care of the Puncture Site

The patient should be instructed to press the gauze on the puncture site for two to five minutes with arm extended to insure that bleeding stops and that a swelling of tissue, or a **hematoma,** does not form. The venipuncturist should check the site to see that it has stopped bleeding before leaving the patient and should apply a bandage if necessary.

## VENIPUNCTURE BY VACUUM TUBE SYSTEM

Blood may also be collected from a vein using a vacuum tube system. This system consists of a special disposable needle, a reusable needle holder or adapter, and blood collecting tubes which have had most of the air evacuated (Figure 3–8). This is the most widely used method of collecting blood. The needle used has two sharp ends; the short end is fitted into the adapter, and the longer end is used to puncture the vein. After the vein is entered, the collecting tube is pushed onto the needle in the adapter and blood is drawn into the tube by vacuum. When the tube is filled, it can be removed from the needle and replaced with another tube. In this manner, several tubes of blood can be collected, using a variety of types of vacuum tubes.

## ANTICOAGULANTS

Vacuum tubes are available in a variety of sizes and with or without anticoagulants added. Most tubes are color-coded so that the color of the stopper denotes which, if any, anticoagulant is present in the tube. Some of the commonly used tubes and their uses are listed in Table 3–1.

### *Precautions*

- Students should only perform a venipuncture under the supervision of a qualified instructor.
- Be sure that the patient is lying down or sitting with the arm firmly supported. Be prepared for the patient who might faint.
- Do not allow the tourniquet to remain in place for more than two minutes.
- Check the pulse to be sure that arterial circulation is not hindered.
- Before performing the puncture, push the plunger all the way to the bottom of the syringe barrel to expel all air from the syringe.

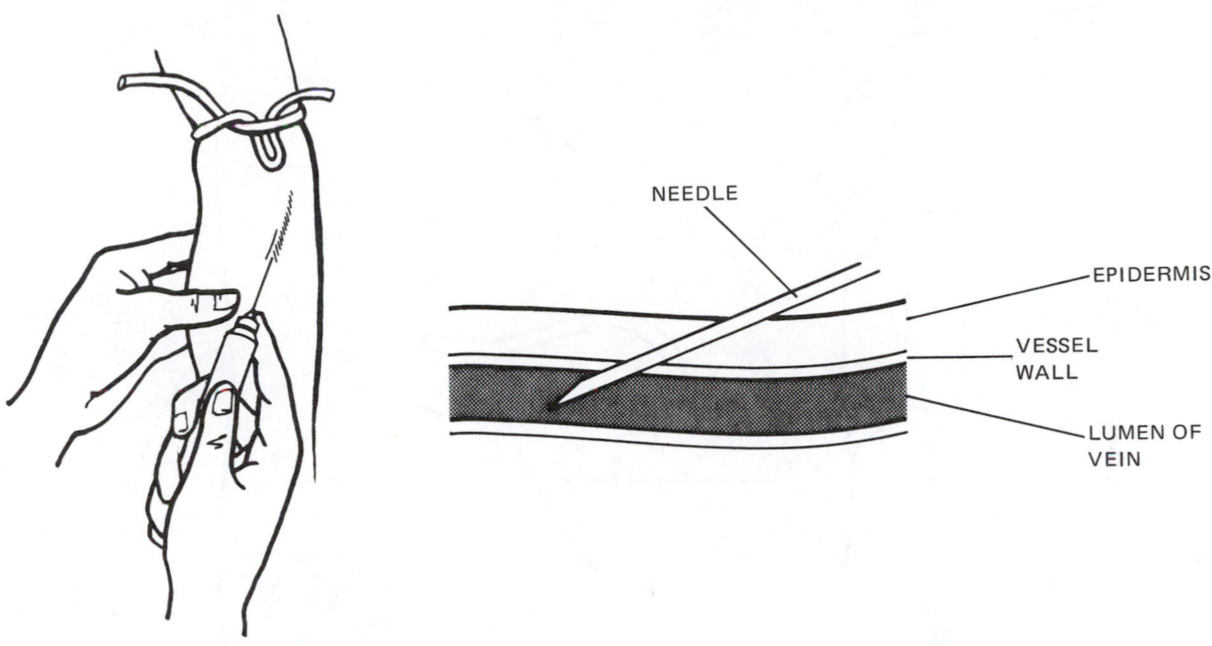


**Figure 3-6.** Performing the puncture

■ Always remove the tourniquet before taking the needle out of the vein to prevent the formation of a hematoma.

■ If difficulty is encountered when entering the vein or if a hematoma or swelling begins to form, release the tourniquet immediately, quickly withdraw the needle, and apply pressure to the wound with gauze.

■ Do not reuse needles or syringes; this prevents possible transmission of disease.

■ Do not throw used needles in a wastebasket; needles should be placed in a special container to avoid the possibility of injury to other workers.

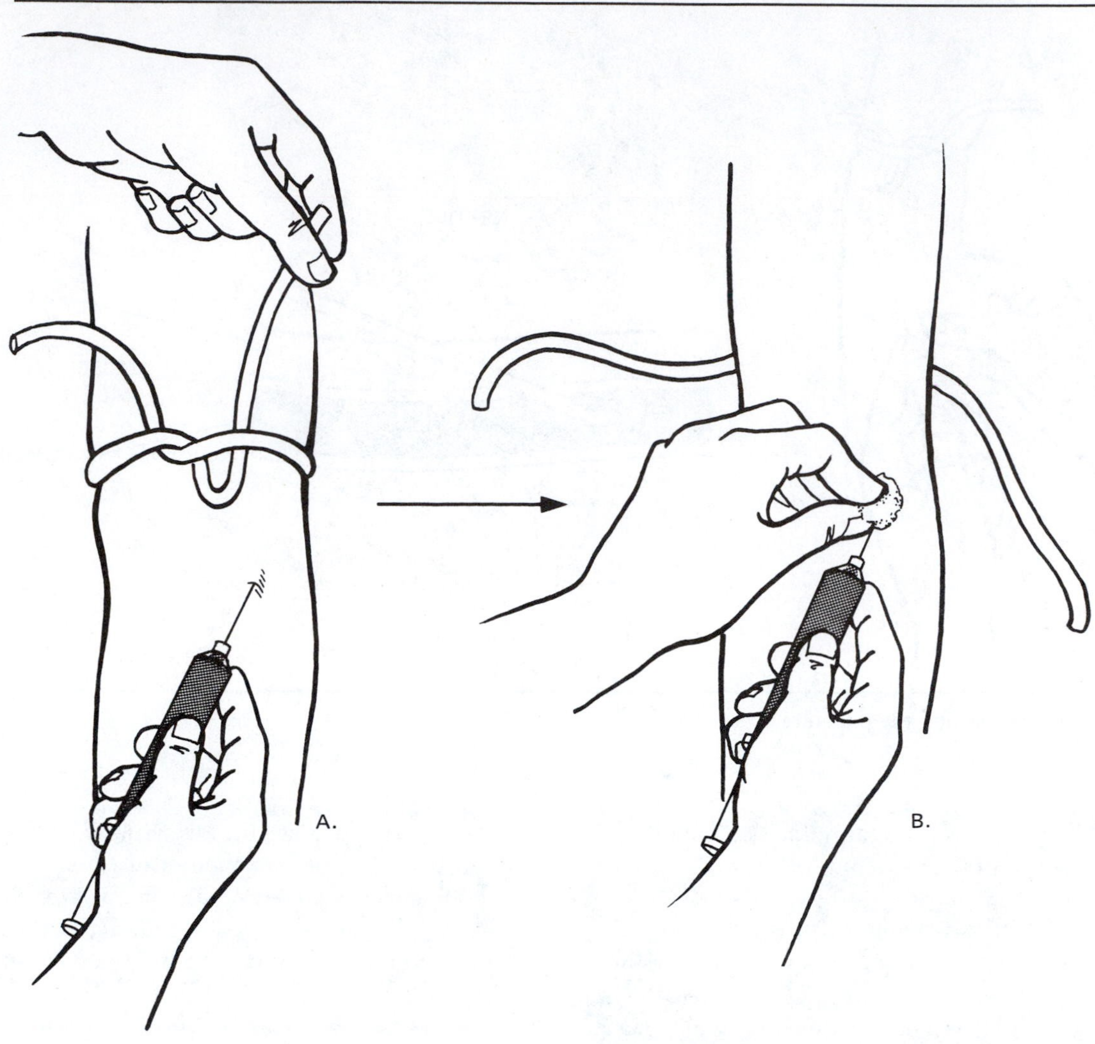


**Figure 3-7.** Withdrawing needle from puncture. A) remove tourniquet, B) withdraw needle and C) apply pressure with sterile cotton

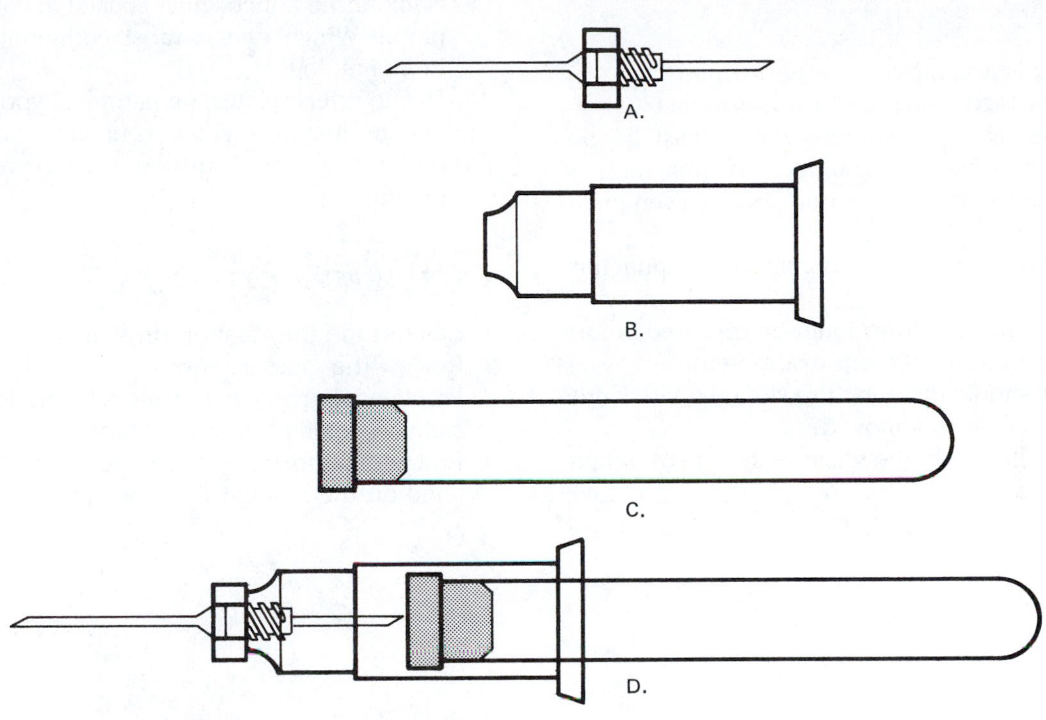


**Figure 3-8.** Vacuum tube blood collecting system. A) needle, B) holder, C), vacuum tube C), and D) assembled unit

**Table 3-1.** Vacuum Tubes: Stopper Colors, Additives, and Uses

| Stopper Color | Anticoagulant in Tube | Uses of Tube |
|---|---|---|
| red | none | used so that blood will clot and serum may be obtained |
| purple | EDTA | used for most hematology studies, examination of blood smears |
| green | heparin | cannot be used for stained smears; used for other tests which require whole blood |
| blue | sodium citrate | used for coagulation studies |

## LESSON REVIEW

1. Why is a venipuncture performed?
2. What is the purpose of a tourniquet?
3. Name five precautions which must be observed when performing a venipuncture.
4. What are the steps in performing a venipuncture?
5. Where is the most common venipuncture site?
6. Why must the tourniquet be removed before taking the needle out of the vein?
7. How should the puncture site be treated after the needle is removed?
8. Explain briefly the vacuum system of obtaining venous blood.
9. Name three anticoagulants used in collecting blood. Which one is most commonly used in hematology?
10. Define artery, gauge, hematoma, hypodermic needle, lumen, median cephalic vein, phlebotomy, syringe, tourniquet, vein, and venipuncture.

## STUDENT ACTIVITIES

1. Re-read the information on venipuncture.
2. Review the glossary terms.
3. Practice applying a tourniquet and locating suitable veins for venipuncture.
4. Practice performing a venipuncture as outlined on the Student Performance Guide.

# Student Performance Guide

NAME ______________________________

DATE ______________________________

## LESSON 3–1 VENIPUNCTURE

### Instructions

1. Practice performing a venipuncture.
2. Demonstrate the procedure for performing a venipuncture satisfactorily for the instructor. All steps must be completed as listed on the instructor's Performance Check Sheet.
3. Complete a written examination successfully.

### Materials and Equipment

- hand disinfectant
- tourniquet
- sterile gauze or cotton
- 70% alcohol
- sterile disposable hypodermic needle, 20–22 gauge
- sterile syringe
- collection tubes
- container for needle disposal
- surface disinfectant
- biohazard container

**Procedure**

S = Satisfactory
U = Unsatisfactory

| You must: | S | U | Comments |
|---|---|---|---|
| 1. Wash hands with hand disinfectant | | | |
| 2. Assemble equipment and materials | | | |
| 3. Place venipuncture equipment and clean gauze within easy reach | | | |
| 4. Identify patient properly | | | |
| 5. Explain venipuncture procedure to patient and position patient properly | | | |

| You must: | S | U | Comments |
|---|---|---|---|
| 6. Obtain a sterile syringe and capped needle | | | |
| 7. Attach the sterile capped needle to the sterile syringe, maintaining sterility (if packed separately) | | | |
| 8. Remove cap and position needle so that the bevel faces in the same direction as the graduations on the syringe | | | |
| 9. Inspect the needle to see that the point is smooth and sharp | | | |
| 10. Slide the plunger up and down in the barrel of the syringe to be sure that it moves freely | | | |
| 11. Push the plunger to the bottom of the barrel so that no air remains in the syringe | | | |
| 12. Place the tourniquet around the patient's arm above the elbow; it should be just tight enough so that the venous circulation is restricted, but not so tight that the arterial circulation is stopped. CAUTION: Do not allow the tourniquet to remain in place for more than two minutes | | | |
| 13. Instruct the patient to open and close the fist a few times in order to increase circulation and to make the veins more noticeable | | | |
| 14. Inspect the bend of the elbow to locate a suitable vein | | | |
| 15. Palpate the vein with the finger tip(s) to determine the direction of the vein, and to estimate its size and depth. *Note:* The vein most frequently used is the median cephalic vein of the forearm | | | |
| 16. Release the tourniquet | | | |
| 17. Cleanse the skin of the puncture site using an alcohol-soaked gauze | | | |
| 18. Allow alcohol to dry | | | |
| 19. Retie the tourniquet, being careful not to touch the sterile puncture site | | | |
| 20. Instruct the patient to straighten the arm and make a fist | | | |
| 21. Hold the syringe in the right hand and be sure that the graduations on the syringe and the bevel of the needle | | | |

| You must: | S | U | Comments |
|---|---|---|---|
| are in full view (facing toward ceiling). With thumb of other hand, hold skin taut | | | |
| 22. Hold the needle at a 30° angle to the arm and insert the needle into the vein. Watch for blood flow into the syringe | | | |
| 23. Instruct the patient to open the fist as soon as the vein has been entered | | | |
| 24. Pull the plunger back slowly with the left hand to withdraw the blood while steadying the syringe and needle with the right hand | | | |
| 25. Release the tourniquet when the desired amount of blood is obtained | | | |
| 26. Place a dry, sterile gauze over the puncture site and withdraw the needle from the vein (do not press down on the needle) | | | |
| 27. Instruct the patient to press the sterile gauze over the wound for three to five minutes with the arm extended | | | |
| 28. Remove the needle from the syringe | | | |
| 29. Fill the collecting tube with blood from the syringe and label the tube properly | | | |
| 30. Discard carefully the used needle and syringe as instructed by the teacher | | | |
| 31. Check patient to be sure that bleeding has stopped; apply bandage if necessary | | | |
| 32. Clean and return equipment to storage | | | |
| 33. Clean work area with surface disinfectant | | | |
| 34. Wash hands with hand disinfectant | | | |

Comments:

Student/Instructor:

Date: ______________________ Instructor: ______________________

# LESSON 3–2

## Erythrocyte Sedimentation Rate

## LESSON OBJECTIVES

After studying this lesson, you should be able to:

- List four properties of blood which affect the erythrocyte sedimentation rate and explain how the rate is affected by each factor.
- Perform a test to measure the erythrocyte sedimentation rate.
- State the normal values for the erythrocyte sedimentation rate.
- List technical factors which may affect the erythrocyte sedimentation rate.
- Define the glossary terms.

## GLOSSARY

**aggregate** / total substances making up a mass; a clustering of particles
**inflammation** / a tissue reaction to injury
**rouleau(x)** / a group of red cells arranged like a roll of coins
**sedimentation** / the process of solid particles settling at the bottom of a liquid
**Wintrobe tube** / a slender thick-walled tube marked from 0–100 mm; used in Wintrobe method of macrohematocrit and erythrocyte sedimentation rate

## INTRODUCTION

The erythrocyte sedimentation rate (ESR) is a simple, frequently performed hematology test. The test is not specific for a particular disease but is used as a general indication of **inflammation** or to follow the course of inflammatory disease.

In a sample of anticoagulated whole blood, the erythrocytes will gradually separate from the plasma and settle to the bottom of the container. The rate at which the erythrocytes fall is known as the erythrocyte sedimentation rate. In the blood of most healthy persons, **sedimentation** takes place slowly. In many diseases, however, the rate is rapid. In some cases, the rate is proportional to the severity of the disease. Measurement of the ESR may be helpful in confirming or following the course of certain diseases.

## WINTROBE METHOD OF MEASURING THE ESR

The Wintrobe method is a common method of measuring the ESR. A **Wintrobe tube** graduated from 0–100 millimeters and with a capacity of one milliliter of blood is used for this method (Figure 3–9). A special rack which holds the tube vertically is also required (Figure 3–10). The sample tested is venous blood with the anticoagulant, EDTA, added.

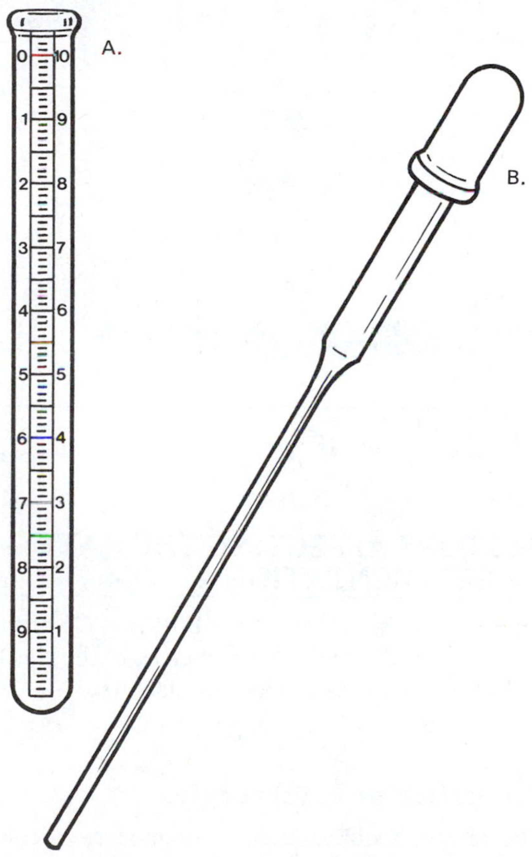


**Figure 3-9.** Materials for erythrocyte sedimentation rate. A) Wintrobe sedimentation tube and B) long-stemmed Pasteur-type pipet used for filling Wintrobe tube

**Table 3-2.** Normal Values for Wintrobe Method of Erythrocyte Sedimentation Rate

| Age/Sex | Normal rate |
|---|---|
| Males | 0–9 mm/hour |
| Females | 0–20 mm/hour |
| Children | 0–13 mm/hour |

A long-tipped Pasteur pipet is used to fill the Wintrobe tube to the zero mark with blood (Figure 3–11). The tube is then placed in the sedimentation rack for one hour. At the end of the hour, the total distance which the erythrocytes have fallen is measured. The rate is recorded in mm/hour (Figure 3–12).

## NORMAL VALUES FOR THE WINTROBE METHOD

Normal values for the ESR vary slightly with age and sex (Table 3–2). Only increased rates are significant. Children usually have a lower ESR than middle-aged adults. Elderly people tend to have a higher ESR. Females have a higher rate than males.

## OTHER METHODS OF MEASURING THE ESR

Other methods of measuring the erythrocyte sedimentation rate are Westergren and Landau-Adams. These methods are based on the same principle as the Wintrobe method but they differ in the amount of sample needed and the size and design of the tubes used for the tests. Each method has its own set of normal values. Therefore, it is necessary to

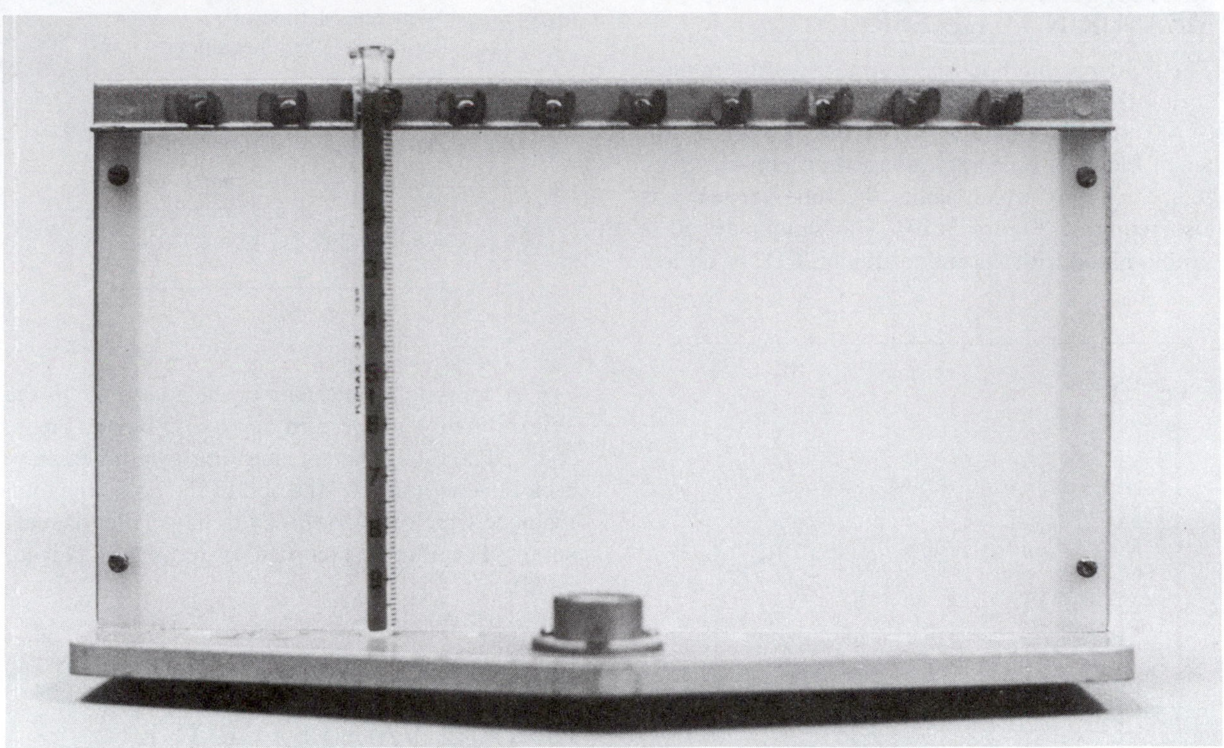

**Figure 3-10.** Wintrobe tube in sedimentation rack (*Photo by John Estridge*)

follow instructions which are specific to each method used.

## RELATIONSHIP OF ESR TO DISEASE

Conditions in which the erythrocyte sedimentation rate is increased include tuberculosis, acute and chronic infections, acute viral hepatitis, cancer, multiple myeloma, lupus erythematosus, and inflammatory processes such as rheumatic fever and rheumatoid arthritis. Pregnant females also have an increased ESR. In polycythemia and sickle cell anemia, the ESR is low or zero.

## FACTORS AFFECTING THE RATE OF SEDIMENTATION

Three factors which affect the ESR are: (1) properties of the erythrocytes, (2) properties of the plasma, and (3) mechanical or technical factors.

### Properties of Erythrocytes

The rate of sedimentation is affected by the size, shape, and number of erythrocytes. In normal blood, erythrocytes suspended in the plasma form few, if any, **aggregates.** The mass of the falling erythrocytes is small and the ESR tends to be low. In abnormal blood, the erythrocytes sometimes aggre-

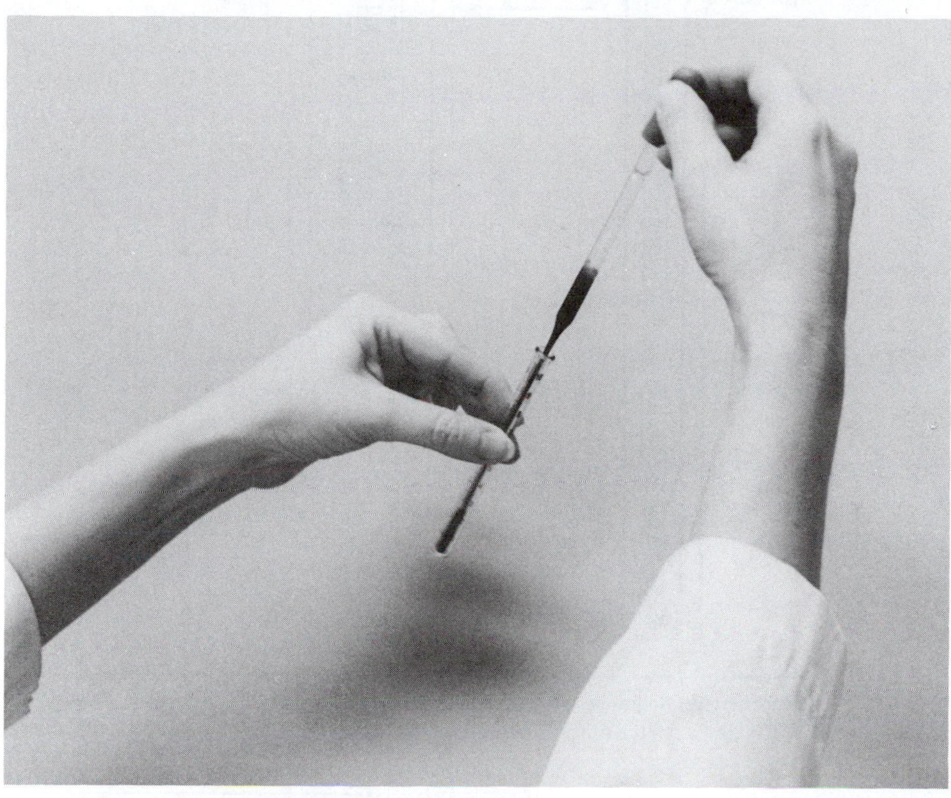

**Figure 3-11.** Filling a Wintrobe sedimentation tube (*Photo by John Estridge*)

gate to form what is called **rouleau.** This phenomenon is called rouleau because the cells form aggregates that look like rolls or stacks of coins (Figure 3–13). This causes an increase in the mass and an increased rate of sedimentation. Changes in the shape of the erythrocytes can also affect the ESR. For example, in sickle cell anemia the irregularly-shaped erythrocytes cannot form rouleaux and the ESR may be slow. The sedimentation rate may be rapid in anemia because there are fewer erythrocytes to interfere with settling. When erythrocytes are increased, as in polycythemia, the erythrocytes settle slowly.

### Properties of the Plasma

The amount and type of plasma proteins present in a blood sample may affect the ESR. If protein levels are elevated, the sedimentation rate may be increased.

### Mechanical or Technical Factors

Mechanical and technical factors such as temperature, time, size of tube, and tilting or vibration of tube during incubation will affect the sedimentation

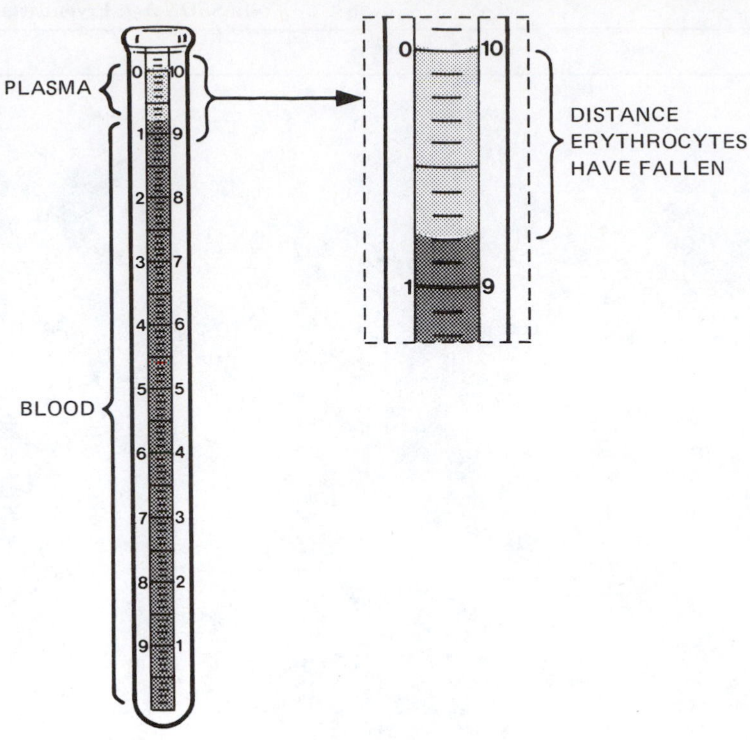


**Figure 3-12.** Sedimentation tube showing settling of cells. Example shown illustrates a sedimentation of 8 mm.

rate. The points listed below should be heeded if the test results are to be correct:

1. The sedimentation tube must be kept exactly vertical; even minor degrees of tilting may greatly increase the ESR.
2. The test should be set up on a counter free from vibration, such as that from a centrifuge, to avoid a falsely increased rate of settling.
3. The temperature in the room should be kept constant while the test is being performed. Low temperatures cause erythrocytes to settle more slowly.
4. The test should be set up within two hours after the blood sample is collected.
5. The length and diameter of the sedimentation tube affect the rate of sedimentation. Therefore, standard tubes should be used in the test.

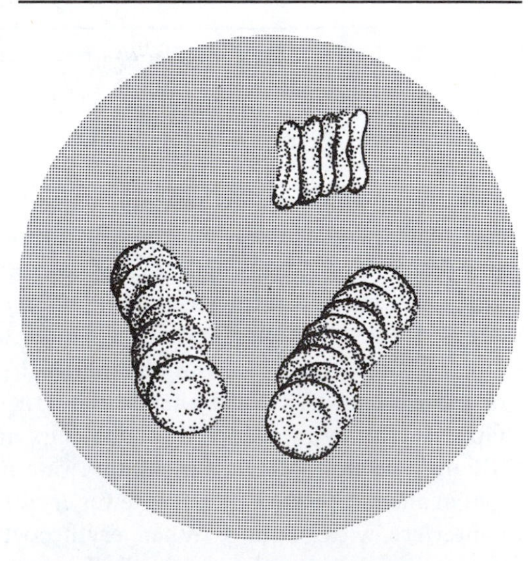

**Figure 3-13.** Erythrocytes forming rouleaux

**6.** The test must be timed carefully. The ESR increases with time.

## LESSON REVIEW

1. Why would an ESR be performed?
2. What four properties of blood affect the ESR? Explain how the ESR is affected by each of these factors.
3. Name five conditions in which the ESR would be increased.
4. What two conditions would have a low ESR?
5. What are the normal values for the ESR using the Wintrobe method?
6. List four technical factors that affect the ESR, and explain what effect each has.
7. Define aggregate, inflammation, rouleau, sedimentation, and Wintrobe tube.

## STUDENT ACTIVITIES

1. Re-read the information on erythrocyte sedimentation rate.
2. Review the glossary terms.
3. Practice performing the erythrocyte sedimentation rate test as outlined on the Student Performance Guide.
4. Evaluate the effect of technical factors on the ESR: set up three ESR tests on a blood sample. Treat one tube correctly, place one in the refrigerator, and place one at an angle at room temperature. Compare the results and explain them.

# Student Performance Guide

NAME ______________________

DATE ______________________

## LESSON 3–2 ERYTHROCYTE SEDIMENTATION RATE

### Instructions

1. Practice performing the procedure to measure the erythrocyte sedimentation rate.
2. Demonstrate the procedure for measuring the erythrocyte sedimentation rate satisfactorily for the instructor. All steps must be completed as listed on the instructor's Performance Check Sheet.
3. Complete a written examination satisfactorily.

### Materials and Equipment

- hand disinfectant
- sample of venous, anticoagulated blood
- long-stem Pasteur pipet with rubber bulb
- Wintrobe sedimentation tube (disposable or reusable)
- sedimentation rack
- timer
- surface disinfectant
- biohazard container

**Procedure**

S = Satisfactory
U = Unsatisfactory

| You must: | S | U | Comments |
|---|---|---|---|
| 1. Wash hands with hand disinfectant | | | |
| 2. Assemble equipment and materials | | | |
| 3. Check the leveling bubble to insure that the rack is level | | | |

| You must: | S | U | Comments |
|---|---|---|---|
| 4. Obtain anticoagulated blood sample | | | |
| 5. Mix blood well and fill Pasteur pipet | | | |
| 6. Fill Wintrobe tube to the "0" mark using the Pasteur pipet, being careful not to overfill. *Note:* Tube must be filled from bottom to avoid getting air bubbles in the tube | | | |
| 8. Place tube in sedimentation rack and set timer for one hour. Be certain the tube is vertical | | | |
| 9. Measure the distance the erythrocytes have fallen (in mm): after one hour, use the scale on the tube to measure the distance from the top of the plasma to the top of the red cells | | | |
| 10. Record the sedimentation rate in mm/hour | | | |
| 11. Clean equipment and return to storage. *Note:* If disposable equipment is used, dispose of in biohazard container | | | |
| 12. Clean work area with surface disinfectant | | | |
| 13. Wash hands with hand disinfectant | | | |

Comments:

Student/Instructor:

Date: ______________________ Instructor: ______________________

# LESSON 3–3

## Reticulocyte Count

### LESSON OBJECTIVES

After studying this lesson, you should be able to:

- Explain why a reticulocyte count is performed.
- Prepare a reticulocyte smear.
- Perform a reticulocyte count.
- Calculate a reticulocyte percentage.
- Name three stains commonly used in the reticulocyte procedure.
- Name two conditions in which the reticulocyte count would be low.
- Name two conditions in which the reticulocyte count would be elevated.
- List the normal reticulocyte count for an adult and a newborn.
- List the precautions that should be observed when performing a reticulocyte count.
- Define the glossary terms.

### GLOSSARY

**reticulocyte** / an immature erythrocyte which has retained basophilic substance in the cytoplasm

**reticulocytopenia** / a decrease below the normal number of reticulocytes

**reticulocytosis** / an increase above the normal number of reticulocytes in the circulating blood

**reticulum** / a network

**supravital stain** / a stain which will color living cells or tissues

### INTRODUCTION

A reticulocyte count is a method of estimating the number of immature erythrocytes in the circulating blood. The test is most commonly used to determine the cause of a decreased red cell count, or anemia. It is also used in following the course of treatment for anemia.

Erythrocytes are produced in the bone marrow.

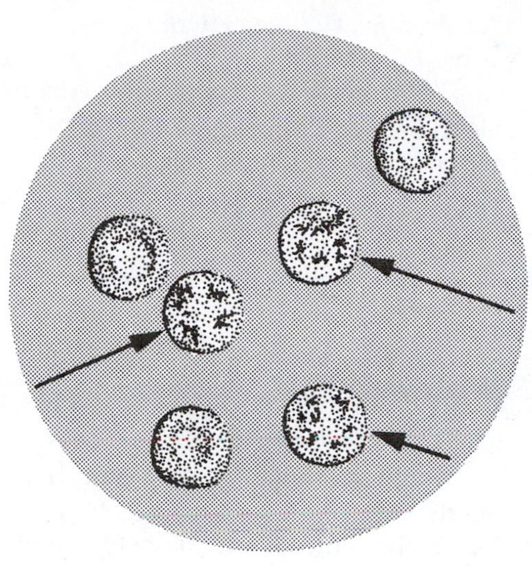

**Figure 3-14.** Reticulocytes showing stained reticulum

After a maturation process, the erythrocytes then enter the circulation where they normally live for 120 days. For the first twenty-four hours after a red cell enters the circulation it retains some evidence of immaturity: the presence of basophilic substance in the cytoplasm. If the cell is exposed to certain stains, the basophilic substance forms granular aggregates or filaments called a **reticulum,** and the cell is called a **reticulocyte** (Figure 3–14). The staining technique is called **supravital** staining, a procedure in which the cell is stained while it is still living. The three most common dyes used for supravital stains are: New Methylene Blue, Brilliant Cresyl Blue, and Nile Blue Sulfate. Reticulocytes appear as blue-tinged erythrocytes with dark bluish-purple granules or filaments. Mature red cells simply appear bluish (see Color Plate 12).

In a healthy adult, approximately 1% of the erythrocytes will stain as reticulocytes when a supravital stain is applied to a blood sample. Reticulocyte counts above 3% in an adult indicate that erythrocytes are being produced at an increased rate. **Reticulocytosis,** an increased number of reticulocytes, may be due to acute blood loss due to hemorrhage, chronic blood loss such as from a bleeding ulcer, or response to treatment of anemia.

Reticulocyte values below 0.5% indicate that the rate of erythrocyte production is decreased. A decrease in reticulocytes, **reticulocytopenia,** may be seen in iron deficiency anemia, vitamin $B_{12}$ or folic acid deficiencies, or aplastic anemia.

## RETICULOCYTE COUNT USING NEW METHYLENE BLUE

A reticulocyte count may be performed using capillary or venous blood. A few drops of blood are mixed with equal parts of New Methylene Blue stain in a small test tube and allowed to stand for fifteen minutes. The blood-stain mixture is then used to prepare blood smears. After the blood smears air dry, they are examined microscopically using the oil immersion objective. A total of 1000 erythrocytes are counted (500 counted per slide) and the number of reticulocytes seen per 1000 erythrocytes is recorded. (A reticulocyte is counted as a red cell.) The percentage of reticulocytes is then calculated.

## CALCULATION

A reticulocyte count is reported as the percentage of erythrocytes that are reticulocytes. This count is not a quantitative count but is only an estimate. The percentage of reticulocytes is calculated using the formula:

$$\frac{\#\text{ reticulocytes counted}}{\#\text{ erythrocytes counted}} \times 100 = \%\text{ reticulocytes}$$

*or*

$$\frac{\#\text{ reticulocytes}}{1000} \times 100 = \%\text{ reticulocytes}$$

*or*

$$\frac{\#\text{ reticulocytes}}{10} = \%\text{ reticulocytes}$$

A sample calculation is shown in Figure 3–15.

I. Count the reticulocytes using two smears:

| | Erythrocytes counted | Reticulocytes seen |
|---|---|---|
| Smear 1 | 500 | 7 |
| Smear 2 | 500 | 5 |
| Total | 1000 | 12 |

II. Calculate the percentage of reticulocytes:

$$\% \text{ retics} = \frac{\#\text{ Reticulocytes counted}}{\#\text{ RBC counted}} \times 100$$

$$\% \text{ retics} = \frac{12}{1000} \times 100$$

$$\% \text{ retics} = \frac{12}{10}$$

$$\% \text{ retics} = 1.2$$

**Figure 3-15.** Sample calculation of reticulocyte percentage

**Table 3-3.** Normal Reticulocyte Percentages

| | **Normal Reticulocyte Count** | **Upper Limit of Normal** |
|---|---|---|
| Adults | 0.5–1.5% | 3% |
| Newborns | 2.5–6.5% | 10% |

## NORMAL VALUES

The normal reticulocyte count varies with age, Table 3-3. Newborn infants have high counts which decrease to the adult level by 2 weeks of age.

### *Precautions*

- The reticulum may be easily overlooked; cells should be examined thoroughly.
- Artifacts may be confused with reticulum.
- Use a definite counting pattern to insure that cells are not counted twice.
- Fresh blood must be used to perform the reticulocyte count.
- The stain must be filtered frequently to prevent stain precipitate from forming on smear and being confused with reticulum.

## *LESSON REVIEW*

1. What is a reticulocyte?
2. Why would a reticulocyte count be performed?
3. What is the normal reticulocyte count for adults—for newborns?
4. What type of stain is used for a reticulocyte count?
5. What are three of the dyes used to stain reticulocytes?
6. What conditions can cause a high reticulocyte count?
7. What conditions can cause a low reticulocyte count?
8. State the formula for calculating a reticulocyte count.
9. List the precautions to be observed when performing a reticulocyte count.
10. Define reticulocyte, reticulocytopenia, reticulocytosis, reticulum, and supravital stain.

## *STUDENT ACTIVITIES*

1. Re-read the information on reticulocyte counts.
2. Review the glossary terms.
3. Practice performing reticulocyte counts and calculating reticulocyte percentages as outlined on the Student Performance Guide.

# Student Performance Guide

NAME ________________________________

DATE ________________________________

## LESSON 3–3
## RETICULOCYTE COUNT

### Instructions

1. Practice performing a reticulocyte count.
2. Demonstrate the procedure for performing a reticulocyte count satisfactorily for the instructor. All steps must be completed as listed on the instructor's Performance Check Sheet.
3. Complete a written examination successfully.

### Materials and Equipment

- hand disinfectant
- microscope
- microscope slides
- lens paper
- immersion oil
- Pasteur pipet with bulb
- New Methylene Blue stain, freshly filtered
- 70% alcohol
- sterile cotton or gauze
- sterile lancet
- capillary tubes, heparinized and plain
- test tube 10 × 75 mm
- tally counter
- surface disinfectant
- biohazard container

**Procedure**

S = Satisfactory
U = Unsatisfactory

| You must: | S | U | Comments |
|---|---|---|---|
| 1. Wash hands with hand disinfectant | | | |
| 2. Assemble equipment and materials | | | |

| You must: | S | U | Comments |
|---|---|---|---|
| 3. Perform a capillary puncture and wipe away the first drop of blood with dry sterile cotton or gauze (or use fresh, well-mixed venous anticoagulated blood to perform the test) | | | |
| 4. Fill one or two heparinized capillary tubes with blood (use plain capillary tubes if using anticoagulated blood) | | | |
| 5. Dispense two to three drops of blood into the bottom of a small test tube | | | |
| 6. Add an equal amount of New Methylene Blue stain to the test tube and mix | | | |
| 7. Allow mixture to stand for fifteen minutes at room temperature | | | |
| 8. Mix contents of tube and fill a plain capillary tube with blood-stain mixture | | | |
| 9. Prepare two blood smears from blood-stain mixture and allow to air dry | | | |
| 10. Place one slide on microscope stage and secure | | | |
| 11. Use low power (10X) objective to find a good area of the smear | | | |
| 12. Place one drop of immersion oil on the slide and carefully rotate oil immersion objective into position | | | |
| 13. Count all erythrocytes in one oil immersion field and record the number of reticulocytes in the field *Note:* A reticulocyte is counted as a red cell | | | |
| 14. Move slide to an adjacent microscopic field | | | |
| 15. Count all erythrocytes in the (adjacent) field and record the number of reticulocytes in the field | | | |
| 16. Continue steps 14–15 until 500 erythrocytes have been counted | | | |
| 17. Repeat steps 10–16 using the second slide | | | |
| 18. Calculate the reticulocyte percentage using the formula: $\frac{\text{\# of retics counted}}{1000} \times 100 = \%$ reticulocytes | | | |

| You must: | S | U | Comments |
|---|---|---|---|
| 19. Record the results | | | |
| 20. Clean oil immersion objective carefully and thoroughly with lens paper | | | |
| 21. Clean any oil from microscope stage with laboratory tissue | | | |
| 22. Return equipment to proper storage | | | |
| 23. Clean work area with surface disinfectant | | | |
| 24. Wash hands with hand disinfectant | | | |
| Comments:<br><br>Student/Instructor: | | | |

Date: ______________________ Instructor: ______________________

# LESSON 3–4
## Platelet Count

## LESSON OBJECTIVES

After studying this lesson, you should be able to:

- Discuss the functions of platelets.
- Name two pathological conditions in which the platelet counts may be abnormal.
- Perform a blood dilution for a platelet count.
- Perform a platelet count.
- Calculate the results of a platelet count.
- List three precautions which must be observed when performing a platelet count.
- Define the glossary terms.

## GLOSSARY

**hemostasis** / process of stopping blood flow
**petri dish** / a shallow covered dish made of plastic or glass
**platelet** / a formed element in the blood which plays an important part in blood clotting; a thrombocyte
**thrombocytopenia** / a decrease below the normal number of platelets in the blood
**thrombocytosis** / an increase above the normal number of platelets in the blood

## INTRODUCTION

The platelet count is one important test used to investigate bleeding disorders, to assess clotting ability, or to monitor drug treatments. Platelets are difficult to count accurately because of their small size and their tendency to clump.

**Platelets,** the smallest of the formed elements in the blood, play an important role in the clotting of blood and in **hemostasis,** the process of stopping bleeding. They help stop bleeding by forming a sticky plug to seal vessel walls and also help initiate a series of enzymatic reactions which result in the formation of the blood clot.

The normal platelet count is 150,000 to 400,000 platelets per cubic millimeter (cu mm or $mm^3$) of blood. An increase in platelets, **thrombocytosis,** may occur in conditions such as polycythemia or after a splenectomy. **Thrombocytopenia,** a decrease in platelets, may occur in some anemias, some leukemias, and following chemotherapy and radiation therapy.

## PROCEDURE FOR PLATELET COUNT

### Diluting the Sample

A platelet count is performed by mixing a blood sample with a diluting fluid of 1% ammonium oxalate in a RBC diluting pipet. Capillary blood may be used but venous anticoagulated blood gives better results. This is because platelets tend to clump rapidly in a capillary sample. The blood is drawn to the 1.0 mark, and the diluting fluid is then drawn to the 101 mark. The resulting dilution for the platelet count is 1:100. The pipet is then shaken for three minutes to mix the sample.

### Filling the Chamber

After mixing, four to five drops are discarded from the stem of the pipet. Both sides of a clean hemacytometer are loaded. Since platelets are so small, they move around easily in the counting chamber. This makes it difficult to count them accurately. To allow time for the platelets to settle and to prevent evaporation of the solution in the counting chamber, the filled hemacytometer is placed in a **petri dish** containing a moist cotton ball for ten minutes (Figure 3–16).

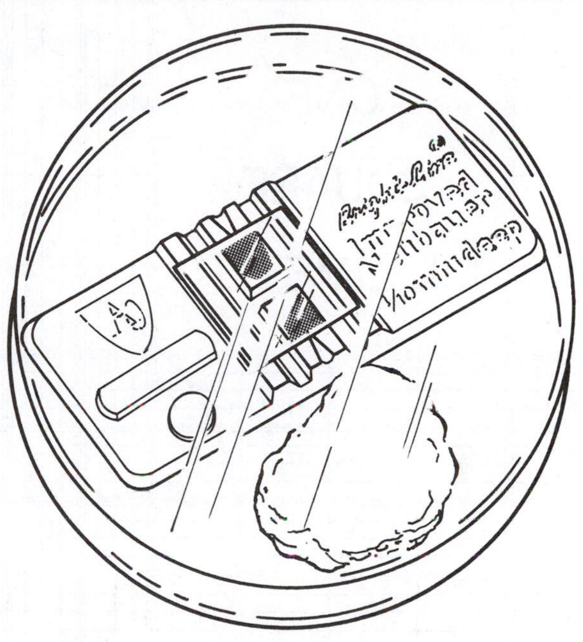

**Figure 3-16.** Hemacytometer in moist chamber (covered petri dish containing moistened cotton)

### Counting the Platelets

To perform the platelet count, the hemacytometer is removed from the moist chamber and placed on the microscope stage. The low power (10X) objective is used to locate the counting area. In a platelet count, the entire center square (1 $mm^2$) is counted (Figure 3–17) using the high power (45X) objective. The platelets may be seen more clearly if the microscope condenser is lowered and the light is decreased (by adjusting the diaphragm). The platelets will appear as shiny refractile objects which darken when the fine adjustment knob is rotated (see Color Plate 15). The platelets in all 25 small squares of the large central square are counted. The count is performed using both sides of the chamber and the average of the two sides is calculated.

### Calculation of Platelet Count

The number of platelets per $mm^3$ of blood is calculated using the general formula:

$$C/mm^3 = \frac{Avg \times D\ (mm) \times DF}{A\ (mm)^2}$$

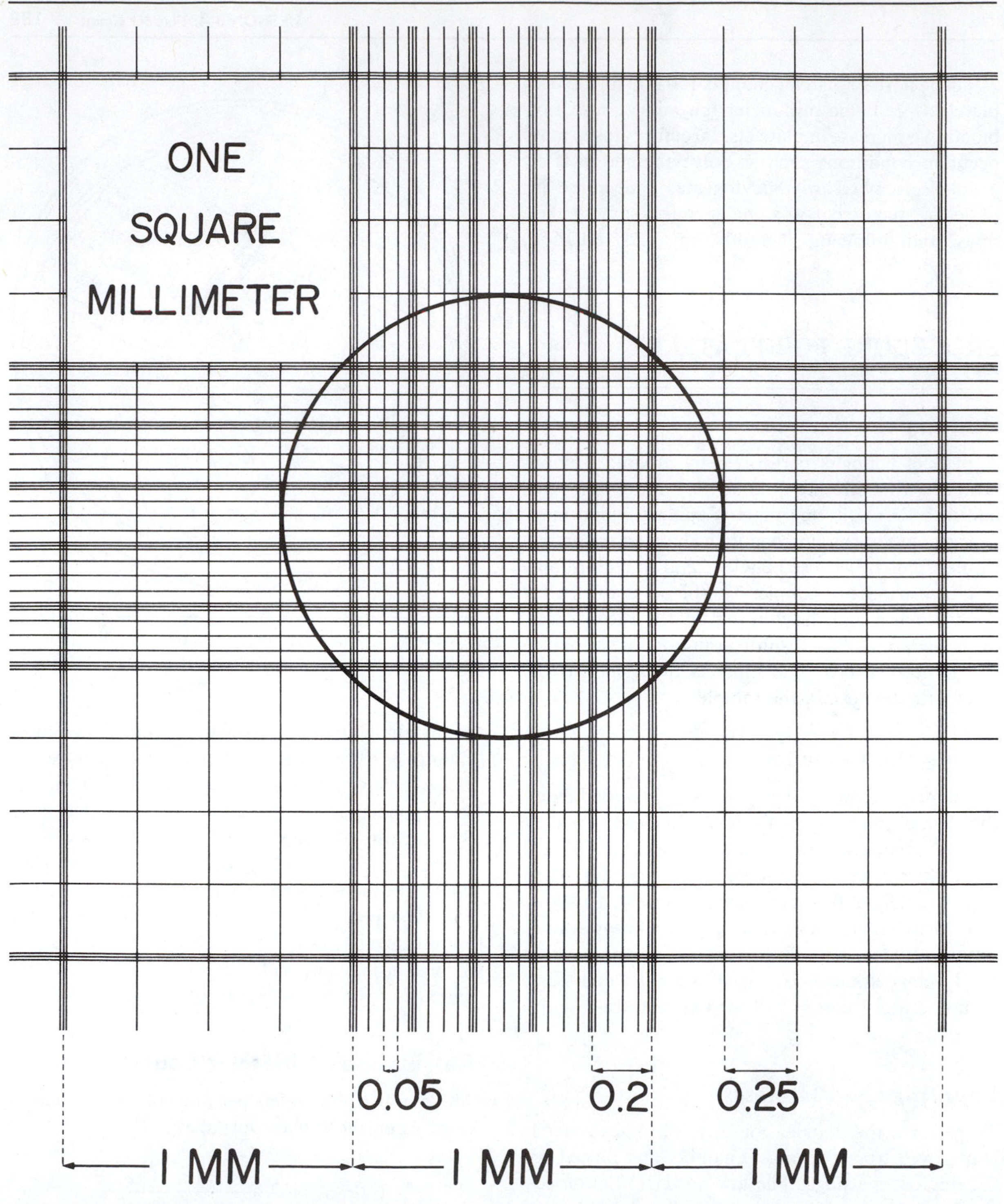


**Figure 3-17.** Platelet counting area (circled)

which is first given on page 100. To simplify, use the following figures.

1. The platelet average is computed using counts from both sides of the chamber.
2. The depth factor (D) is 10.
3. The dilution factor (DF) is 100.
4. The area (A) counted is 1 $mm^2$.

These numbers are substituted into the formula as follows:

$$\frac{\text{Average \# platelets} \times 10 \times 100}{1} = \text{average \# platelets} \times 1000 = \frac{\text{platelets}}{mm^3}$$

Therefore, the platelet count can be determined by simply multiplying the average number of platelets by 1000 (or by adding three zeroes). A sample calculation of a platelet count is shown in Figure 3–18.

## UNOPETTE® MICROCOLLECTION SYSTEM

The most acceptable manual method of counting platelets is the use of self-filling, self-diluting systems such as Unopette®. Such a system provides greater accuracy than the pipet method, and the components are disposable (Figure 3–19).

Unopette® systems consist of a reservoir, a capillary pipet, and a pipet shield. The reservoir contains a pre-measured volume of diluting fluid. The capillary pipet is made to contain a specific volume. The shield protects the pipet and is used to puncture the diaphragm which seals the reservoir. The Unopette® system used for platelet counts contains 1.98 ml of diluting fluid in the reservoir. A 20 $\mu$l capillary pipet is used to measure the sample. When the sample is diluted in the reservoir, the resulting dilution is 1:100. This blood dilution is then loaded into a hemacytometer and the platelets are counted as in the manual pipet method.

## AUTOMATION

Platelet counts are still performed by hand in many laboratories. However, there are instruments which have been used for several years which have the ability to perform platelet counts. The platelet counter may be a part of a system which performs several other procedures, such as cell counts and hemoglobin measurements, or it may perform only platelet counts.

1. Count the platelets in the entire large center square (1 $mm^2$):
   Side 1 = 156 Side 2 = 180
2. Compute the average:
   A. 156 + 180 = 336 platelets
   B. 336 ÷ 2 = 168 average
3. Calculate the count:

$$\text{platelets}/mm^3 = \frac{\text{average \# platelets} \times \text{depth factor (mm)} \times \text{dilution factor}}{\text{area counted } (mm^2)}$$

$$\text{platelets}/mm^3 = \frac{168 \times 10 \times 100}{1}$$

$$\text{platelets}/mm^3 = 168 \times 1000$$

$$\text{platelets}/mm^3 = 168{,}000 \text{ (or } 1.68 \times 10^5\text{)}/mm^3$$

**Figure 3-18.** Sample calculation of platelet count

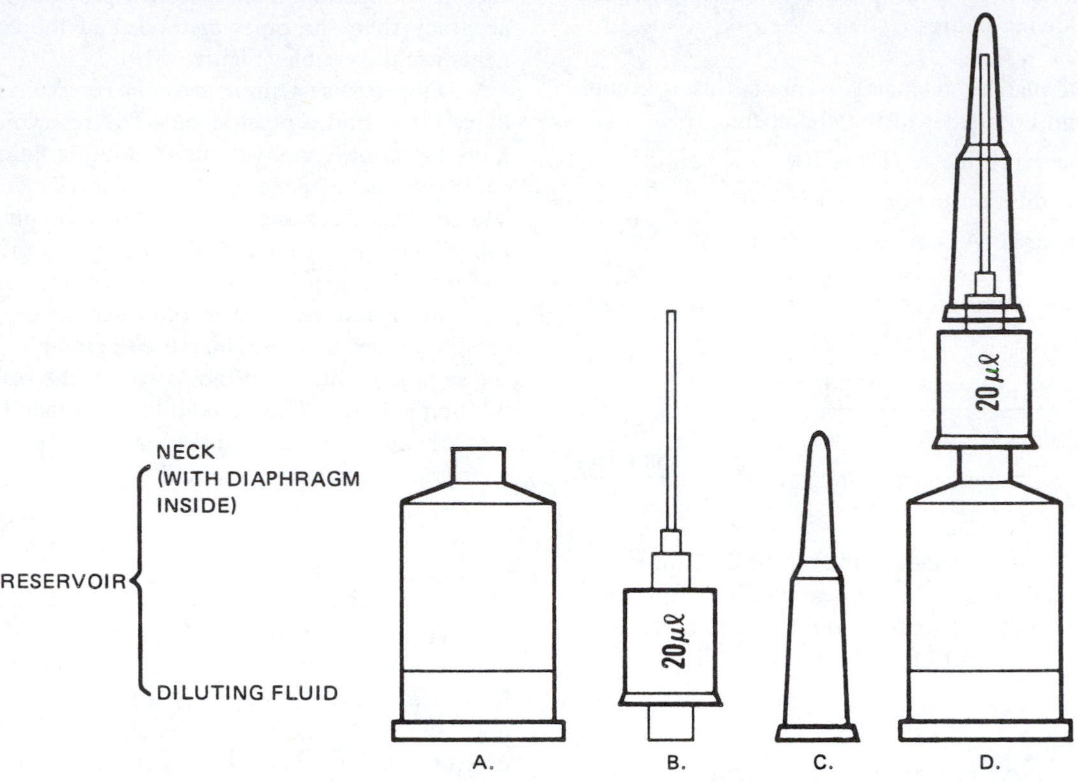


**Figure 3-19.** Unopette® microcollection system

### *Precautions*

■ The hemacytometer must be free of dirt and debris which might be confused with platelets.

■ The platelet count must be performed within 30 minutes of dilution of the sample.

■ Platelets clump easily; therefore, counts performed from capillary blood are usually lower than those performed on an anticoagulated sample.

■ The microscope light must be low to provide good contrast and to enable platelets to be seen.

■ If platelets are clumped or are distributed unevenly in the counting chamber, the chamber should be cleaned and refilled (after remixing pipet contents). If clumps are still present, a new sample should be obtained.

■ The moist cotton ball must not come into contact with the coverglass or the fluid in the hemacytometer.

## *LESSON REVIEW*

1. Explain the function of platelets.
2. Name a condition in which thrombocytosis may occur.
3. Name a cause of thrombocytopenia.

4. Why is it important to thoroughly clean the coverglass and hemacytometer before performing the platelet count?
5. What is the purpose of the moist chamber?
6. What area of the hemacytometer is used to count platelets?
7. State the formula for calculating a platelet count.
8. How is a blood dilution performed for a platelet count?
9. Define hemostasis, petri dish, platelet, thrombocytopenia, and thrombocytosis.

## *STUDENT ACTIVITIES*

1. Re-read the information on platelet counts.
2. Review the glossary terms.
3. Practice performing a platelet count as outlined on the Student Performance Guides, using the worksheet.
4. Prepare a stained blood smear from the blood sample used for the platelet count. Compare the number of platelets in the stained smear with the number counted, as in Lesson 2–10.

# Student Performance Guide

NAME ______________________________

DATE ______________________________

## LESSON 3–4
## PLATELET COUNT (PIPET METHOD)

### Instructions

1. Practice performing and calculating a platelet count.
2. Perform the platelet count procedure satisfactorily for the instructor. All steps must be completed as listed on the instructor's Performance Check Sheet.
3. Complete a written examination successfully.

### Materials and Equipment

- hand disinfectant
- RBC pipet
- rubber tubing and mouthpiece
- blood sample, anticoagulated with EDTA
- hemacytometer with coverglass
- test tube rack or beaker to hold blood sample
- platelet diluting fluid: 1% ammonium oxalate (store in refrigerator and filter before using)
- microscope
- petri dish
- cotton ball (slightly moistened with water)
- lens paper
- alcohol (70% ethanol)
- pipet shaker (optional)
- hand tally counter
- surface disinfectant
- biohazard container

**Procedure**

S = Satisfactory
U = Unsatisfactory

| You must: | S | U | Comments |
|---|---|---|---|
| 1. Wash hands with hand disinfectant | | | |
| 2. Assemble equipment and materials | | | |
| 3. Clean and polish the hemacytometer and coverglass carefully with alcohol and lens paper | | | |
| 4. Attach rubber tubing with mouthpiece to the end of the RBC pipet which has the 101 mark | | | |
| 5. Mix the tube of blood by inverting tube thirty times (if anticoagulated blood is unavailable, obtain blood by capillary puncture) | | | |
| 6. Position the mouthpiece between the lips | | | |
| 7. Tilt the sample so that the blood flows near the lip of the tube and insert the pipet tip into the tube | | | |
| 8. Draw the blood exactly to the 1.0 mark on the pipet | | | |
| 9. Replace the blood sample tube into test tube rack | | | |
| 10. Wipe the blood from the outside of the pipet stem with soft tissue | | | |
| 11. Aspirate platelet diluting fluid to the 101 mark | | | |
| 12. Mix the pipet contents for three minutes gently (or place on pipet shaker) | | | |
| 13. Prepare a moist chamber: Place a slightly moist cotton ball into a petri dish leaving enough space for the hemacytometer | | | |
| 14. Discard four to five drops from the pipet and wipe the stem | | | |
| 15. Fill both sides of the hemacytometer | | | |
| 16. Place the hemacytometer into the petri dish. Do not allow the cotton ball to touch the hemacytometer | | | |
| 17. Place the cover on the petri dish and allow the preparation | | | |

| You must: | S | U | Comments |
|---|---|---|---|
| to stand ten minutes (this permits the platelets to settle in the chamber) | | | |
| 18. Place the hemacytometer on the microscope stage carefully and secure. Do not wait longer than thirty minutes to complete the platelet count | | | |
| 19. Use the low power (10X) objective to bring the ruled area into focus | | | |
| 20. Locate the large central square (Figure 3–17) | | | |
| 21. Rotate the high power objective (45X) into position carefully and focus with the fine adjustment knob until lines are clear | | | |
| 22. Lower the condenser and reduce the light by partially closing the diaphragm for best contrast. Platelets should appear as round or oval particles which are refractile and are smaller than red blood cells (Color Plate 15) | | | |
| 23. Count the platelets in the entire center square of the ruled area (all twenty-five small squares) using the left-to-right, right-to-left counting pattern and record results | | | |
| 24. Repeat the procedure on the other side of the hemacytometer | | | |
| 25. Average the results from the two sides | | | |
| 26. Calculate the platelet count: $\text{platelets/mm}^3 = \frac{\text{Avg} \times \text{D (mm)} \times \text{DF}}{\text{A (mm}^2)}$ or $\text{platelets/mm}^3 = \text{average \# platelets} \times 1000$ | | | |
| 27. Record the result | | | |
| 28. Clean and dry hemacytometer | | | |
| 29. Wash and dry pipet | | | |
| 30. Return equipment to proper storage | | | |
| 31. Clean work area with surface disinfectant | | | |

| You must: | S | U | Comments |
|---|---|---|---|
| 32. Wash hands with hand disinfectant | | | |

Comments:

Student/Instructor:

Date: ______________________ Instructor: ______________________

# Student Performance Guide

NAME ____________________

DATE ____________________

## LESSON 3–4 PLATELET COUNT (UNOPETTE® METHOD)

### Instructions

1. Practice performing and calculating a platelet count using the Unopette®.
2. Perform the platelet count procedure satisfactorily for the instructor. All steps must be completed as listed on the instructor's Performance Check Sheet.
3. Complete a written examination successfully.

### Materials and Equipment

- hand disinfectant
- blood sample, anticoagulated with EDTA
- hemacytometer with coverglass
- test tube rack or beaker to hold blood sample
- Unopette® for platelet count (reservoir and pipet assembly)
- microscope
- petri dish
- cotton ball (moistened slightly with water)
- lens paper
- alcohol (70% ethanol)
- hand tally counter
- surface disinfectant
- biohazard container

*Note:* The following is a general procedure for the use of the Unopette® system. Consult the package insert for specific instructions.

## Procedure

S = Satisfactory
U = Unsatisfactory

| You must: | S | U | Comments |
|---|---|---|---|
| 1. Wash hands with hand disinfectant | | | |
| 2. Assemble equipment and materials | | | |
| 3. Place a clean hemacytometer coverglass over a clean hemacytometer | | | |
| 4. Puncture the diaphragm of the Unopette® reservoir. Hold the reservoir firmly on a flat surface with one hand and use the tip of the pipet shield to puncture the diaphragm. *Note:* The opening must be made large enough to easily accommodate the pipet | | | |
| 5. Remove the shield from the pipet assembly | | | |
| 6. Fill the capillary pipet using blood from capillary puncture or tube of well-mixed EDTA anticoagulated blood. The pipet will fill by capillary action and will stop filling automatically. *Note:* Keep pipet horizontal or at a slight (5°) angle to avoid overfilling | | | |
| 7. Wipe excess blood from the outside of the capillary pipet with soft laboratory tissue. *Note:* Do not allow tissue to touch pipet tip | | | |
| 8. Squeeze the reservoir slightly, being careful not to expel any of the liquid | | | |
| 9. Maintain the pressure on the reservoir and insert the capillary pipet into the reservoir, seating the pipet firmly into the neck of the reservoir. Do not expel any of the liquid | | | |
| 10. Release the pressure on the reservoir, drawing the blood out of the capillary pipet into the diluent | | | |
| 11. Squeeze the reservoir gently three to four times to rinse the remaining blood from the capillary pipet. *Note:* Do not allow the blood–diluent mixture to flow out the top | | | |
| 12. Mix the contents of the reservoir thoroughly by gently swirling the reservoir and/or turning it side to side | | | |

| You must: | S | U | Comments |
|---|---|---|---|
| 13. Let stand at least ten minutes until red cells are completely destroyed. *Note:* Do not allow to stand longer than 2 hours | | | |
| 14. Prepare a moist chamber: place a slightly moist cotton ball into a petri dish, leaving enough space for the hemacytometer | | | |
| 15. Withdraw the capillary pipet from the reservoir and place into the neck of the reservoir in reverse position (the pipet tip should now project upward from the reservoir) | | | |
| 16. Mix the contents of the reservoir thoroughly. Invert the reservoir and gently squeeze to discard 4–5 drops onto gauze or paper towel | | | |
| 17. Fill both sides of the hemacytometer | | | |
| 18. Place the hemacytometer into the petri dish. Do not allow the cotton ball to touch the hemacytometer | | | |
| 19. Place the cover on the petri dish and allow the preparation to stand ten minutes (this permits the platelets to settle in the chamber) | | | |
| 20. Place the hemacytometer on the microscope stage carefully and secure. Do not wait longer than 30 minutes to complete the platelet count | | | |
| 21. Use the low power (10X) objective to bring the ruled area into focus | | | |
| 22. Locate the large central square (Figure 3–17) | | | |
| 23. Rotate the high power (45X) objective into position carefully and focus with the fine adjustment knob until lines are clear | | | |
| 24. Lower the condenser and reduce the light by partially closing the diaphragm for best contrast. Platelets should appear as round or oval particles which are refractile and are smaller than red blood cells | | | |
| 25. Count the platelets in the entire center square of the ruled area (all twenty-five small squares) using the left-to-right, right-to-left counting pattern and record results | | | |

| You must: | S | U | Comments |
|---|---|---|---|
| 26. Repeat the procedure on the other side of the hemacytometer | | | |
| 27. Average the results from the two sides | | | |
| 28. Calculate the platelet count: $\text{platelets/mm}^3 = \frac{\text{Avg} \times \text{D (mm)} \times \text{DF}}{\text{A (mm}^2\text{)}}$ or $\text{platelets/mm}^3 = \text{average \# platelets} \times 1000$ | | | |
| 29. Record the result | | | |
| 30. Clean and dry hemacytometer | | | |
| 31. Wash and dry pipet | | | |
| 32. Return equipment to proper storage | | | |
| 33. Clean work area with surface disinfectant | | | |
| 34. Wash hands with hand disinfectant | | | |

Comments:

Student/Instructor:

Date: ______________________ Instructor: ______________________

# Worksheet

NAME ______________________________ DATE ____________

SPECIMEN NO. ____________

## LESSON 3–4 PLATELET COUNT

Platelets counted:

Side 1 ____________

Side 2 ____________

Total ____________

Average (Total ÷ 2) _____

Calculations:

$$\text{platelets/mm}^3 = \frac{\text{average \# platelets counted} \times \text{depth factor (mm)} \times \text{dilution factor}}{\text{area counted (mm}^2)}$$

$$\text{platelets/mm}^3 = \text{average \# platelets counted} \times 1000$$

$\text{platelets/mm}^3 =$ ______________________________

* Normal platelet count = 150,000 − 400,000/$mm^3$

# LESSON 3–5
## The Spectrophotometer

## LESSON OBJECTIVES

After studying this lesson, you should be able to:

- Explain the principle of the spectrophotometer.
- List the parts of the spectrophotometer.
- State Beer's Law.
- Use the spectrophotometer.
- Construct a standard curve.
- List precautions that should be observed when using a spectrophotometer.
- Define the glossary terms.

## GLOSSARY

**absorbance** / the light absorbed (not transmitted) by a liquid containing colored molecules; designated in formulas by "A"; also called optical density (O.D.)

**blank** / reagent blank; solution which contains some or all of the reagents used in the test but does not contain the substance being measured

**cuvette** / a small test tube used to hold liquids to be examined in the spectrophotometer; must be manufactured to certain standards for clarity and lack of distortion in the glass

**diffraction grating** / a device which disperses a light beam into a spectrum

**galvanometer** / instrument which measures electrical current

**monochromatic** / consisting of one color; light which is one wavelength

**monochromator** / device which allows only one color of light to reach the cuvette

**percent transmittance** / the percentage of light which passes through a liquid sample

**photoelectric cell** / a device which detects light and converts it into electricity

**spectrophotometer** / an instrument which can be used to determine the concentration of a solution by measuring the light transmitted or absorbed by the solution

**standard curve** / a graph which shows the relationship between the concentration of a solution and the absorbance or percent transmittance of a solution

## INTRODUCTION

A **spectrophotometer** is an instrument used to determine the concentration of colored solutions (Figure 3–20). This determination is made by passing a beam of light through the solution. The portion of light which passes through the colored solution is the **percent transmittance.** The light which does not pass through the solution is absorbed and is measured as **absorbance.** Concentrated solutions allow less light to pass through than dilute solutions. Thus, it can be said that the more concentrated the solution the greater its absorbance and the less its transmittance. Either the absorbance or the percent transmittance can be read from most spectrophotometers. For most colored solutions the absorbance increases with the concentration. These solutions are said to follow Beer's Law which states that the absorbance of a colored substance is directly

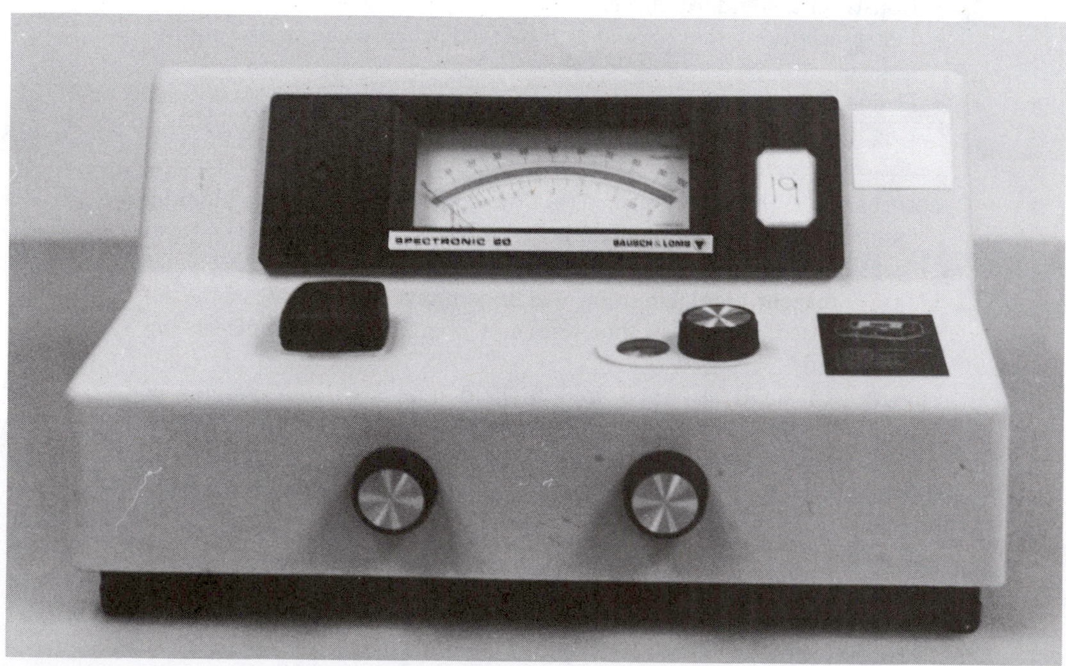


**Figure 3-20.** An example of a spectrophotometer (*Photo by John Estridge*)

proportional to its concentration. This relationship is linear. For most colored solutions the percent transmittance decreases as the concentration increases; this relationship is geometric (non-linear).

### Parts of the Spectrophotometer

Spectrophotometers may vary in external design but all have essentially the same internal parts (Figure 3-21). Each of these parts has a definite function in the measurement of a solution's concentration. A light source in the spectrophotometer provides a beam of light which passes to a **monochromator** (Figure 3-21). This monochromator has a **diffraction grating** which disperses the light into a spectrum. It also contains a slit which isolates a beam of **monochromatic light** (light of one wavelength or color). This monochromatic light is directed toward the sample well in which a **cuvette** (holding the colored solution) is placed. The cuvette is a special glass tube manufactured to precise specifications. Depending on the concentration of the solution a portion of the light will be absorbed and a portion of light will pass through the solution. The light which passes through is detected by a **photoelectric cell** which converts it to electricity. This electrical current is then measured and recorded by a **galvanometer.** The information can be presented as either absorbance (A) units or percent transmittance (%T) on the readout dial of the spectrophotometer.

## STANDARD CURVES

**Standard curves** can be used to determine the concentrations of colored solutions which follow Beer's Law. The solutions are prepared by making specific dilutions of a standard of known concentration. The absorbances, or percent transmittances, of the dilutions are read on the spectrophotometer. The readings are plotted versus the concentrations of the dilutions. Absorbance is plotted using linear graph paper. If percent transmittance is measured, semilog

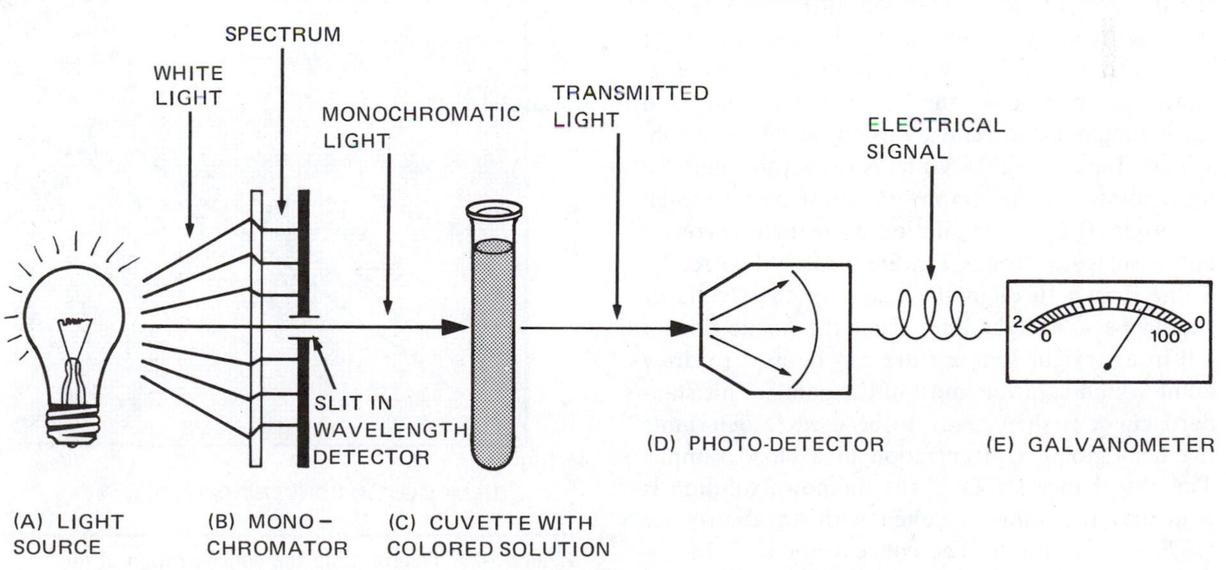


**Figure 3-21.** Diagram of internal parts of a spectrophotometer

paper must be used to obtain a straight line. This graph, the standard curve, may then be used to find the concentration of unknown samples of the same solution. A standard curve must be prepared for each spectrophotometer and each test procedure.

## Preparation of a Hemoglobin Standard Curve

A standard curve for hemoglobin can be made using dilutions of a hemoglobin standard of known concentration. Dilutions of a standard hemoglobin solution containing 20 g/dl are made with Drabkin's reagent. The tubes should contain concentrations of 5, 10, 15, and 20 g/dl. (Standards are available in various concentrations and manufacturer's instructions should be followed in preparing the required dilutions.) Drabkin's reagent is the chemical solution which is mixed with blood in the hemoglobin test. A wavelength of 540 nm is selected on the spectrophotometer, and the absorbance is set to zero using Drabkin's (in a cuvette) as a blank. A **blank** is a solution which contains some or all of the reagents but none of the substance being measured. Each dilution is transferred to a cuvette and the absorbance is determined. The absorbance, or percent transmittance, of each is plotted. The absorbances are plotted on the "Y" axis (ordinate) and the hemoglobin concentrations on the "X" axis (abscissa) (Figure 3–22). A line is drawn through the four points on the graph and must pass through the origin (0, 0). If the dilutions were made correctly and absorbances (or %T) were measured correctly, a line drawn through the points of the standards should be a straight line. If all the points do not fall in a straight line, a ruler can be used to draw a line which connects most of the points. This standard curve is then ready to be used to determine the hemoglobin concentration in a blood sample. The absorbance (%T) of the unknown solution is read and the value matched with an absorbance (%T) on the graph. The concentration of the unknown can then be read directly from the graph (Figure 3–23). This method of measurement is valid only when the substance follows Beer's Law.

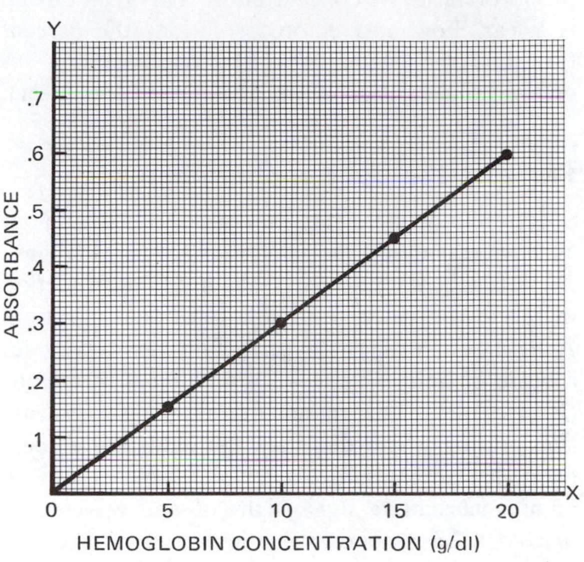


**Figure 3-22.** Illustration of a hemoglobin standard curve showing absorbance vs concentration

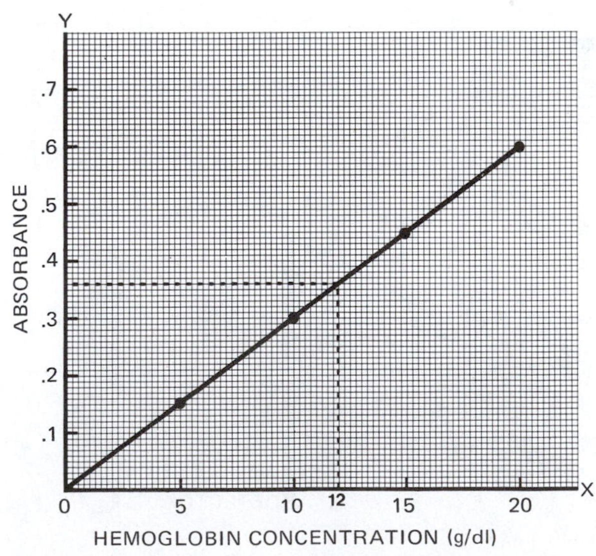


**Figure 3-23.** Determining the concentration of an unknown using a standard curve. The absorbance of the unknown is .360; the concentration of the unknown is read as 12.0 g/dl from the standard curve.

## QUALITY CONTROL

Quality control procedures should be performed on spectrophotometers periodically according to manufacturer's instructions. The spectrophotometer should be checked for stray light before each use. This is done by verifying that the percent transmittance reads zero when the light path is blocked. To insure that results from a spectrophotometer are reliable, a standard curve must be constructed for each instrument at the beginning of each work day and when new reagents are used. Controls must also be used with every set of determinations.

## CARE OF SPECTROPHOTOMETER AND CUVETTES

The spectrophotometer should be kept covered when not in use to protect it from dust. Jarring the instrument or spilling reagents onto the spectrophotometer should be avoided. The same precautions that are followed when using electrical instruments should be observed.

Cuvettes should be optically matched and kept free from scratches. They should be washed carefully, avoiding the use of abrasives, rinsed in distilled water, and air-dried. Cuvettes should be inverted when stored to avoid dust. They should be held only by the upper edge and the outside of the cuvette should be wiped free of fingerprints before using.

### *Precautions*

- Use Drabkin's reagent cautiously; do not mouth pipet. CAUTION: Drabkin's reagent contains cyanide and is poisonous.
- Allow the spectrophotometer to warm up before using.
- Check the spectrophotometer daily with standards and controls.
- Use cuvettes which are clean and free of fingerprints.
- Avoid air bubbles in the cuvette.
- Avoid spilling reagents onto the spectrophotometer.
- Set the instrument to zero absorbance (100%T) with the reagent blank before measuring a sample.

## *LESSON REVIEW*

1. Diagram and name the parts of the spectrophotometer.
2. Explain the principle of the spectrophotometer.
3. State Beer's Law.
4. What kind of solution is used to set the instrument at 100%T or zero absorbance?
5. Show in a simple sketch a standard curve.
6. List the precautions that should be observed when using a spectrophotometer.
7. Define absorbance, blank, cuvette, diffraction grating, galvanometer, monochromatic, monochromator, photoelectric cell, spectrophotometer, standard curve, and transmittance.

## *STUDENT ACTIVITIES*

1. Re-read the information on the spectrophotometer.
2. Review the glossary terms.
3. Practice the procedure for preparing and constructing a standard curve as outlined on the Student Performance Guide, using the worksheet.

# Student Performance Guide

NAME ______________________

DATE ______________________

## LESSON 3–5 THE SPECTROPHOTOMETER

### Instructions

1. Practice the procedure for preparing a standard curve for hemoglobin.
2. Demonstrate the procedure for preparing a standard curve for hemoglobin satisfactorily for the instructor. All steps must be completed as listed on the instructor's Performance Check Sheet.
3. Complete a written examination successfully.

### Materials and Equipment

- hand disinfectant
- spectrophotometer
- cuvettes (use matched cuvettes for clinical work)
- standard hemoglobin solution (20 grams/dl)
- graduated pipets: 5 ml, 10 ml
- soft laboratory tissue
- distilled water
- Drabkin's reagent
- test tubes, 13 × 100 mm
- safety bulbs for pipets
- parafilm
- surface disinfectant

*Note:* The following is a general procedure for use of a spectrophotometer. Consult the operating manual for proper use of the spectrophotometer being used.

**Procedure**

S = Satisfactory
U = Unsatisfactory

| You must: | S | U | Comments |
|---|---|---|---|
| 1. Wash hands with hand disinfectant | | | |
| 2. Turn on spectrophotometer to warm up (use time suggested by manufacturer, usually 10 to 30 minutes) | | | |
| 3. Set wavelength at 540 nm | | | |
| 4. Assemble materials | | | |
| 5. Label five (5) test tubes: 0 (blank), 5, 10, 15, and 20 | | | |
| 6. Using a 5 ml pipet and safety bulb (do not mouth pipet), dispense Drabkin's reagent into the tubes as follows:<br>Tube<br>0 = 6.0 ml<br>5 = 4.5 ml<br>10 = 3.0 ml<br>15 = 1.5 ml<br>20 = 0 ml | | | |
| 7. Dispense the hemoglobin standard into the same tubes as follows, using a clean 5 ml pipet with a safety bulb:<br>Tube:<br>0 = 0 ml<br>5 = 1.5 ml<br>10 = 3.0 ml<br>15 = 4.5 ml<br>20 = 6.0 ml | | | |
| 8. Observe tubes to see that each contains the same volume and mix each tube well | | | |
| 9. Transfer contents of the "O" tube to a clean cuvette and place in cuvette well of spectrophotometer *Note:* Wipe all fingerprints from cuvette with soft tissue before inserting any cuvette into spectrophotometer | | | |
| 10. Set absorbance to zero using control knob and with the cap over the top of the cuvette well | | | |
| 11. Remove the "O" tube from well | | | |
| 12. Transfer contents of the "5" tube to a clean cuvette and place in cuvette well | | | |

| You must: | S | U | Comments |
|---|---|---|---|
| 13. Record absorbance. *Note:* Do not adjust control knob | | | |
| 14. Remove cuvette from the sample well | | | |
| 15. Repeat steps 12–14 for tubes 10, 15, and 20 | | | |
| 16. Record the results on worksheet | | | |
| 17. Draw the "X" and "Y" axes as shown in Figure 3–22 | | | |
| 18. Label the "X" axis in units of concentration: 0, 5, 10, 15, and 20 g/dl | | | |
| 19. Label the "Y" axis in absorbance (A) units 0–1.0 using intervals of 0.10 | | | |
| 20. Plot the absorbances of tubes 5, 10, 15, and 20 | | | |
| 21. Draw the best straight line through the points, being sure it passes through the origin (0, 0) | | | |
| 22. Save this graph for use in determining the hemoglobin concentration of a blood sample (Lesson 3–6) | | | |
| 23. Clean the equipment and return to proper storage | | | |
| 24. Clean work area with surface disinfectant | | | |
| 25. Wash hands with hand disinfectant | | | |

Comments:

Student/Instructor:

Date: ______________________ Instructor: ______________________

# Worksheet

NAME ______________________________ DATE ______________

## LESSON 3–5 SPECTROPHOTOMETER

I. Record results from spectrophotometer:

| *Standard Concentration* | *A (or %T)* |
|---|---|
| 0 (blank) | ___ |
| ___ | ___ |
| ___ | ___ |
| ___ | ___ |
| ___ | ___ |

II. Plot A vs. concentration using the graph below. Draw a line connecting the points. The line should pass through the origin (0, 0). (If %T is used, semi-log paper must be used to obtain a straight line.)

# LESSON 3–6

## Hemoglobin Determination

## LESSON OBJECTIVES

After studying this lesson, you should be able to:

- List the two main components of hemoglobin.
- State the function of hemoglobin.
- List two methods for determining hemoglobin and explain each.
- List the normal hemoglobin values for children and adults.
- Determine the hemoglobin concentration in a blood sample using the cyanmethemoglobin method.
- Read a hemoglobin value from a standard curve.
- List precautions to be observed when measuring hemoglobin.
- Define the glossary terms.

## GLOSSARY

**cyanmethemoglobin** / a stable compound formed when hemoglobin is combined with Drabkin's reagent

**Drabkin's reagent** / a diluting reagent used for hemoglobin determination; contains iron, potassium, cyanide, and sodium bicarbonate

**globin** / the portion of the hemoglobin molecule composed of protein

**heme** / the portion of the hemoglobin molecule containing iron

**hemoglobin** / a red blood cell constituent which is composed of heme and globin and which carries oxygen; abbreviated "Hb" or Hgb"

**Sahli pipet** / a pipet with a volume of 0.02 ml, used for manual hemoglobin determinations

**synthesis** / the combining of elements to produce a compound

## THE HEMOGLOBIN MOLECULE

**Hemoglobin** is the main constituent of the red blood cells. This molecule gives the characteristic red color to the erythrocytes and to the blood. The main purpose of hemoglobin is to transport oxygen ($O_2$) to the tissue cells and to carry away the carbon dioxide ($CO_2$) from the tissues.

Determining hemoglobin concentration in the

blood can be performed as part of a CBC or as an individual test. The test is used to indirectly evaluate the oxygen-carrying capacity of the blood. The test may be performed on venous or capillary blood.

The hemoglobin molecule is composed of two substances, **heme** and **globin.** The heme portion of the molecule requires iron for its **synthesis.** If the diet is deficient in iron-rich foods, the red cells will not contain enough hemoglobin and the oxygen-carrying capacity of the blood will be reduced.

## Methods of Determining Hemoglobin

Various methods of determining hemoglobin have been used through the years. Most of these methods utilized the addition of acid or alkali to a blood sample. Procedures based on various principles have been developed. Two that are commonly used are the specific gravity technique and the cyanmethemoglobin method.

***Specific Gravity Technique.*** This method gives only an estimate of hemoglobin concentration and requires no special instrument. A drop of blood is dropped into a pre-prepared copper sulfate ($CuSO_4$) solution of a particular density or specific gravity. If the drop falls to the bottom of the container rapidly, the specific gravity of the blood is greater than the specific gravity of the copper sulfate. Blood with the normal amount of hemoglobin should fall rapidly. Blood with a low hemoglobin concentration does not fall rapidly. This test is commonly used for screening blood donors.

***Cyanmethemoglobin.*** This is the most widely-used hemoglobin method. A dilution of the blood is made by adding 20 $\mu$l of whole blood from a **Sahli pipet** (Figure 3–24) to 5 ml of **Drabkin's reagent.** The red cells are broken down (lysed), releasing the hemoglobin into the solution. The chemicals in Drabkin's reagent react with the released hemoglobin to form a stable pigment. The minimum time for

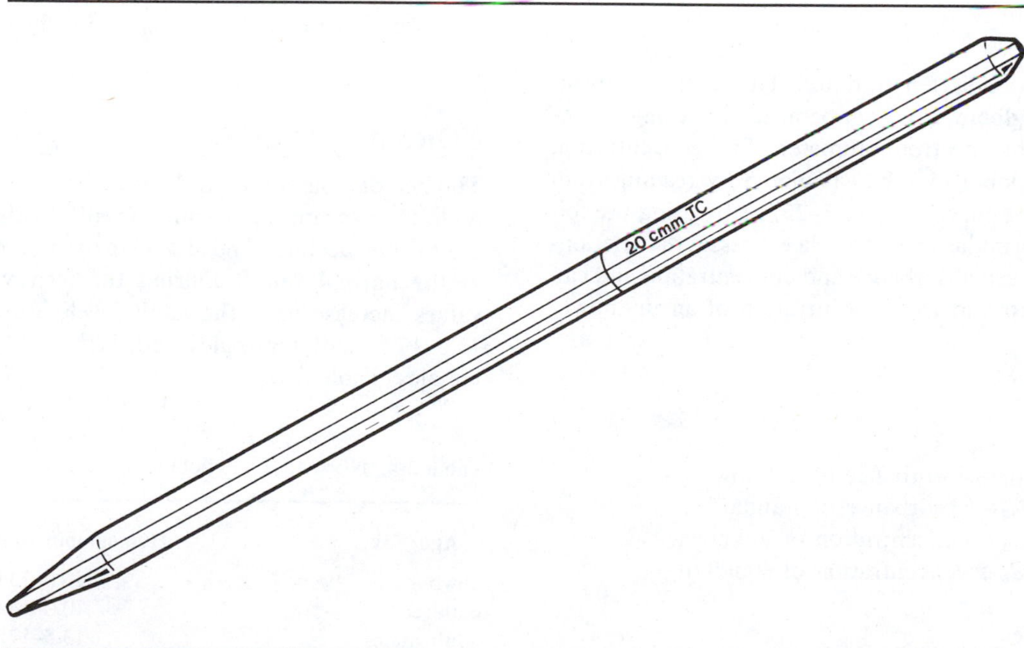


**Figure 3-24.** Sahli pipet

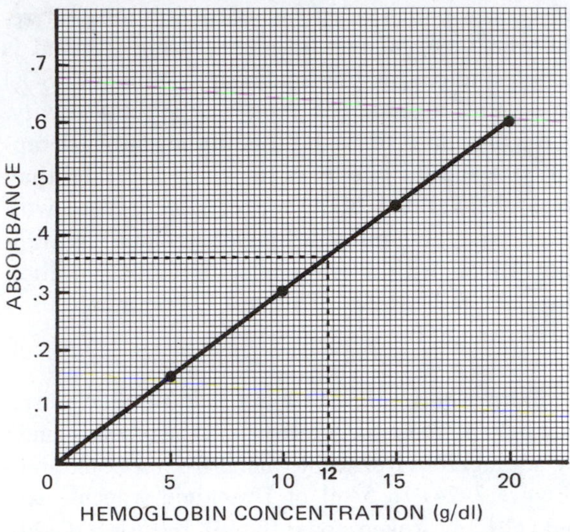


**Figure 3-25.** Determination of the concentration of hemoglobin in a sample by reading from a standard curve. The absorbance of the unknown is .360; the hemoglobin concentration of the unknown is read as 12.0 g/dl from the standard curve.

this reaction is ten minutes. This pigment, **cyanmethemoglobin,** can then be measured using a photometer or spectrophotometer. The concentration of hemoglobin may be calculated by reading from a standard curve (Figure 3–25) or by using the following formula. This formula expresses the relationship between absorbance and concentration and can be used to find the concentration of an unknown.

$$\frac{C_u}{C_s} = \frac{A_u}{A_s}$$

Where: $A_u$ = absorbance of unknown
$A_s$ = absorbance of standard
$C_u$ = concentration of unknown
$C_s$ = concentration of standard

Therefore:

$$C_u = \frac{A_u}{A_s} \times C_s$$

Given the following values, use the absorbance formula to find the hemoglobin concentration of the unknown:

$$A_s = 0.600$$
$$A_u = 0.300$$
$$C_s = 20 \text{ g/dl}$$

Use the absorbance formula:

$$\frac{C_u(\text{g/dl})}{C_s(\text{g/dl})} = \frac{A_u}{A_s}$$

Substitute the values given:

$$\frac{C_u(\text{g/dl})}{20 \text{ g/dl}} = \frac{0.300}{0.600}$$

$C_u$ = 10.0 g/dl. Therefore, the unknown hemoglobin = 10.0 g/dl.

**Figure 3-26.** Sample calculation of hemoglobin using the absorbance formula

A sample hemoglobin calculation is shown in Figure 3–26.

Once formed, the cyanmethemoglobin is stable several months if stored properly. This stability has made it possible to have reliable standards and controls for this method of determining hemoglobin.

## NORMAL VALUES

The hemoglobin values at birth are normally quite high, 16–23 grams per deciliter (g/dl). In childhood, that value declines and 10–14 g/dl is considered in the normal range. During the teen years the values increase until the adult levels are reached: 13.5–17.5 g/dl for males and 12.5–15.5 g/dl for females, Table 3–4.

**Table 3-4.** Normal Hemoglobin Values

| Age/Sex | Hemoglobin Range (g/dl) |
|---|---|
| newborn | 16.0–23.0 |
| children | 10.0–14.0 |
| adult males | 13.5–17.5 |
| adult females | 12.5–15.5 |

## FACTORS AFFECTING THE HEMOGLOBIN LEVELS

There are various factors which affect the hemoglobin level in the blood. The diet must contain enough iron for adequate levels of hemoglobin to be produced. If the diet is deficient in iron, iron-deficiency anemia will result. The age and sex of the individual affects the hemoglobin value. Normally, males have a higher hemoglobin value than females and newborns have a higher hemoglobin value than children and adults. Living at high altitudes increases the hemoglobin level because the body produces more red cells for a greater oxygen-carrying capacity. A bleeding problem in a patient will reduce the hemoglobin level.

## AUTOMATION

There are some situations and localities in which hemoglobin determinations may be performed manually. However, in most laboratories these tests are performed by instrumentation. The instrumentation may be as simple as an automatic diluter which aspirates the correct amount of blood and dispenses the correct amount of Drabkin's reagent. Or, instrumentation may be as complex as a system which draws up the blood sample from a tube and performs the hemoglobin test as a part of the CBC.

### *Precautions*

- Do not mouth pipet the Drabkin's reagent; it contains cyanide and is poisonous.
- Always use clean cuvettes.
- Insure that the dilution is made correctly.
- Set the wavelength at 540 nm.
- Mix the blood ten to twenty times before sampling.
- Do not squeeze the finger hard at the capillary puncture site.

## *LESSON REVIEW*

1. What is the function of hemoglobin?
2. Name two methods of determining hemoglobin.
3. Give the normal hemoglobin values for newborns, children, adult males, and adult females.
4. What is the compound formed when Drabkin's reagent is added to blood?
5. List two components of hemoglobin.
6. Define cyanmethemoglobin, Drabkin's reagent, globin, heme, hemoglobin, Sahli pipet, and synthesis.

## *STUDENT ACTIVITIES*

1. Re-read the information on hemoglobin.
2. Review the glossary terms.
3. Practice the procedure for determining hemoglobin as listed on the Student Performance Guide.
4. Perform hemoglobin determinations on several samples. Read the value of each determination from the standard curve prepared in Lesson 3–5.

# Student Performance Guide

NAME ______________________

DATE ______________________

## LESSON 3–6 HEMOGLOBIN DETERMINATION

### Instructions

1. Practice the procedure for determining hemoglobin concentration.
2. Demonstrate the procedure for hemoglobin determination satisfactorily for the instructor. All steps must be completed as listed on the instructor's Performance Check Sheet.
3. Complete a written examination successfully.

### Materials and Equipment

- hand disinfectant
- spectrophotometer
- graduated pipet, 5 ml
- cuvette
- blood sample
- Sahli pipet
- Drabkin's reagent
- rubber tubing and mouthpiece
- test tubes
- standard hemoglobin solution (20 g/dl)
- standard curve for hemoglobin
- safety bulb for pipet
- parafilm
- surface disinfectant
- biohazard container

*Note:* Consult operating manual for specific instructions for spectrophotometer.

## Procedure

S = Satisfactory
U = Unsatisfactory

| You must: | S | U | Comments |
|---|---|---|---|
| 1. Wash hands with hand disinfectant | | | |
| 2. Assemble equipment and materials | | | |
| 3. Turn on spectrophotometer | | | |
| 4. Set wavelength at 540 nm | | | |
| 5. Label two test tubes: blank and unknown | | | |
| 6. Dispense 5.0 ml of Drabkin's reagent into each test tube using a safety bulb and a 5 ml pipet | | | |
| 7. Attach rubber tubing with mouthpiece to Sahli pipet | | | |
| 8. Draw blood up to 0.02 ml (20 cu mm) mark on the pipet | | | |
| 9. Wipe excess blood from exterior of pipet with tissue | | | |
| 10. Deliver blood sample into the unknown tube by gentle blowing | | | |
| 11. Rinse the pipet at least 3 times with the solution in the tube by alternately aspirating the solution into the pipet and gently blowing it out | | | |
| 12. Mix contents of test tube thoroughly and let it stand for at least ten minutes (tubes can be mixed by inverting after placing parafilm over the top of tube) | | | |
| 13. Transfer contents of the blank tube to a cuvette; place cuvette in the well of spectrophotometer; set absorbance to zero following manufacturer's instructions | | | |
| 14. Transfer contents of unknown tube to a cuvette; place cuvette in the well of spectrophotometer | | | |
| 15. Read the absorbance and record results | | | |
| 16. Pipet 5.0 ml of the 20 gm/dl hemoglobin standard into a cuvette; read the absorbance and record | | | |
| 17. Calculate the hemoglobin concentration by methods a and b: | | | |

| You must | S | U | Comments |
|---|---|---|---|
| a. Use the following formula to calculate hemoglobin concentration and record results $$\frac{A_{unk}}{A_{std}} \times conc_{std} = Conc_{unk}(g/dl)$$ | | | |
| b. Read the hemoglobin concentration from the standard curve constructed in Lesson 3–5 on spectrophotometry; record the results | | | |
| 18. Compare the results of the two methods of calculations | | | |
| 19. Clean equipment and return to proper storage | | | |
| 20. Clean work area with surface disinfectant | | | |
| 21. Wash hands with hand disinfectant | | | |

Comments:

Student/Instructor:

Date: ______________________ Instructor: ______________________

# LESSON 3–7
## Erythrocyte Indices

## LESSON: OBJECTIVES

After studying this lesson, you should be able to:

- State the procedure for determining the erythrocyte indices.
- Write the formulas for each of the three indices.
- Perform the calculations necessary to determine the erythrocyte indices.
- Explain the uses of the erythrocyte indices values.
- List the normal values for the erythrocyte indices.
- Define the glossary terms.

## GLOSSARY

**indices** / plural of index; indexes; erythrocyte indices are values which compare a blood sample to standard values

**mean corpuscular hemoglobin** / MCH; average red cell hemoglobin concentration; an estimate of the hemoglobin in a red cell in a blood specimen; measured in picograms (pg)

**mean corpuscular hemoglobin concentration** / MCHC; compares the weight of hemoglobin in a red cell to the size of the cell; reported in percentage or g/dl

**mean corpuscular volume** / MCV; average red cell volume; an estimate of the volume of a red cell in a blood specimen; measured in femtoliters (fl) or cubic microns ($\mu^3$)

**micron** / a unit of measurement, $1 \times 10^{-6}$ meter or one micrometer

**picogram** / micromicrogram; $1 \times 10^{-12}$ gram; pg

## INTRODUCTION

The erythrocyte **indices** are calculations which yield information concerning the size and the hemoglobin content of the red cells. They are also called the mean corpuscular values. The three indices are: the **mean corpuscular volume (MCV),** the **mean corpuscular hemoglobin (MCH),** and the **mean corpuscular**

$$MCV = \frac{\text{hematocrit (in percent)}}{\text{RBC (in millions)}} \times 10$$

Using a hematocrit of 36% and an RBC of 4.0 million/$mm^3$:

$$MCV = \frac{36}{4.0} \times 10$$

$$MCV = 90 \text{ fl (or } \mu^3)$$

**Figure 3-27.** Calculation of mean corpuscular volume (MCV)

**hemoglobin concentration (MCHC).** These indices aid in classifying the anemias.

The indices are calculated by formulas using the red cell count, the hemoglobin, and the hematocrit. The validity of the indices results depends on the accuracy of those three values.

## Calculation of Mean Corpuscular Volume

The mean corpuscular volume (MCV) is calculated by using the hematocrit percentage and the red blood cell count (Figure 3–27). The result is reported in femtoliters (fl), formerly cubic **microns,** and gives the average volume of a red cell in an individual blood sample. The formula for the MCV is:

$$MCV = \frac{\text{Hematocrit}}{\text{RBC}} \times 10$$

## Calculation of Mean Corpuscular Hemoglobin

The mean corpuscular hemoglobin (MCH) is calculated from the hemoglobin and red cell count values. This result estimates the weight of hemoglobin in a red cell in an individual blood sample. It is expressed in **picograms** (pg). One picogram is equivalent to $10^{-12}$ gram. The formula for the MCH is:

$$MCH = \frac{\text{hemoglobin (in grams)}}{\text{RBC (in millions)}} \times 10$$

Using a hemoglobin value of 15 g/dl and an RBC of 5.2 million/$mm^3$:

$$MCH = \frac{15.0}{5.2} \times 10$$

$$MCH = 28.8 \text{ pg}$$

**Figure 3-28.** Calculation of mean corpuscular hemoglobin (MCH)

$$MCH = \frac{\text{Hemoglobin}}{\text{RBC}} \times 10$$

A sample calculation is shown in Figure 3–28.

## Mean Corpuscular Hemoglobin Concentration

The mean corpuscular hemoglobin concentration (MCHC) is calculated from the hemoglobin and hematocrit results. The MCHC expresses the concentration of hemoglobin in the red cells relative to cell size. It is reported in percentage or g/dl since it actually is a comparison of hemoglobin to the hematocrit. The formula is:

$$MCHC = \frac{\text{Hemoglobin}}{\text{Hct}} \times 100$$

A sample calculation is shown in Figure 3–29.

$$MCHC = \frac{\text{hemoglobin (in grams)}}{\text{hematocrit}} \times 100$$

Using a hemoglobin value of 15 g/dl and a hematocrit of 44%:

$$MCHC = \frac{15}{44} \times 100$$

$$MCHC = 34\% \text{ or } 34 \text{ g/dl}$$

**Figure 3-29.** Calculation of mean corpuscular hemoglobin concentration (MCHC)

**Table 3-5.** Normal Values for Erythrocyte Indices

| | Normal Values |
|---|---|
| MCV | 80–100 fl |
| MCH | 27–32 pg |
| MCHC | 33–38% |

## NORMAL VALUES (TABLE 3-5)

The normal range for the MCV is 80–100 femtoliters (fl). A cell with an MCV below 80 fl is said to be *microcytic. Macrocytic* cells are those having an MCV greater than 100 fl.

The normal range for the MCH is 27–32 picograms (pg). A value below 27 pg indicates a low weight of hemoglobin in the red cells and could be found in microcytes or normocytes. A value greater than 32 pg could be found in macrocytes.

The normal range for the MCHC is 33–38% (or g/dl). This relationship compares the concentration of hemoglobin to the packed volume of red cells. It gives the concentration (percentage) of hemoglobin in the red cells. The normal range is 32–37%. Values less than 32% indicate less hemoglobin than is normal for that red cell population. This is referred to as *hypochromia.* A value greater than normal is not possible since it would indicate that the cell is supersaturated or contains more hemoglobin than it can actually hold.

## FACTORS WHICH AFFECT THE INDICES

The indices results can be used to classify the anemias. In iron deficiency anemia, which is characterized by hypochromia and microcytes, all three indices values will be decreased. In the macrocytic anemias, such as pernicious anemia or $B_{12}$ deficiency anemia, the MCV and the MCH are increased.

### Sources of Error

There is much chance for error in the calculation of the erythrocyte indices. All of the calculations rely on the results obtained from the red blood cell counts, the hematocrits, and the hemoglobins. Any error in those results will in turn cause error in the indices results.

## AUTOMATION

Almost all medical laboratories now have instrumentation to perform the complete blood count (CBC). These instruments use the values from the hemoglobin, red blood cell count, and hematocrit to calculate the erythrocyte indices. In a physician's office, such automation is not usually available. In such cases, the indices are calculated manually or using an indices calculator, and are performed infrequently.

***Precautions***

- The Hgb, Hct, and RBC values inserted in the formulas must be accurate.
- The correct values must be inserted in the formulas.
- The calculations must be performed correctly.

## *LESSON REVIEW*

1. Results from which three hematology procedures are used to calculate the indices?
2. State one use of the indices.
3. What is the normal value for the MCV?

4. In what units are the MCH and the MCHC reported?
5. What does an MCV greater than 100 cubic microns indicate?
6. Give the normal values for the MCH and MCHC.
7. Define indices, MCV, MCH, MCHC, micron, and picogram.

## *STUDENT ACTIVITIES*

1. Re-read the information on erythrocyte indices.
2. Review the glossary terms.
3. Practice calculating erythrocyte indices as outlined on the Student Performance Guide, using the worksheet.

# Student Performance Guide

NAME ____________________

DATE ____________________

## LESSON 3–7
## ERYTHROCYTE INDICES

### Instructions

1. Practice the procedure for calculating the erythrocyte indices.
2. Demonstrate the procedure for performing Hgb, Hct, and RBC on a sample and calculating the erythrocyte indices satisfactorily for the instructor. All steps must be completed as listed on the instructor's Performance Check Sheet.
3. Complete a written examination successfully.

### Materials and Equipment

- hand disinfectant
- tube of venous blood, anticoagulated (or use capillary blood)
- materials for capillary puncture (optional)
- worksheet
- surface disinfectant
- biohazard container

Materials for RBC count:

- RBC blood diluting pipets
- rubber tubing and mouthpiece
- RBC diluting fluid
- hemacytometer and coverglass
- lens paper
- alcohol
- microscope

Materials for hemoglobin determination:

- spectrophotometer
- Drabkin's reagent
- Sahli pipet
- cuvettes
- test tubes

Materials for hematocrit:

- capillary tubes
- sealing clay
- microhematocrit centrifuge
- microhematocrit reader

## Procedure

S = Satisfactory
U = Unsatisfactory

| You must: | S | U | Comments |
|---|---|---|---|
| 1. Wash hands with hand disinfectant | | | |
| 2. Assemble appropriate equipment and materials for Hgb, Hct, and RBC procedures | | | |
| 3. Perform Hgb, Hct, and RBC from either capillary puncture or well-mixed tube of previously-drawn blood, and record results | | | |
| 4. Calculate the MCV on the worksheet and record the result | | | |
| 5. Calculate the MCH on the worksheet and record the result | | | |
| 6. Calculate the MCHC on the worksheet and record the result | | | |
| 7. Dispose of sharp objects in a biohazard container | | | |
| 8. Clean equipment and return to proper storage | | | |
| 9. Clean work area with surface disinfectant | | | |
| 10. Wash hands with hand disinfectant | | | |

Comments:

Student/Instructor:

Date: ______________________ Instructor: ______________________________

# Worksheet

NAME ______________________________ DATE ______________

SPECIMEN NO. ______________

## LESSON 3–7 ERYTHROCYTE INDICES

RBC/$mm^3$ = _______

Hb (g/dl) = _______

Hct (%) = _______

**1.** Calculate the MCV:

**2.** Calculate the MCH:

**3.** Calculate the MCHC:

# LESSON 3–8

## Bleeding Time

## LESSON OBJECTIVES

After studying this lesson, you should be able to:

- State the purpose of the bleeding time test.
- Name three components that interact to cause hemostasis.
- Name and describe two methods used to determine the bleeding time and list the normal values of each.
- List three conditions in which the bleeding time will be prolonged.
- Perform a bleeding time test.
- Name the puncture sites used in the Ivy and Duke bleeding time tests.
- Report the results of a bleeding time.
- List the precautions to be observed in performing a bleeding time.
- Define the glossary terms.

## GLOSSARY

**coagulation factors** / proteins present in plasma which interact to form the fibrin clot

**dysfunction** / impaired or abnormal function

**hemorrhage** / excessive or uncontrolled bleeding

**vasoconstriction** / a contracting or narrowing of a vessel

## INTRODUCTION

The bleeding time test is a screening procedure used to evaluate some aspects of the body's ability to stop bleeding. The bleeding time test is performed by making a small standardized incision of the capillaries. The length of time required for the bleeding to stop is then measured.

## HEMOSTASIS

*Hemostasis,* the cessation of bleeding, involves a series of complex interactions. The components which must interact are (1) the blood vessels, (2) the blood platelets, and (3) the plasma proteins called **coagulation factors.** The blood vessels must have the ability to constrict and slow blood flow after an injury. This property is known as **vasoconstriction.** The platelets react within seconds after an injury to form a plug and to release certain chemical activators. The coagulation factors, proteins in the plasma, are activated by the platelets and the injured tissue.

When all the hemostasis components interact and function properly, a clot is formed and bleeding stops. The failure of the clotting mechanism can be due to the absence, deficiency, or improper function of any of the components. Failure of the hemostatic or clotting mechanism may result in **hemorrhage.**

Several laboratory tests can be performed which will detect deficiencies of the hemostatic system. The bleeding time is one of these tests. It is influenced by the number and function of platelets and the condition of the vessels. The bleeding time may be prolonged in thrombocytopenia, platelet **dysfunction,** and after ingestion of aspirin. The bleeding time is usually normal when there is a deficiency of only one of the coagulation factors.

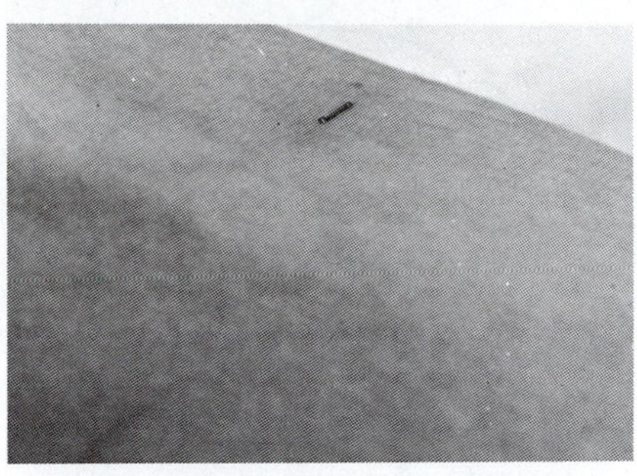

**Figure 3-30.** Puncture site in Ivy bleeding time (*Photo courtesy of General Diagnostics Division of Warner Lambert*)

## METHODS OF MEASURING BLEEDING TIME

Two methods for measuring the bleeding time are the Ivy method and the Duke method. The Ivy method, although more difficult to perform correctly, is the preferred method because it is more sensitive. Both of these tests and other coagulation tests must be performed carefully and accurately by well-trained technicians.

### Ivy Bleeding Time

The Ivy bleeding time is performed by incising the forearm and measuring the time required for bleeding to stop. A blood pressure cuff is placed around the patient's arm above the elbow, and the pressure is increased to 40 mm of mercury to standardize the pressure in the capillaries. This pressure is held constant for the entire procedure. The forearm is cleansed with 70% alcohol. A 3 mm deep incision is made in an area that is free of large superficial blood vessels (Figure 3–30). A stopwatch is started when the first drop of blood appears. At thirty second intervals, the blood is blotted with filter paper without touching the puncture site (Figure 3–31). When the bleeding ceases, the time is noted and

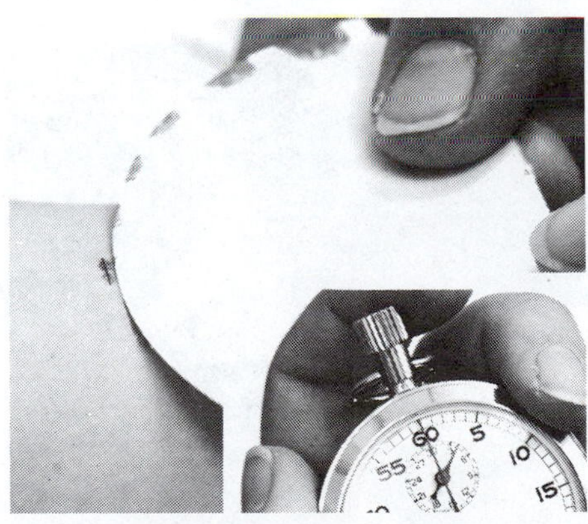


**Figure 3-31.** Blotting blood with filter paper in Ivy bleeding time (*Photo courtesy of General Diagnostics Division of Warner Lambert*)

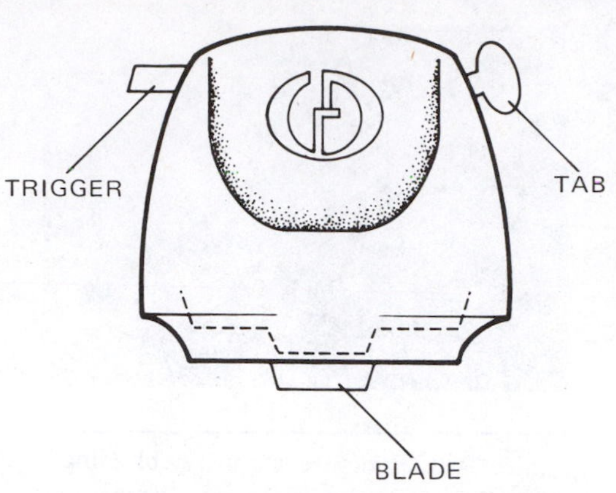


**Figure 3-32.** Simplate® device used in performing bleeding time test

the pressure cuff is removed. The time between the first appearance of blood and the stopping of blood flow is the bleeding time. The normal bleeding time by the Ivy method is one to seven minutes. This method may also be performed using a device called a Simplate® which makes a more standardized incision than a lancet or blade (Figures 3–32 and 3–33).

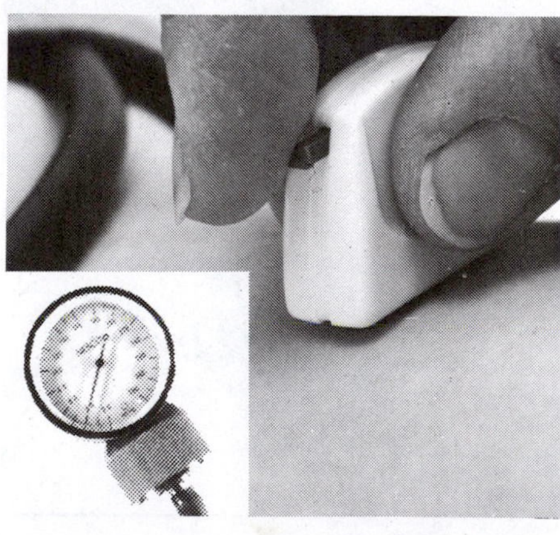

**Figure 3-33.** Performing a bleeding time test using a Simplate® (*Photo courtesy of General Diagnostics Division of Warner Lambert*)

## Duke Bleeding Time

The Duke bleeding time is performed by incising the earlobe and measuring the time required for bleeding to cease. The earlobe is cleansed with alcohol and allowed to dry. A 2–3 mm deep puncture is made with a sterile lancet (Figure 3–34) and timing is begun when the first drop of blood appears. The blood is blotted every thirty seconds with filter paper and without touching the puncture site. The watch is stopped when bleeding ceases. The time elapsed is reported as the bleeding time. The normal bleeding time by the Duke method is one to three minutes.

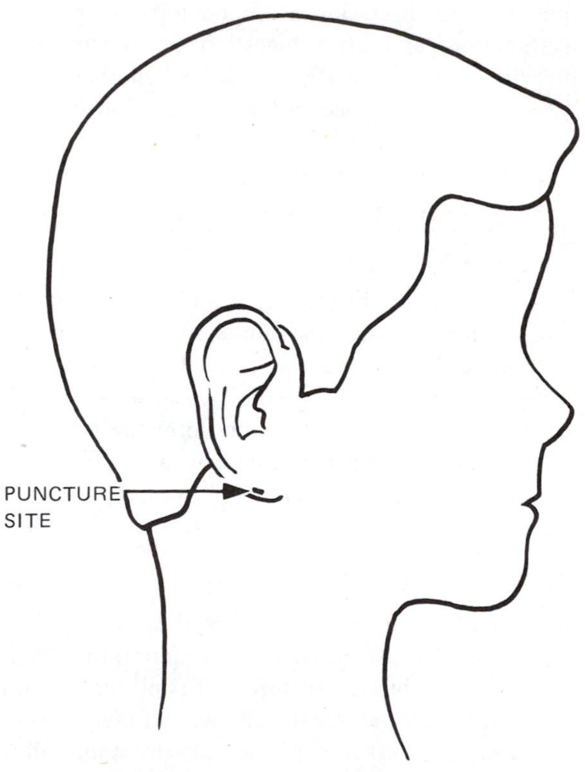


**Figure 3-34.** Puncture site for Duke bleeding time

### *Precautions*

- Do not perform the bleeding time test if the patient has taken aspirin within seven days of the test.
- The puncture site should be warm to ensure that circulation is good.
- The puncture site should be in an area free of superficial veins, so that only capillaries are punctured.
- The puncture site must be dry before the incision is made.
- The first drop of blood that appears after the puncture is not wiped away.
- If bleeding continues more than ten minutes (Duke) or fifteen minutes (Ivy), stop the test and apply pressure to the wound.
- When blotting the blood with filter paper, the paper should not touch the puncture site, to insure that clot formation is not disturbed.

## *LESSON REVIEW*

1. What does the bleeding time measure?
2. What three components interact to cause hemostasis?
3. Name three conditions in which the bleeding time will be prolonged.
4. Explain the procedure for the Ivy bleeding time.
5. Explain the procedure for the Duke bleeding time.
6. State the normal ranges for bleeding times by the Ivy method and the Duke method.
7. List four precautions which should be observed when performing a bleeding time test.
8. What puncture site is used for the Ivy bleeding time—for the Duke bleeding time?
9. Define coagulation factors, dysfunction, hemorrhage, and vasoconstriction.

## *STUDENT ACTIVITIES*

1. Re-read the information on bleeding time.
2. Review the glossary terms.
3. Practice explaining the bleeding time procedure to a patient.
4. Practice performing a bleeding time, by the Duke method, as outlined on the Student Performance Guide.

# Student Performance Guide

NAME ____________________

DATE ____________________

## LESSON 3–8
## BLEEDING TIME

### Instructions

1. Practice performing a bleeding time test (Duke method).
2. Demonstrate the procedure for the bleeding time test satisfactorily for the instructor. All steps must be completed as outlined on the instructor's Performance Check Sheet.
3. Complete a written examination successfully.

### Materials and Equipment

- hand disinfectant
- sterile cotton balls or gauze
- 70% alcohol or alcohol swabs
- blood lancets
- filter paper
- stopwatch
- clean microscope slide
- surface disinfectant
- biohazard container

**Procedure**

S = Satisfactory
U = Unsatisfactory

| You must: | S | U | Comments |
|---|---|---|---|
| 1. Wash hands with hand disinfectant | | | |
| 2. Assemble equipment and materials | | | |
| 3. Explain the procedure to the patient | | | |
| 4. Cleanse the earlobe with 70% alcohol and allow to dry (or wipe dry with dry sterile gauze) | | | |

| You must: | S | U | Comments |
|---|---|---|---|
| 5. Puncture the earlobe with a sterile lancet and start the stopwatch | | | |
| 6. *Do not* wipe away the first drop of blood | | | |
| 7. Blot the blood with filter paper every thirty seconds by lightly touching the edge of the drop. Do not touch puncture site with filter paper | | | |
| 8. Stop the watch when blood is no longer absorbed onto the filter paper | | | |
| 9. Report the bleeding time to the nearest thirty seconds | | | |
| 10. Treat the puncture site by cleansing gently without disturbing the clot | | | |
| 11. Clean equipment and return to proper storage | | | |
| 12. Clean work area with surface disinfectant | | | |
| 13. Wash hands with hand disinfectant | | | |
| Comments: | | | |
| Student/Instructor: | | | |

Date: ______________________ Instructor: ______________________

# LESSON 3–9

## Capillary Coagulation

### LESSON OBJECTIVES

After studying this lesson, you should be able to:

- List the component of the hemostatic mechanism which is tested by the capillary coagulation procedure.
- List a situation in which the capillary coagulation procedure would be performed.
- Perform a capillary coagulation procedure.
- List the normal capillary coagulation time.
- Name three conditions that may cause a prolonged capillary coagulation time.
- List the precautions to observe when performing the capillary coagulation procedure.
- Define the glossary terms.

### GLOSSARY

**coagulation** / formation of a fibrin clot which aids in stopping bleeding

**fibrin** / protein filaments formed in the coagulation process, resulting from the action of the enzyme, thrombin, on the plasma protein, fibrinogen

## INTRODUCTION

The capillary coagulation test is a simple procedure. It is used to screen for problems in the blood clotting or **coagulation** mechanism. It measures the amount of time needed for the blood to form a **fibrin** clot. This procedure tests the function of the coagulation factors rather than of the platelets or blood vessels. Delayed clotting or lack of clotting can be due to a deficiency in any one or more of the coagulation factors.

The capillary coagulation test is not a specific test. Thus, it has been largely replaced by other tests which are newer and more specific. However, the capillary coagulation test may still be used to screen pediatric patients before surgical procedures such as tonsillectomy or adenoidectomy.

## PERFORMING THE PROCEDURE

The capillary coagulation test is performed by making a capillary puncture of the fingertip with as little trauma to the tissue as possible. The first drop of blood is wiped away using a sterile cotton or gauze. A stopwatch is started when the second drop of blood appears. At least three special capillary coagulation tubes are filled three-fourths full and laid horizontally on the counter top. The tubes are left undisturbed until two minutes have passed from the starting of the watch. Meanwhile, place a gauze over the puncture site and have the patient apply pressure. When two minutes have passed, the first tube filled is picked up and one-half inch of the tube is carefully broken off at one end (Figure 3–35). The two broken ends are gently pulled apart (about one-quarter to one-half inch) to look for the fibrin thread. If a fibrin thread is not seen, breaks are made in the same tube every thirty seconds until a fibrin thread has formed and is observed. If the thread is not observed in the first tube, the second and third tubes are broken in the same manner. The stopwatch is stopped when the fibrin thread is first seen (Figure 3–36). The capillary coagulation time is the time on the stopwatch (or the time elapsed between the appearance of the second drop of blood and the formation of fibrin).

## NORMAL VALUES

The normal time for a fibrin thread to appear in the capillary coagulation time test is two to six minutes. There are various factors which can affect the coagulation time. Many of the coagulation factors are produced in the liver and are affected by any disease of or damage to the liver. Production of some of the factors is dependent on vitamin K and

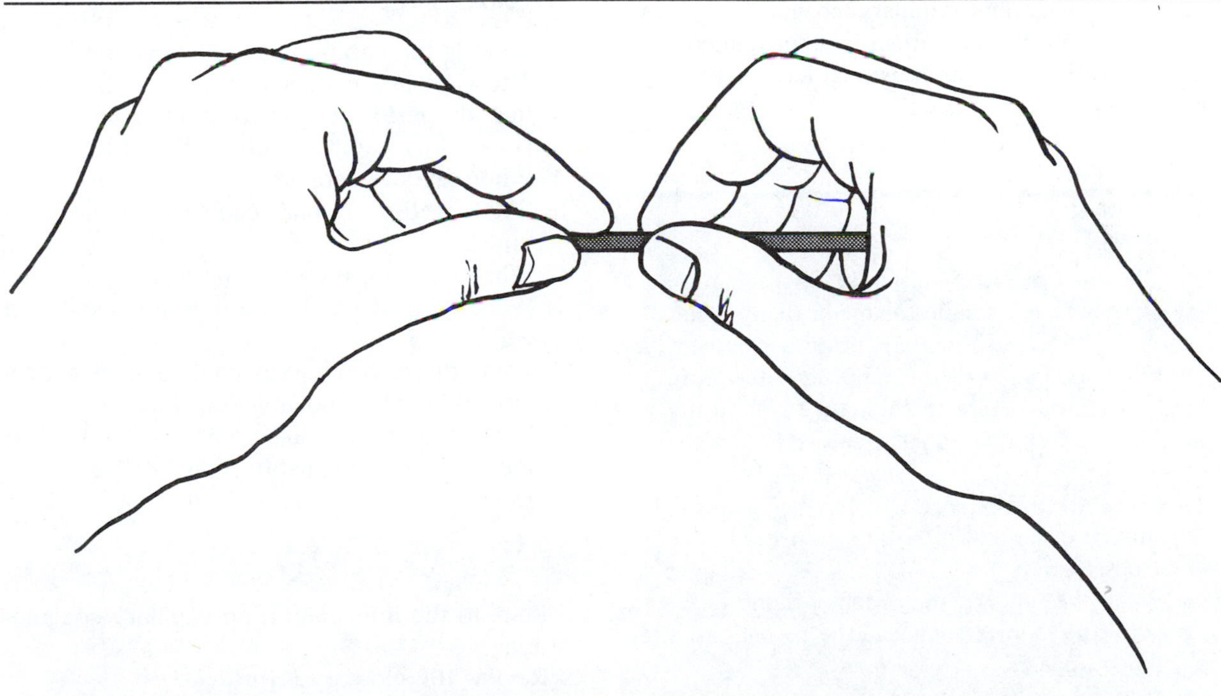

**Figure 3-35.** Capillary coagulation: breaking the capillary tube

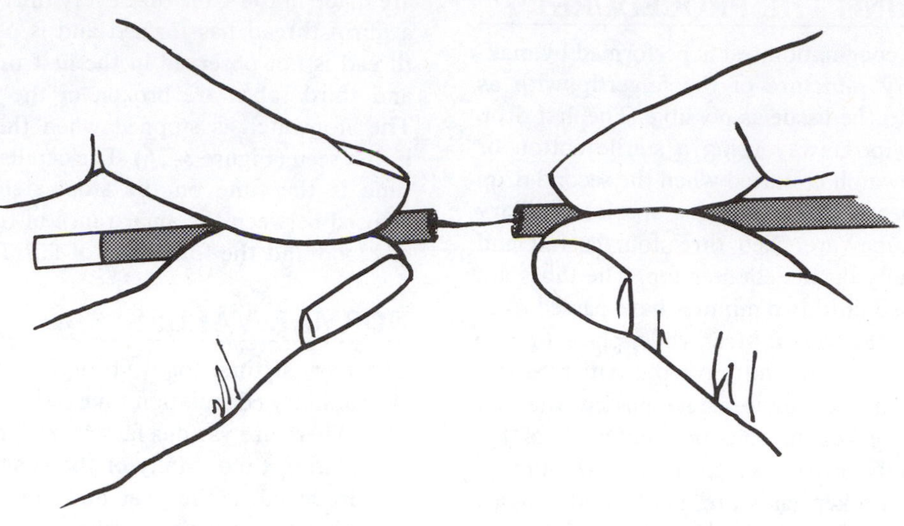

**Figure 3-36.** Capillary coagulation: appearance of the fibrin thread

a deficiency of that vitamin can prolong the coagulation time. Abnormal capillary coagulation times may also occur when a patient is taking anticoagulant medication, or if an individual has a deficiency of one or more factors.

### *Precautions*

- Use only tubes made specially for coagulation tests; they have a smaller diameter than regular capillary tubes and contain no anticoagulant.
- Fill at least two or three tubes since the fibrin may not form before the first tube is used up.
- The finger should not be squeezed hard when filling the tubes.
- Break the tubes carefully to avoid cutting the fingers or destroying the fibrin thread before it is observed.
- Break the tubes in the order of filling.
- Start the stopwatch when the second drop of blood appears.
- Stop the watch when the fibrin thread is first observed.

## *LESSON REVIEW*

1. What is the capillary coagulation time?
2. The capillary coagulation time is most frequently performed on what age patient?
3. How many capillary tubes should be filled?
4. When are the capillary tubes broken?
5. What is the normal capillary coagulation time?
6. What signals the end of the test?
7. What type of capillary tubes are used and why?
8. What three conditions could cause a prolonged capillary coagulation time?
9. What component of hemostasis is tested in the capillary coagulation time?
10. Define coagulation and fibrin.

## *STUDENT ACTIVITIES*

1. Re-read the information on capillary coagulation.
2. Review the glossary terms.
3. Practice performing a capillary coagulation time as outlined on the Student Performance Guide.

# Student Performance Guide

NAME ______________________

DATE ______________________

## LESSON 3–9
## CAPILLARY COAGULATION

### Instructions

1. Practice the procedure for capillary coagulation.
2. Demonstrate the procedure for performing the capillary coagulation time satisfactorily for the instructor. All steps must be completed as listed on the instructor's Performance Check Sheet.
3. Complete a written examination successfully.

### Materials and Equipment

- hand disinfectant
- capillary puncture materials
- stopwatch
- capillary coagulation tubes
- surface disinfectant
- biohazard container

### Procedure

S = Satisfactory
U = Unsatisfactory

| You must: | S | U | Comments |
|---|---|---|---|
| 1. Wash hands with hand disinfectant | | | |
| 2. Assemble equipment and materials | | | |
| 3. Perform capillary puncture using proper procedure | | | |
| 4. Wipe away the first drop of blood with sterile gauze | | | |
| 5. Start the stopwatch when the second drop of blood | | | |

| You must: | S | U | Comments |
|---|---|---|---|
| appears and fill one capillary coagulation tube three-fourths full | | | |
| 6. Place the filled capillary tube on the counter top | | | |
| 7. Fill two additional tubes and place them on the counter top in the order in which they were filled | | | |
| 8. Place gauze over puncture site and have patient apply pressure | | | |
| 9. Observe the stopwatch until two minutes have passed (from start) | | | |
| 10. Pick up the first tube filled (at the two-minute time) and gently break approximately one-half inch from end | | | |
| 11. Look carefully for a fibrin thread. If a thread is not observed, continue breaking a segment every thirty seconds | | | |
| 12. Break one-half inch segments from the second tube every thirty seconds if a thread is not seen in the first tube | | | |
| 13. Continue breaking the segments every thirty seconds until a fibrin thread is observed | | | |
| 14. Stop the stopwatch when the fibrin thread is observed | | | |
| 15. Record the total time elapsed as the capillary coagulation time | | | |
| 16. Dispose of lancets and capillary tubes in a biohazard container for sharp objects | | | |
| 17. Clean equipment and return to proper storage | | | |
| 18. Clean work area with surface disinfectant | | | |
| 19. Wash hands with hand disinfectant | | | |

Comments:

Student/Instructor:

Date: ______________________ Instructor: ______________________

# UNIT 4

# Introduction To Serology

## UNIT OBJECTIVES

After studying this unit, you should be able to:

- Perform ABO slide typing.
- Perform ABO tube typing.
- Perform Rh slide typing.
- Perform a slide test for pregnancy.
- Perform a slide test for infectious mononucleosis.

## OVERVIEW

Immunology is the study of the body's responses which protect us from disease or provide immunity. Most of us think of immunity as the production of antibodies in response to foreign substances which are called antigens. Serology, a branch of immunology, is a term used for laboratory procedures which utilize the antigen-antibody reaction in the tests. Serology was named because early laboratories used serum for testing. Today, most serological procedures use serum, whole blood, or urine for testing.

Modern serology laboratories detect, identify, and measure antibodies found in diseases such as infectious mononucleosis and rheumatoid arthritis. Other serological procedures may use antibodies to identify substances such as hormones, as in the pregnancy test.

Immunohematology, or blood banking, is a specialized branch of immunology which uses serological procedures to study and identify the blood groups. Procedures in blood banking may be simple, such as routine ABO and Rh blood typing. Or, blood banking may involve more complex procedures such as identifying tissue antigens for organ transplantation.

The exercises in Unit 4 are an introduction to new techniques, such as agglutination and agglutination inhibition, which are commonly used in laboratories and require minimum equipment and time.

# LESSON 4–1

## ABO Slide Typing

### LESSON OBJECTIVES

After studying this lesson, you should be able to:

- Name the four blood groups in the ABO system.
- State the frequency of the four blood groups.
- Name the blood group antigens and antibodies found in each of the four groups.
- Explain forward typing.
- Perform an ABO slide typing on a blood sample.
- Interpret the results of an ABO slide typing.
- List the precautions to be observed in an ABO slide typing.
- Define the glossary terms.

### GLOSSARY

**agglutination** / clumping of cells or particles; in serology due to reaction of the particle with antibody

**antiserum** / serum containing antibodies

**blood group antibody** / a serum protein that reacts specifically with a blood group antigen

**blood group antigen** / a substance or structure on the red cell membrane which causes antibody formation and reacts with that antibody

**serology** / laboratory study of serum and the reactions between antigens and antibodies

### INTRODUCTION

ABO typing may be performed using a slide test or a tube test. The slide method is quick, easy, and requires no special equipment. However, the tube test (Lesson 4–2) is the preferred method and is used most commonly in medical laboratories.

The ABO system is the major human blood group system. A patient's ABO group (or type) must be determined before a blood transfusion can be given. Blood groups must also be considered in organ transplantation, questions of paternity, forensic investigations, and genetic studies.

**Table 4-1.** Table of ABO Antigens and Antibodies

| ABO group | Antigen on Red Blood Cells | Antibody in Serum |
|---|---|---|
| A | A | anti–B |
| B | B | anti–A |
| AB | A and B | neither anti–A nor anti–B |
| O | neither A nor B | both anti–A and anti–B |

## A AND B ANTIGENS

**Serology** is the laboratory study of serum and the reactions between antigens and antibodies. *Immunohematology,* a branch of serology, is the study of the blood groups. The ABO blood group system, which is the major human blood group system, was discovered around 1900. All humans can be placed into one of four major groups: A, B, AB, or O. This grouping is based on the presence or absence of two **blood group antigens,** which are substances found on the surface of the red blood cells. The ability to produce these antigens is an inherited characteristic. These antigens are named A and B. Individuals are grouped according to the antigens present on their cells: a person who is type A has A antigen; a person who is type B has B antigen; a person who is type AB has A and B antigens; and a person who is type O has neither A nor B antigen (Table 4–1). The slide test is a procedure which detects A and/or B antigen on the red blood cells, a procedure called *forward* or *direct typing.*

## ANTIBODIES

The discovery of the A and B antigens was accompanied by the discovery of the corresponding **blood group antibodies** in human blood. An *antibody* is a serum protein molecule that reacts with an antigen. If the antigen is on a particle such as a cell, the antibody can cause **agglutination** or clumping of the cells. This reaction can be easily seen. Antibodies are named according to the antigen they react with: an antibody that reacts with A antigen (A red cells) is called anti–A; an antibody that reacts with B antigen (B red cells) is called anti–B. Since O cells are named because they have no A or B antigen, there is no anti–O antibody.

Blood group antibodies occur naturally in serum. If an antigen is missing from an individual's cells, the antibody specific for the missing antigen will be present. For example, an individual who is type A will have anti–B antibody in their serum. A person who is type O will have anti–A and anti–B antibodies since O cells have neither A nor B antigen (Table 4–1). Testing serum for the presence of the blood group antibodies is called *reverse* or *indirect typing.*

### Frequency of ABO Groups

The blood group antigens are products of inherited genes. In the United States, about forty-five percent of the population is O and forty-one percent is A. Only ten percent of the population is B and four percent is AB.

### Importance of ABO Typing

ABO typing is performed so that blood may be matched if a transfusion is necessary. An individual should be transfused with blood of the same ABO group. The rule to follow in transfusing blood is to avoid giving the patient an antigen they do not already have. In an emergency, O blood may be used because it contains neither A nor B antigen. For this reason, people of blood group O have been called universal donors.

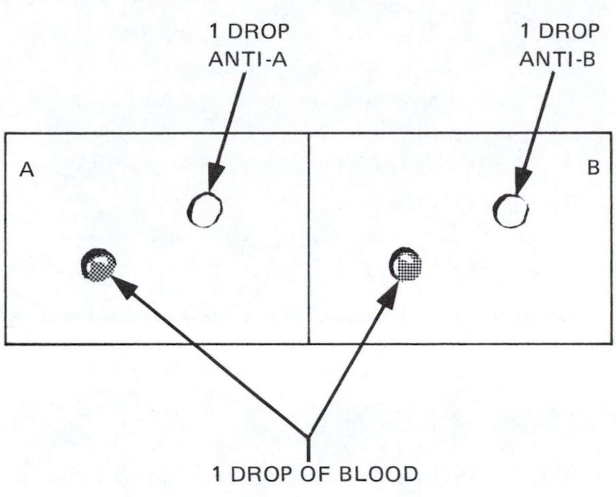


**Figure 4-1.** ABO slide typing: microscope slide with antisera and blood added

## PRINCIPLE OF SLIDE TYPING

The slide test detects the A or B antigens on red cells by using the principle of agglutination. This procedure may be called direct or forward typing and is accomplished by combining cells of unknown type with a known **antiserum** and observing for agglutination. If the antigen present on the cells corresponds to the antibody in the antiserum, agglutination will occur. If the antigen is not present on the cells, no agglutination will be observed.

## PERFORMING ABO SLIDE TYPING

Slide typing is performed using a clean microscope slide which has been marked into two halves using a wax pencil. One drop of anti–A is added to the left side and one drop of anti–B to the right side. A small drop of well-mixed blood, capillary or venous, is placed on each side of the slide (Figure 4–1). The anti–A is mixed with one drop of the blood using a wooden applicator stick. The procedure is repeated using a clean applicator stick for anti–B and the other drop of blood (Figure 4–2).

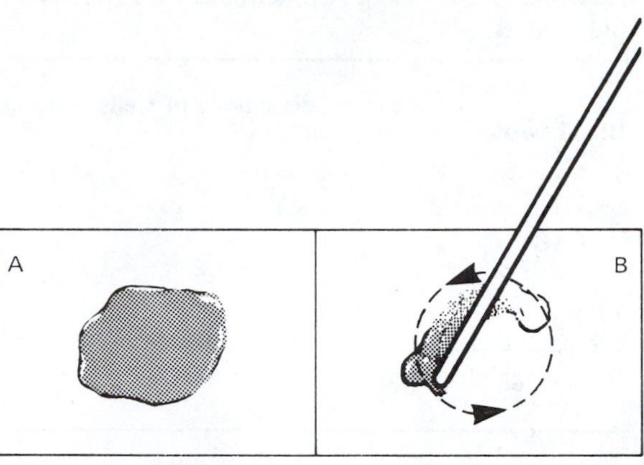


**Figure 4-2.** ABO slide typing: mixing antisera and blood

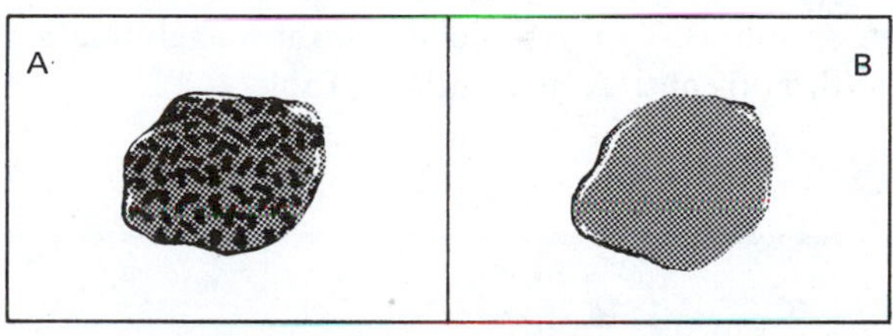


**Figure 4-3.** Agglutination of blood cells by anti–A in ABO typing. Reaction shown indicates type A blood.

The slide is then rocked gently for two minutes and observed under good light for agglutination. Agglutination will appear as a clumping together of the red cells (Figure 4–3). The results should be recorded as positive (+) or negative (0) for each antibody.

## INTERPRETATION OF SLIDE TYPING RESULTS

If only the A antigen is present on the red cells, the cells will agglutinate with anti–A but not with

**Table 4-2.** Reactions of ABO Groups with Anti–A and Anti–B

| Blood Group | Reactions of Cells with: anti–A | anti–B |
|---|---|---|
| A | + | 0 |
| B | 0 | + |
| AB | + | + |
| O | 0 | 0 |

+ = agglutination
0 = no agglutination

anti–B. If only B antigen is present, the cells will agglutinate with anti–B but not with anti–A. Type O blood will show no agglutination with either anti–A or anti–B. Type AB blood will show agglutination with both anti–A and anti–B (Table 4–2).

### *Precautions*

- All reagents must be in date and equipment must be clean.
- Manufacturer's instructions for the use of antisera should be observed.
- Care should be taken to prevent contamination of antisera.
- If capillary blood is used, the slide typing must be completed before clotting occurs.
- Timing should be observed carefully; drying around the edges of the cell mixture should not be confused with agglutination.
- Reactions should be observed under good lighting conditions.
- Results should be recorded as soon as they are observed to avoid error.
- Forward typing should be confirmed by reverse typing.

## *LESSON REVIEW*

1. What antigens present on red blood cells determine the ABO groups?
2. Name the four groups in the ABO system and give the frequency of each.
3. What antibody is present in the serum of a person who is type B—type O?
4. What agglutination results would be observed when testing type A blood with anti–A and anti–B—when testing type AB blood?
5. What is being tested in forward typing?
6. Define agglutination, antiserum, blood group antibody, blood group antigen, and serology.

## *STUDENT ACTIVITIES*

1. Re-read the information on ABO typing.
2. Review the glossary terms.
3. Practice performing ABO slide typing as outlined on the Student Performance Guide, using the worksheet.

# Student Performance Guide

NAME ______________________

DATE ______________________

## LESSON 4–1
## ABO SLIDE TYPING

### Instructions

1. Practice performing ABO slide typing.
2. Demonstrate the procedure for ABO slide typing satisfactorily for the instructor. All steps must be completed as listed on the instructor's Performance Check Sheet.
3. Complete a written examination successfully.

### Materials and Equipment

- hand disinfectant
- blood samples, anticoagulated venous
- anti–A serum
- anti–B serum
- pasteur pipets and bulb
- clean microscope slides (or typing slides)
- wax pencil
- wooden applicator sticks
- light source
- blood typing worksheet
- stopwatch
- surface disinfectant
- biohazard container

*Note:* Package insert should be consulted for specific instructions before test is performed.

**Procedure** — S = Satisfactory, U = Unsatisfactory

| You must: | S | U | Comments |
|---|---|---|---|
| 1. Wash hands with hand disinfectant | | | |
| 2. Assemble equipment and materials | | | |
| 3. Place a clean microscope slide on the work area | | | |

| You must: | S | U | Comments |
|---|---|---|---|
| 4. Mark the slide into two halves using a wax pencil | | | |
| 5. Label the left side "A" and the right side "B" | | | |
| 6. Place one drop of anti–A on the "A" side (do not allow dropper to touch slide) | | | |
| 7. Place one drop of anti–B on the "B" side (do not allow dropper to touch slide) | | | |
| 8. Add one drop of well-mixed blood to each side of the slide using the pasteur pipet (the drop of blood should be no larger than the drop of antibody) | | | |
| 9. Mix the blood and antiserum on side A into a smooth round circle about the size of a quarter using a clean wooden applicator stick | | | |
| 10. Repeat the same procedure on side B using a clean applicator stick | | | |
| 11. Rock the slide gently for two minutes and look for agglutination using strong light | | | |
| 12. Record agglutination results on worksheet: + = agglutination, 0 = no agglutination | | | |
| 13. Determine the blood group and record | | | |
| 14. Repeat steps 3–13 on additional blood samples | | | |
| 15. Discard specimens appropriately | | | |
| 16. Clean equipment and return to proper storage | | | |
| 17. Clean work area with disinfectant | | | |
| 18. Wash hands with hand disinfectant | | | |

Comments:

Student/Instructor:

Date: ______________________ Instructor: ______________________

# Worksheet

NAME ______________________________ DATE ______________

## LESSON 4–1 ABO SLIDE TYPING

| Sample # | Agglutination Results* anti–A | anti–B | Interpretation ABO Group |
|---|---|---|---|
| ______ | ____ | ____ | ________ |
| ______ | ____ | ____ | ________ |
| ______ | ____ | ____ | ________ |
| ______ | ____ | ____ | ________ |
| ______ | ____ | ____ | ________ |

* Record results as:
0 = no agglutination
+ = agglutination

# LESSON 4–2
## ABO Tube Typing

### LESSON OBJECTIVES

After completion of this lesson, you should be able to:

- Explain reverse or indirect typing.
- Perform ABO forward and reverse typing by the tube method.
- Interpret the results of tube typing tests.
- List the precautions to be observed in performing ABO tube typing.
- Define the glossary terms.

### GLOSSARY

**blood bank** / place where blood is typed, tested, and stored until it is needed for transfusion

## INTRODUCTION

Tube typing is a more sensitive and reliable method of determining a patient's blood type than slide typing. Tube typing is widely used in **blood banks** and in clinical laboratories. Tube typing consists of (1) direct or forward typing, which identifies the antigens on the cells, and (2) confirmatory or reverse typing, which identifies the blood group antibodies in the serum. A centrifuge or serofuge may be used to speed up the reaction. A serofuge is a specialized centrifuge which spins small test tubes at a high—usually fixed—speed.

## TUBE TYPING

Tube typing refers to typing carried out in a test tube rather than on a slide. With tube typing, the cells that are used must be a 2–5% saline suspension of red blood cells, instead of the whole blood used in slide typing.

### Direct or Forward Typing

Forward or direct typing identifies the antigens present on a patient's red blood cells by reacting a suspension of the patient's cells with anti–A and anti–B and observing agglutination after centrifugation. If a centrifuge is not available the reactions may be observed after allowing the tubes to sit at room temperature for fifteen to thirty minutes.

A 2–5% cell suspension is made by adding eighteen to nineteen drops of saline to one drop of the patient's blood. Two tubes labeled "A" and "B" are set up: one drop of anti–A is placed in the "A" tube and one drop of anti–B is placed in

**Table 4-3.** Forward and Reverse Typing Results for ABO Blood Groups

| | Forward Typing Reaction of Cells with: | | Reverse Typing Reaction of Serum with: | | |
|---|---|---|---|---|---|
| **ABO Group** | **anti–A** | **anti–B** | **A cells** | **B cells** | **O cells** |
| O | 0 | 0 | + | + | 0 |
| A | + | 0 | 0 | + | 0 |
| B | 0 | + | + | 0 | 0 |
| AB | + | + | 0 | 0 | 0 |

0 = no agglutination
+ = agglutination

the "B" tube. One drop of the patient's 2–5% cell suspension is added to each tube and the contents are mixed. The tubes are centrifuged for thirty seconds to enhance the reaction. The tubes are then removed from the centrifuge. They are shaken gently to remove the cells from the bottom of the tube and are observed for agglutination. A clumping of the cells indicates the antigen present on the cells corresponds to the antibody placed in the test tube.

## Reverse or Indirect Typing

Reverse (or indirect or confirmatory) typing identifies the antibodies present in a patient's serum or plasma by reacting the patient's serum with a 2–5% suspension of group A cells and a 2–5% suspension of group B cells and observing agglutination. Two drops of the patient's serum are added to each of three tubes marked "a," "b," and "control." One drop of the group A cell suspension is added to the tube "a," one drop of group B cell suspension is added to tube "b," and one drop of a 2–5% suspension of patient cells to "control" tube. The contents of the tubes are mixed and the tubes are centrifuged for thirty seconds. The tubes are then shaken gently to remove the cells from the bottom of the tubes. The tubes are then observed for agglutination. A positive test, agglutination, indicates that antibody is present in the serum which corresponds to the antigen on cells added to the tube. The control tube should always be negative for agglutination since it contains only the patient's serum and cells. The results of forward and reverse typing should be compared to insure that they agree (Table 4–3). (Reverse typing should confirm the results of forward typing.)

### *Precautions*

- Follow manufacturer's directions regarding the use of all reagents.
- Cells used for tube typing must be a 2–5% cell suspension.

## *LESSON REVIEW*

1. What is reverse typing?
2. What antibodies would be present in the serum of a person who is type A—type AB?
3. How is a 2–5% cell suspension made?
4. How are the results of tube typing tests interpreted?
5. Define blood bank.

## *STUDENT ACTIVITIES*

1. Re-read the information on ABO tube typing.
2. Review the glossary terms.
3. Practice performing ABO tube typings as outlined on the Student Performance Guide, using the worksheet.

# Student Performance Guide

NAME ____________________

DATE ____________________

## LESSON 4–2 ABO TUBE TYPING

### Instructions

1. Practice performing ABO tube typing.
2. Demonstrate ABO tube typing satisfactorily for the instructor. All steps must be completed as listed on the instructor's Performance Check Sheet.
3. Complete a written examination successfully.

### Materials and Equipment

- hand disinfectant
- specimens for typing: requires a serum and EDTA anticoagulated specimen for each individual typed
- physiological saline (0.85% or .15M NaCl)
- pasteur pipets and rubber bulb
- anti–A serum
- anti–B serum
- A cells (2–5% saline suspension)
- B cells (2–5% saline suspension)
- serofuge or centrifuge capable of spinning 13 × 75 mm tubes at 2000–2500 rpm (optional)
- test tubes, 13 × 75 mm
- test tube racks
- blood typing worksheet
- surface disinfectant
- biohazard container

*Note:* Package insert should be consulted for specific instructions before test is performed.

## Procedure

S = Satisfactory
U = Unsatisfactory

| You must: | S | U | Comments |
|---|---|---|---|
| 1. Wash hands with hand disinfectant | | | |
| 2. Assemble equipment and materials | | | |
| 3. Obtain a blood sample and perform ABO forward tube typing following steps 4–13 | | | |
| 4. Place one drop of well-mixed blood into a test tube; add eighteen to nineteen drops of saline, and label the tube "patient cells" (2–5%) | | | |
| 5. Label two test tubes "A" and "B" | | | |
| 6. Place one drop of anti–A in tube "A" | | | |
| 7. Place one drop of anti–B in tube "B" | | | |
| 8. Place one drop of the 2–5% patient cell suspension in each tube and mix | | | |
| 9. Place tubes in serofuge and spin thirty seconds. *Note:* Balance the serofuge by placing tubes opposite each other. (If no centrifuge is available, allow tubes to stand at room temperature for 15–30 minutes and go to step 11) | | | |
| 10. Allow the serofuge to come to a complete stop and remove tubes | | | |
| 11. Shake each tube gently to remove cells from bottom of tube and observe for agglutination using good light | | | |
| 12. Record results from each tube on worksheet: 0 = no agglutination, + = agglutination | | | |
| 13. Determine the blood group of the sample and record | | | |
| 14. Obtain a blood sample and perform ABO reverse typing following steps 15–25 | | | |
| 15. Centrifuge the blood sample, remove serum from sample, and place in a clean test tube (plasma may be used for practice) | | | |
| 16. Label three test tubes "a," "b," and "control" | | | |
| 17. Place two drops of serum (or plasma) into each tube | | | |

| You must: | S | U | Comments |
|---|---|---|---|
| 18. Place one drop of a 2–5% suspension of A cells into tube "a" and mix | | | |
| 19. Place one drop of a 2–5% suspension of B cells into tube "b" and mix | | | |
| 20. Place one drop of patient's 2–5% cell suspension into "control" tube and mix | | | |
| 21. Place tubes in serofuge, balance, and spin thirty seconds | | | |
| 22. Remove the tubes from the serofuge after it stops completely | | | |
| 23. Shake each tube gently and observe for agglutination | | | |
| 24. Record the results from each tube on worksheet: 0 = no agglutination, + = agglutination | | | |
| 25. Determine the blood group of the sample and record | | | |
| 26. Compare results of forward typing of the sample with results of reverse typing of the same sample. Reverse typing should confirm results of forward typing | | | |
| 27. Discard specimens appropriately | | | |
| 28. Clean equipment and return to proper storage | | | |
| 29. Clean work area with surface disinfectant | | | |
| 30. Wash hands with hand disinfectant | | | |

Comments:

Student/Instructor:

Date: ______________________ Instructor: ______________________

# Worksheet

NAME ______________________________ DATE ____________

## LESSON 4–2 ABO TUBE TYPING

| Specimen No. | Direct (Forward) Typing* anti–A | Direct (Forward) Typing* anti–B | Interpretation ABO Group | Indirect (Reverse) Typing A cells | Indirect (Reverse) Typing B cells | Indirect (Reverse) Typing Control | Interpretation ABO Group |
|---|---|---|---|---|---|---|---|
| | | | | | | | |
| | | | | | | | |
| | | | | | | | |
| | | | | | | | |
| | | | | | | | |

* Record results as:
0 = no agglutination
\+ = agglutination

# LESSON 4–3

## Rh Slide Typing

### LESSON OBJECTIVES

After studying this lesson, you should be able to:

- Explain the importance of the Rh blood group system.
- Name the most important antigen in the Rh system.
- Name two ways in which immunization to the Rh D antigen may occur.
- Name two problems which may occur as a result of immunization to the D antigen.
- Explain why Rh (D) immune globulin is used.
- Perform Rh slide typing.
- Interpret the results of Rh slide typing.
- Explain the significance of the $D^u$ antigen.
- List the precautions which should be observed while performing the Rh slide typing procedure.
- Define the glossary terms.

### GLOSSARY

**hemolytic disease of the newborn (HDN)** / a disease in which antibody from the mother destroys the red cells of the fetus

**immunization** / process by which an antibody is produced in response to an antigen

**Rh (D) immune globulin** / a concentrated, purified solution of human anti–D, used for injection; RhIG

### INTRODUCTION

Testing for antigens of the Rh system is a routine procedure in blood banks and clinical laboratories. These antigens may be detected by the slide method or the tube method. The slide method is discussed in this lesson.

## ANTIGENS OF THE Rh SYSTEM

The Rh blood group, discovered in the 1940s, is the second most important human blood group system. The system is named Rh because the rhesus monkey was being used in the experiments when the system was discovered.

The antigens of the Rh system are products of inherited genes and are present on the surface of red blood cells. The major antigen in the Rh system is the D antigen. Red blood cells that possess the D antigen are called Rh positive. Cells that lack the D antigen are called Rh negative. Eighty-five percent of the U.S. population is Rh positive (Rh+) and the other fifteen percent of the population is Rh negative (Rh−). There are now several other known antigens which are part of the Rh system. However, the D antigen is the strongest of the antigens and is the only one that is tested for routinely.

## ANTIBODIES OF THE Rh SYSTEM

Unlike the ABO system, the Rh system does not have antibodies which occur naturally. However, anti–D may be produced if an Rh negative person is immunized or sensitized with the D antigen.

**Immunization** to the D antigen and subsequent production of anti–D may occur if an Rh negative person is transfused with Rh positive blood. If the Rh negative person is transfused a second time with Rh positive blood, a severe transfusion reaction may occur when the anti–D reacts with the D positive transfused cells.

When an Rh negative mother gives birth to an Rh positive baby, immunization sometimes occurs followed by production of anti–D by the mother. The effect may be seen in subsequent Rh positive pregnancies when the mother's antibodies may enter the fetus' bloodstream and attack the unborn baby's red blood cells, a condition called **hemolytic disease of the newborn,** or **HDN.** The effects on the fetus may be mild or severe and may range from mild jaundice to anemia or brain damage. In severe cases, stillbirth or miscarriage may occur.

It is now possible to prevent most cases of Rh hemolytic disease of the newborn by administering **Rh (D) immune globulin** (RhIG) to the mother. RhIG is a concentrated solution of human anti–D antibody which, when injected into the mother, will prevent her from making the anti–D antibody. This injection must be given within seventy-two hours after delivery of an Rh D positive baby or after termination of pregnancy. Expectant mothers should be typed during the first trimester of pregnancy. This helps to identify mothers who are at risk of having a baby with HDN so that the fetus may be monitored for signs of stress.

## NOMENCLATURE

The two commonly used methods of naming the antigens in the Rh system are the Fisher-Race method and the Wiener method. The names of the antigen and antibody in both systems are given in Table 4–4. Manufacturers of blood bank reagents may use one or both systems in labeling reagents.

## WEAK D ANTIGEN: $D^u$

Some individuals have a form of the D antigen which is weak. This weak antigen is called the $D^u$ antigen. Blood cells containing the $D^u$ antigen may give a negative reaction in routine slide or tube typing. All blood samples that are negative by routine slide or tube typing should be tested for the $D^u$

**Table 4-4.** Fisher-Race and Wiener Nomenclature for Rh System

| Nomenclature | Antigen | Antibody |
|---|---|---|
| Fisher-Race | D | anti–D |
| Wiener | $Rh_o$ | anti–$Rh_o$ |

antigen before assuming that the sample is Rh negative. The $D^u$ test will not be covered in this lesson for two reasons: (1) most laboratories will not allow non-certified workers to perform the test, and (2) the test involves techniques and principles not covered in this text.

## IMPORTANCE OF Rh TYPING

It is important to test for the D antigen in all patients who are to receive transfusions so that the proper type of blood will be given. Rh negative patients should always be transfused with Rh negative blood. Testing for the D antigen is also a way of identifying females who might be at risk of giving birth to an infant with HDN. Since the blood group antigens are inherited, identification of these antigens may aid in establishing parentage in legal or civil cases.

## Rh SLIDE TYPING PROCEDURE

The D antigen may be identified using a slide typing technique. A control should always be run as part of the test, since the patient's serum contains no natural antibody for reverse or confirmatory typing.

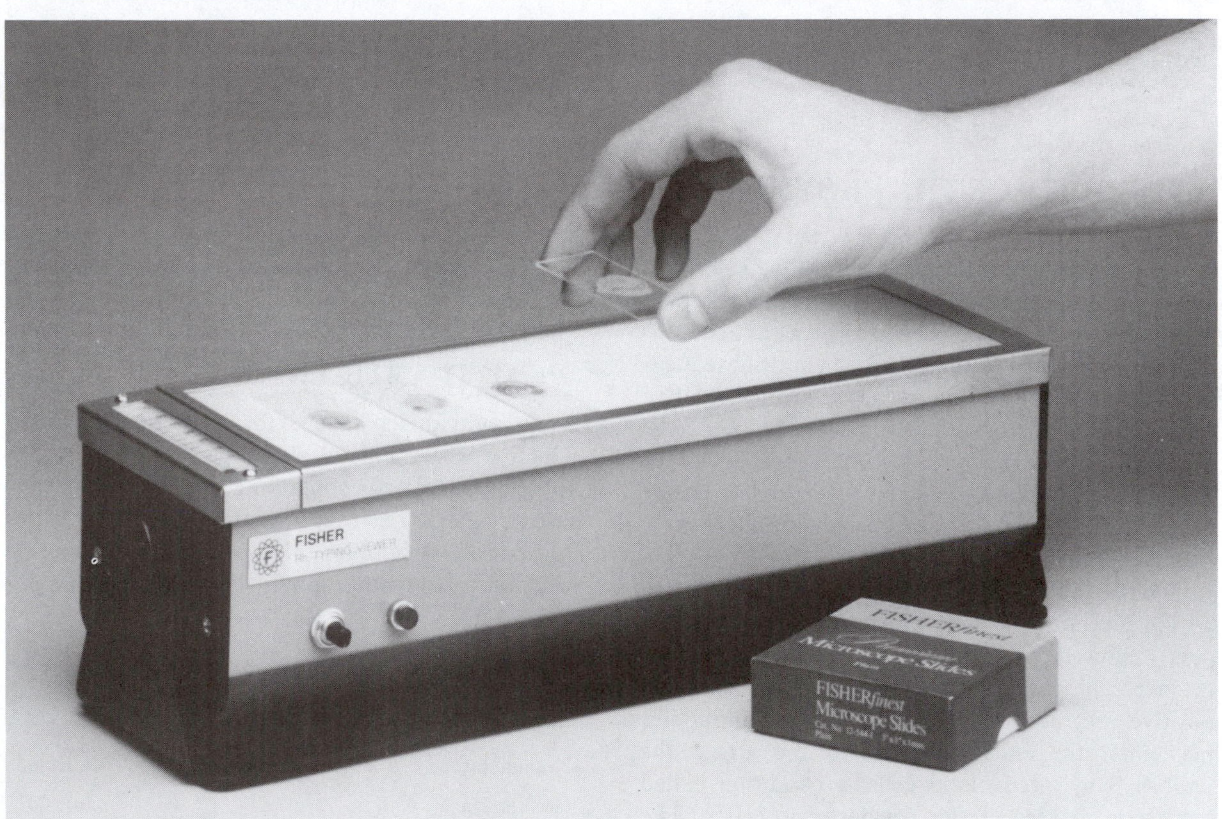


**Figure 4-4.** Rh slide typing using viewbox (*Photo courtesy of Fisher Scientific Co.*)

**Table 4-5.** Interpretation of Results of Rh Slide Typing

| Reaction of cells with: anti–D | control serum | Interpretation |
|---|---|---|
| + | 0 | Rh (D) positive |
| 0 | 0 | Rh (D) negative (confirm with $D^u$ test) |
| + | + | unable to interpret; repeat test using another method |

+ = agglutination
0 = no agglutination

Slide typing is performed by (1) mixing one drop of anti–D with one drop of blood on a microscope slide and (2) mixing one drop of control serum, usually 22% or 30% bovine albumin, with one drop of blood on another slide. The slides are placed on a heated, lighted viewbox to heat them to 37°C, and are rocked gently (Figure 4–4). The slides are observed for two minutes for agglutination and the results are recorded and interpreted. It is important to follow the manufacturer's directions in the use of anti–D.

## INTERPRETATION OF RESULTS

If the cells are Rh positive, agglutination should be observed on the anti–D slide only. If the cells are Rh negative, no agglutination should be seen in either slide (Table 4–5). The control slide should always be negative for agglutination. If positive results are observed in the control, the test cannot be interpreted and should be repeated by the tube method. Positive control results may be due to contaminated control serum or abnormalities in the patient blood sample. Rh negative results should be confirmed by a tube test and a $D^u$ test.

### *Precautions*

- Always follow manufacturer's instructions for use of reagents.
- Do not observe heated slides for more than two minutes before interpreting results.
- Rh slide typing should always be performed at 37°C, using a lighted viewbox.
- Negative slide typing results should be confirmed with a tube test and a $D^u$ test.

## *LESSON REVIEW*

1. What is the major antigen in the Rh system?
2. What circumstances must exist before anti–D is produced by an individual?
3. What is the weak D antigen?
4. Explain how hemolytic disease of the newborn occurs.
5. Why is Rh D typing performed?
6. What two problems may occur after immunization to the D antigen?
7. Define hemolytic disease of the newborn, immunization, and Rh (D) immune globulin.

## *STUDENT ACTIVITIES*

1. Re-read the information on Rh slide typing.
2. Review the glossary terms.
3. Practice performing Rh slide typing on several blood samples as outlined on the Student Performance Guide, using the worksheet.

# Student Performance Guide

NAME ______________________________

DATE ______________________________

## LESSON 4–3
## Rh SLIDE TYPING

### Instructions

1. Practice performing Rh slide typing.
2. Demonstrate the procedure for Rh slide typing satisfactorily for the instructor. All steps must be completed as listed on the instructor's Performance Check Sheet.
3. Complete a written examination successfully.

### Materials and Equipment

- hand disinfectant
- clean microscope slides
- wooden applicator sticks
- anti–D serum (anti–$Rh_o$)
- Rh control serum (22% or 30% bovine albumin)
- blood specimen
- lighted viewbox
- blood typing worksheet
- wax pencil
- stopwatch
- surface disinfectant
- biohazard container

*Note:* Package insert should be consulted for specific instructions before test is performed.

**Procedure**

S = Satisfactory
U = Unsatisfactory

| You must: | S | U | Comments |
|---|---|---|---|
| 1. Wash hands with hand disinfectant | | | |
| 2. Assemble equipment and materials | | | |
| 3. Turn on viewbox | | | |

| You must: | S | U | Comments |
|---|---|---|---|
| 4. Label two clean microscope slides "D" and "C" (control) | | | |
| 5. Place one drop of anti–D serum on the "D" slide | | | |
| 6. Place one drop of Rh control serum (albumin) on the "C" slide | | | |
| 7. Place one large drop of well-mixed whole blood on each slide | | | |
| 8. Mix blood and anti–D well with an applicator stick, spreading the mixture over two-thirds of the slide | | | |
| 9. Repeat procedure for the control slide using a clean applicator stick | | | |
| 10. Place slides on the lighted viewbox | | | |
| 11. Tilt the viewbox slowly back and forth for two minutes to mix the contents on the slides | | | |
| 12. Observe for agglutination at the end of two minutes | | | |
| 13. Record results on worksheet: + = agglutination, 0 = no agglutination | | | |
| 14. Determine Rh type and record on worksheet | | | |
| 15. Repeat steps 4–14 on at least two other blood samples | | | |
| 16. Discard specimens appropriately | | | |
| 17. Clean equipment and return to proper storage | | | |
| 18. Clean work area with surface disinfectant | | | |
| 19. Wash hands with hand disinfectant | | | |

Comments:

Student/Instructor:

Date: ______________________ Instructor: ______________________

# Worksheet

NAME ______________________________ DATE ____________

## LESSON 4–2 Rh SLIDE TYPING

| Sample # | Agglutination Results* anti–D | Control (albumin) | Interpretation Rh type |
|---|---|---|---|
| ________ | ______ | ______________ | ___________ |
| ________ | ______ | ______________ | ___________ |
| ________ | ______ | ______________ | ___________ |
| ________ | ______ | ______________ | ___________ |
| ________ | ______ | ______________ | ___________ |

* Record results as:
0 = no agglutination
\+ = agglutination

# LESSON 4–4

## Urine Pregnancy Test

## LESSON OBJECTIVES

After studying this lesson, you should be able to:

- Name the hormone present in pregnant females.
- State when the hormone first appears in urine.
- Explain the principle of agglutination inhibition.
- Perform a slide test for pregnancy.
- Interpret the results of a urine pregnancy test.
- Name a cause of a false positive urine pregnancy test.
- List precautions to observe when performing a slide test for pregnancy.
- Define the glossary terms.

## GLOSSARY

**agglutination inhibition** / interference of agglutination

**HCG** / human chorionic gonadotropin, a hormone found in pregnant women; sometimes called uterine chorionic gonadotropin (UCG)

### INTRODUCTION

Most pregnancy tests are designed to detect human chorionic gonadotropin, or **HCG,** a hormone normally found in the serum and urine of pregnant women. It is sometimes called uterine chorionic gonadotropin, or UCG. The urine test is most commonly used because urine is easily available for testing.

### TYPES OF PREGNANCY TESTS

Most pregnancy tests may be classified as either tube tests or slide tests. Tube tests are carried out in test tubes and the results are usually available after two hours. Slide tests are carried out on a glass or cardboard slide and results are usually available within a few minutes. The slide test is rapid, sensitive, and easy to perform.

### PRINCIPLE OF PREGNANCY TESTS

Most pregnancy tests employ serological methods to detect the HCG hormone. These tests are usually based on the principle of **agglutination inhibition.**

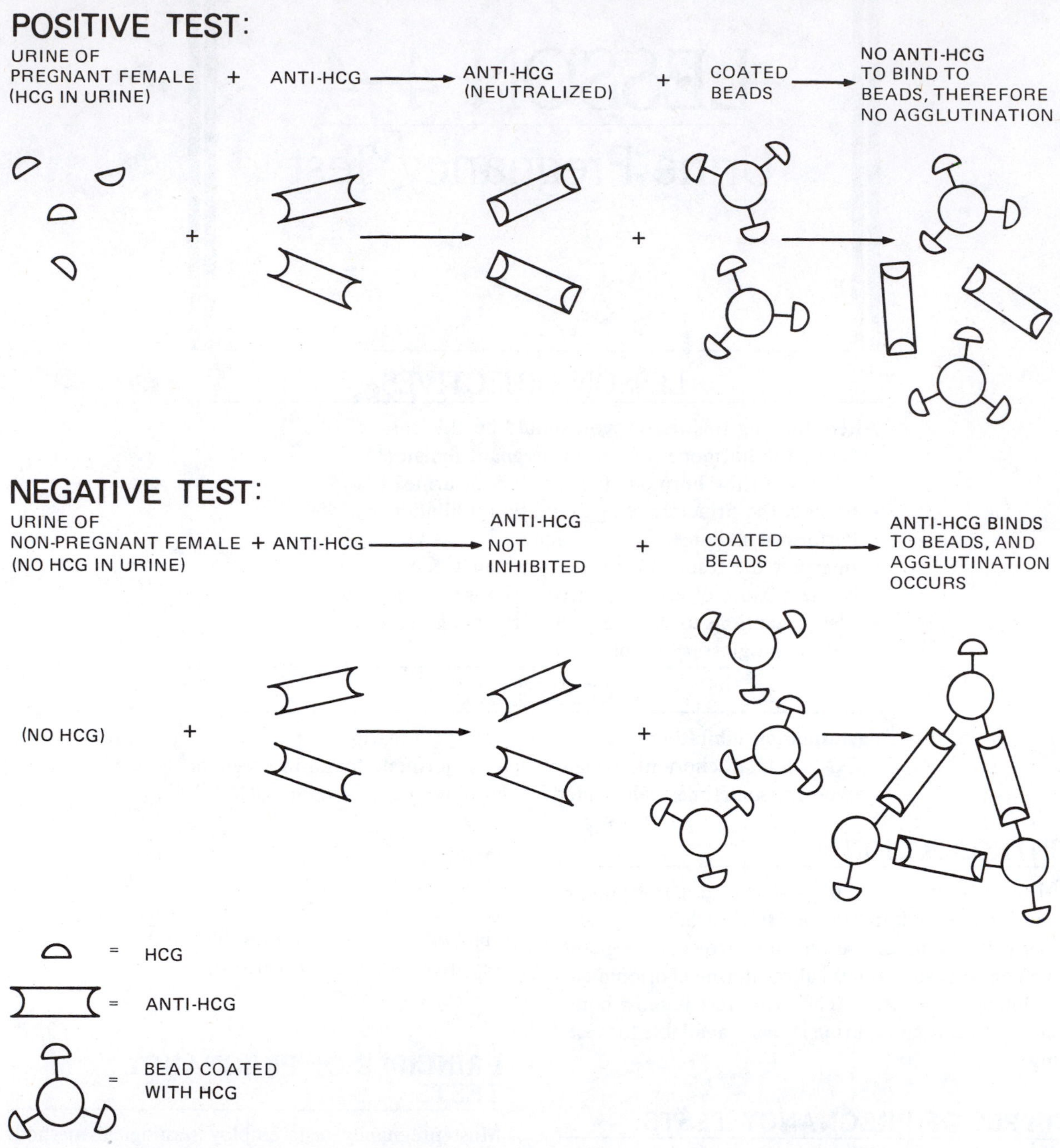


**Figure 4-5.** Principle of agglutination inhibition test for pregnancy

| | | | | | | | | |
|---|---|---|---|---|---|---|---|---|
| Urine of Pregnant Female (HCG in urine) | + | anti–HCG | → | anti–HCG neutralized | + | coated beads | → | no anti–HCG to bind to beads, therefore no agglutination |
| Urine of Non-pregnant female (no HCG in urine) | + | anti–HCG | → | anti–HCG not inhibited | + | coated beads | → | anti–HCG binds to beads, and agglutination occurs |

**Fig. 4-5 (cont.)**

In an agglutination inhibition test, the substance being tested, when present, will inhibit agglutination. Absence of agglutination is a positive test result. If the substance being tested is not present, agglutination will occur and will be interpreted as a negative test.

## SPECIMEN

The urine sample tested should be the first urine voided in the morning since the hormone will be more concentrated then. The hormone HCG appears in the urine and serum about one week after the missed onset of menstruation. The level of HCG rises during early pregnancy, begins to decline about the third month of pregnancy, and disappears a few days after delivery.

## COMPONENTS OF HCG TESTS

Urine test kits are available from a variety of manufacturers. The majority of the kits rely on the following test components:

1. *HCG hormone.* Present in the urine of pregnant females.
2. *Anti–HCG.* This is an antibody which will react with HCG. It is produced by inoculating HCG into an animal so that the animal will produce antibodies against the HCG. The serum is then harvested from the animal, purified, packaged, and sold as the source of anti-HCG for a variety of pregnancy tests.
3. *Indicator particles.* Suspensions of latex beads or cells (usually red cells) which are coated with HCG hormone.

## GENERAL PROCEDURE FOR AGGLUTINATION INHIBITION TEST FOR PREGNANCY

A portion of a urine sample is mixed with anti–HCG. If HCG is present in the urine (if the patient is pregnant), the HCG will bind to the antibody (anti–HCG) and "neutralize" or inhibit the activity of the antibody. This reaction is not visible. If the urine sample is from a non-pregnant female, no reaction will occur with the antibody, since the urine will have no HCG.

After the urine and the anti-HCG antibody are mixed together, HCG-coated particles are added to the mixture to make the reaction visible. If the patient is pregnant, the antibody will have been inhibited by the patient's HCG, will be unable to bind to the HCG-coated beads, and no agglutination will be seen. If the patient is not pregnant, the antibody will combine with the HCG-coated particles and cause agglutination or clumping of the particles (Figure 4–5).

### Precautions

- Control samples (positive and negative urines) should always be tested at the same time as the patient sample to be certain that reagents are reacting properly.
- Many early pregnancies (the first one to two weeks) have undetectable levels of HCG. Therefore, negative tests should be repeated in one to two weeks.
- Specimens should be tested within 24 hours and kept refrigerated until tested.
- Serological tests for HCG may give false positive results due to elevated levels of pituitary hormones, and rare conditions such as choriocarcinoma and hydatiform mole.

## LESSON REVIEW

1. What hormone is tested for in most pregnancy tests?
2. What two types of specimens can be used in a pregnancy test?
3. Describe the principle of agglutination inhibition.
4. When does the HCG hormone first appear in pregnancy? When does it disappear?
5. What precautions should be observed in performing the slide test for pregnancy?
6. Define agglutination inhibition and HCG.

## STUDENT ACTIVITIES

1. Re-read the information on the pregnancy test.
2. Review the glossary terms.
3. Practice performing a slide test for pregnancy as outlined on the Student Performance Guide.

# Student Performance Guide

NAME ____________________

DATE ____________________

## LESSON 4–4
## URINE PREGNANCY TEST

### Instructions

1. Practice performing a slide test for pregnancy.
2. Demonstrate the slide test procedure for pregnancy satisfactorily for the instructor. All steps must be completed as listed on the instructor's Performance Check Sheet.
3. Complete a written examination successfully.

### Materials and Equipment

- hand disinfectant
- urine specimen
- stopwatch
- positive and negative urine controls
- slide test kit for pregnancy (kit should include slide, dispensers, stirrers, reagents)
- surface disinfectant
- biohazard container

*Note:* The procedure should be modified to conform to the manufacturer's instructions of the kit being used.

| **Procedure** | | | S = Satisfactory<br>U = Unsatisfactory |
|---|---|---|---|
| **You must:** | **S** | **U** | **Comments** |
| 1. Wash hands with hand disinfectant | | | |
| 2. Assemble equipment and materials | | | |
| 3. Place one drop of antiserum in the center of the slide | | | |
| 4. Obtain urine sample. Insert tip of dispenser into urine sample, squeeze, and release pressure to draw up specimen | | | |
| 5. Hold dispenser perpendicular over slide and squeeze to release one drop of urine beside the drop of antiserum | | | |
| 6. Mix urine and antiserum with stirrer provided | | | |
| 7. Rock slide to mix for appropriate time interval | | | |
| 8. Apply one drop of indicator particles to mixture on slide | | | |
| 9. Using same stirrer mix indicator particles with antiserum and spread mixture over entire circled area of slide | | | |
| 10. Rock slide slowly in a figure-eight motion for appropriate time interval | | | |
| 11. Observe slide for agglutination at the end of the time interval and record results | | | |
| 12. Repeat steps 3–11 using a positive urine control and a negative urine control | | | |
| 13. Discard used supplies in biohazard container | | | |
| 14. Clean work area with surface disinfectant | | | |
| 15. Wash hands with hand disinfectant | | | |

Comments:

Student/Instructor:

Date: ______________________________ Instructor: ______________________________

# LESSON 4–5

## Slide Test for Infectious Mononucleosis

## LESSON OBJECTIVES

After studying this lesson, you should be able to:

- Name the cause of infectious mononucleosis.
- List five clinical symptoms of infectious mononucleosis.
- Name two types of tests which are performed to diagnose infectious mononucleosis.
- Perform a slide test for infectious mononucleosis.
- Interpret the results of a slide test for infectious mononucleosis.
- Define the glossary terms.

## GLOSSARY

**heterophile antibody** / antibody which is increased in infectious mononucleosis

**lymphocytosis** / an increase above normal in the number of lymphocytes in the blood

## INTRODUCTION

Infectious mononucleosis is a contagious disease which may have vague clinical symptoms and may mimic other diseases. Serological tests are often the basis for an early diagnosis of the disease, and may also be used to follow the course of the disease. The most common serological test used is a rapid slide test which tests serum for the presence of antibodies called **heterophile antibodies.** The slide test gives quick, reliable results and is simple to perform.

### Symptoms of Infectious Mononucleosis

Infectious mononucleosis (IM) is commonly called "mono" or "kissing disease." IM is a viral disease which affects mostly the fifteen to twenty-five year-old age group. The disease is a result of infection of the lymphocytes by the Epstein-Barr virus (EBV). Clinically, the symptoms are nonspecific and may include fatigue, fever, sore throat, weakness, headache, and swollen lymph nodes. In order to properly diagnose IM, hematological and serological test results must be considered along with the clinical symptoms.

## HEMATOLOGICAL TEST FOR IM

The hematological test for IM includes a white cell count and evaluation of the patient's lymphocytes. In IM, a **lymphocytosis,** or increase in lymphocytes, usually occurs and the lymphocytes have an unusual or "atypical" appearance.

## SEROLOGICAL TEST FOR IM

Persons with IM produce an antibody called **heterophile antibody** by the sixth to tenth day of the illness. Detection of this heterophile antibody combined with the hematological and clinical findings can provide the basis for the diagnosis of IM. The serological test is usually positive after the first week of illness. However, if a negative test results, the test may be repeated in another week if clinical symptoms are still present.

## SLIDE TEST FOR INFECTIOUS MONONUCLEOSIS

The procedure for detecting the heterophile antibody of IM discussed in this lesson is the one developed by Ortho Diagnostics and marketed under the name Monospot.® Several other tests are available which follow the same general principles as this one. Manufacturer's instructions for each kit should be strictly followed.

Serological kits for infectious mononucleosis usually provide all necessary reagents, materials, and controls. The laboratory must provide the specimen to be tested, which is usually a small sample of the patient's serum.

The slide test is a rapid method of detecting heterophile antibody in serum. The procedure is based on agglutination of horse erythrocytes by the heterophile antibody present in IM. There are other antibodies which will also react with horse erythrocytes. Therefore, the serum is reacted with absorbents to remove these other antibodies before it is reacted with the horse cells.

The test is performed using a glass slide which has two squares (I and II) etched on the slide. The reagents are mixed thoroughly and a drop of indica-

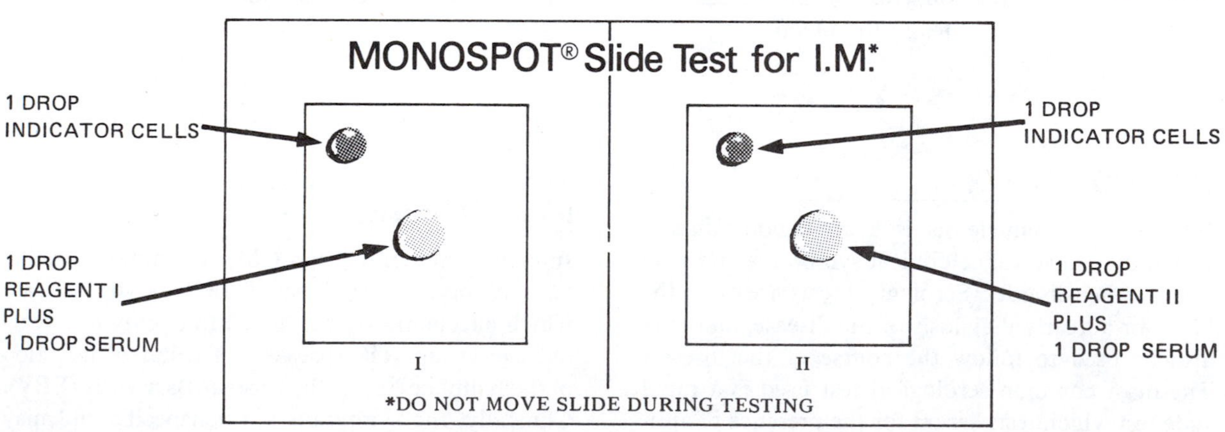


**Figure 4-6.** Monospot® slide with reagents added

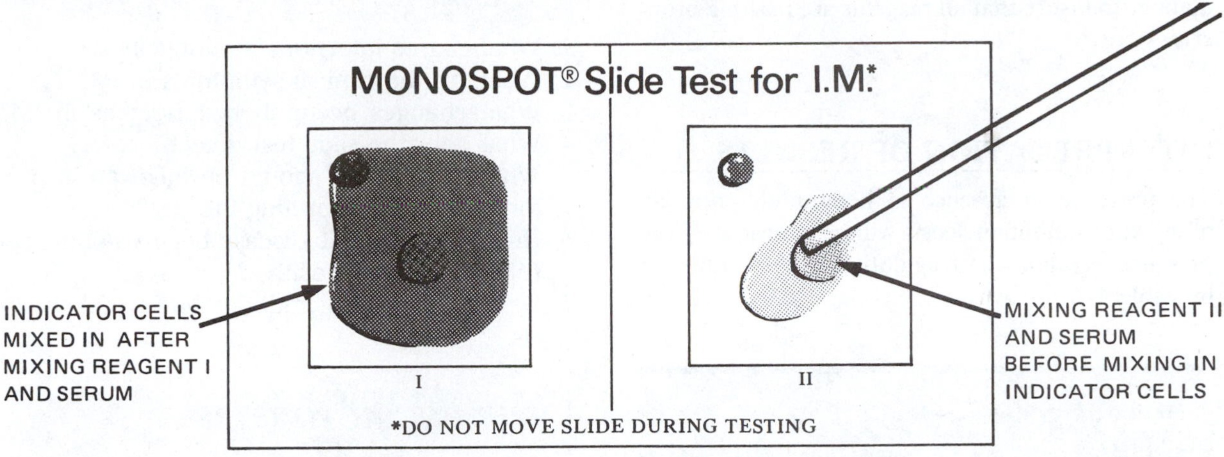


**Figure 4-7.** Mixing reagents on Monospot® slide using wooden applicator

tor cells (horse erythrocytes) is added to a corner of each square using the capillary pipet provided. One drop of Reagent I is then placed in the center of square I and one drop of Reagent II is placed in the center of square II. One drop of serum is placed in the center of each square using the plastic pipet provided in the kit (Figure 4–6). The serum and reagent I are mixed using at least ten stirring motions with a clean wooden applicator stick. The cells are blended in so that the entire surface of the square is covered. The contents of square II are mixed in the same manner as square I (Figure 4–7). A timer is started as soon as mixing is completed and the slide is observed for one minute for agglutination of the horse cells. During this time the slide should not be moved or picked up. At the end of one minute the results are recorded and interpreted. Positive and negative serum controls

**Table 4-6.** Interpretation of Results of Monospot® Test

| **Positive test:** | **Negative test:** |
|---|---|
| Agglutination pattern is stronger on the left side of the slide (square I) than on the right side of the slide (square II) | A. Agglutination pattern is stronger on the right side of the slide (square II) than in square I<br>*or*<br>B. No agglutination appears in either square<br>*or*<br>C. Agglutination is equal in both squares of the slide |

provided with the kit should be tested in the same manner to insure that all reagents are reacting properly.

## INTERPRETATION OF RESULTS

The presence or absence of heterophile antibody of infectious mononucleosis will be indicated by the presence or absence of agglutination, as indicated in Table 4–6.

### *Precautions*

- Slide should not be moved during the one-minute incubation period.
- Agglutination appearing after one minute or when the slide is picked up should not be interpreted as a positive result.
- Manufacturer's instructions for kits must be adhered to.

## *LESSON REVIEW*

1. What causes infectious mononucleosis?
2. What are the clinical symptoms of IM?
3. What changes occur in lymphocytes in IM?
4. What does the slide test detect?
5. What precautions should be followed in performing and interpreting the test?
6. How soon after the disease begins will the serological test be positive?
7. Define heterophile antibody and lymphocytosis.

## *STUDENT ACTIVITIES*

1. Re-read the information on the slide test for infectious mononucleosis.
2. Review the glossary terms.
3. Practice performing the slide test for infectious mononucleosis as outlined on the Student Performance Guide.

# Student Performance Guide

NAME ______________________

DATE ______________________

## LESSON 4–5 SLIDE TEST FOR INFECTIOUS MONONUCLEOSIS

### Instructions

1. Practice performing the slide test for infectious mononucleosis.
2. Demonstrate the procedure for the slide test for infectious mononucleosis satisfactorily for the instructor. All steps must be completed as listed on the instructor's Performance Check Sheet.
3. Complete a written examination successfully.

### Materials and Equipment

- hand disinfectant
- serum
- stopwatch
- surface disinfectant
- test kit for infectious mononucleosis (kit should include instructions, slide, serum dispensers, stirrers, reagents)
- biohazard container

*Note:* Procedure given is for Monospot® test by Ortho Diagnostics. Package insert should be consulted before test is performed. If another kit is used, the manufacturer's instructions should be followed.

| **Procedure** | | | S = Satisfactory<br>U = Unsatisfactory |
|---|---|---|---|
| **You must:** | **S** | **U** | **Comments** |
| 1. Wash hands with hand disinfectant | | | |
| 2. Assemble equipment and materials | | | |
| 3. Place the Monospot® slide on the work surface | | | |
| 4. Mix the reagent vials several times by inversion | | | |
| 5. Fill the capillary pipet to the top mark:<br>a. Place the rubber bulb on the end of the capillary pipet with the heavy black line<br>b. Insert the pipet into the vial of indicator cells<br>c. Allow the pipet to fill by capillary action to the top mark | | | |
| 6. Place the index finger over the hole in the bulb and squeeze gently to dispense one-half the cells onto a corner of square I of the slide (the level of the cells should now be at the lower mark on the pipet) | | | |
| 7. Deliver the remaining cells to a corner of square II | | | |
| 8. Place one drop of thoroughly-mixed Reagent I in the center of square I | | | |
| 9. Place one drop of thoroughly-mixed Reagent II in the center of square II | | | |
| 10. Add one drop of serum to the center of each square using the disposable plastic pipet provided | | | |
| 11. Mix Reagent I with the serum using *at least ten* stirring motions with a clean wooden applicator stick | | | |
| 12. Blend in the indicator cells in square I with the applicator stick using *no more than ten* stirring motions, and spreading the mixture over the entire surface of the square | | | |
| 13. Repeat steps 11–12 using Reagent II in square II, using a clean applicator stick | | | |
| 14. Start the stopwatch upon completion of the mixing of both squares | | | |

| You must | S | U | Comments |
|---|---|---|---|
| 15. Observe for agglutination at the end of one minute (no longer) without moving the slide or picking it up | | | |
| 16. Record the agglutination in each square and interpret the results: if the agglutination pattern is stronger in square I than in square II, the test is positive for the heterophile antibody of infectious mononucleosis. Any other combination of reactions is negative | | | |
| 17. Record test results as positive or negative | | | |
| 18. Repeat test procedure (steps 3–17) using positive and negative control sera | | | |
| 19. Dispose of specimen appropriately | | | |
| 20. Clean work area with surface disinfectant | | | |
| 21. Wash hands with hand disinfectant | | | |
| Comments: | | | |
| Student/Instructor: | | | |

Date: ______________________ Instructor: ______________________________

# UNIT 5

# Urinalysis

## UNIT OBJECTIVES

After completion of this unit, you should be able to:

- Describe proper urine collection and preservation methods.
- Perform a physical examination of urine.
- Perform a chemical examination of urine.
- Identify components of urine sediment.
- Perform a microscopic examination of urine sediment.

## OVERVIEW

The urinary system is an excretory system consisting of the kidney, ureters, bladder, and urethra. The kidney is the organ in which urine is formed. Three processes are involved in urine formation: (1) filtration of waste products, salts, and excess fluid from the blood, (2) reabsorption of water and solutes from the filtrate, and (3) secretion of ions and certain drugs into the urine.

The filtering unit is called the *glomerulus.* The part which secretes substances, reabsorbs substances and concentrates the filtrate is called the *tubule.* Together, these two parts form the *nephron.* There are approximately one million nephrons in each kidney. Each minute more than 1000 ml of blood flows through the kidney to be cleansed. In the glomerulus, certain substances are filtered out of the blood. The remaining filtrate then passes into the tubule where various changes occur. Some tubular cells reabsorb certain constituents such as glucose. Other tubular cells have the ability to secrete certain substances such as potassium and hydrogen ions. In another part of the tubule most of the water in the filtrate is reabsorbed. The portion which is not reabsorbed forms the *urine.* This urine passes out of the kidney into the bladder through a tube called the *ureter.* The *bladder* is used for temporary storage of the urine until it is excreted by the body through a tube called the *urethra.*

An examination of the urine, a urinalysis, may be performed for two purposes: (1) to check for certain metabolic end products which indicate particular diseases, or (2) to observe physical, chemical, and microscopic characteristics which indicate disease or damage to the urinary tract itself. In this unit, through demonstration and practice, you will understand that the urinalysis test results can and do make a difference in the diagnosis and treatment of the patient.

# LESSON 5–1

## Collection and Preservation of Urine

## LESSON OBJECTIVES

After studying this lesson, you should be able to:

- Explain how to correctly collect a clean-catch urine.
- Explain how to correctly collect a mid-stream urine.
- List causes of contamination in urine specimens.
- List various methods of preserving urine specimens.
- State the normal 24-hour urine volume for adults.
- Name the factors that influence urine volume.
- Instruct a male and female patient to properly collect a clean-catch urine.
- Define the glossary terms.

## GLOSSARY

**anuria** / absence of urine production

**clean-catch urine** / a urine sample collected after the urethral opening and surrounding tissues have been cleansed

**mid-stream urine** / a urine sample collected in the middle of voiding

**nocturia** / excessive urination at night

**oliguria** / decreased production of urine

**polyuria** / excessive production of urine

## INTRODUCTION

Examination of a urine specimen can yield many results which are helpful in the diagnosis and treatment of patients. However, proper collection of the sample is essential in order for the test results to be valid.

## PREFERRED SPECIMEN

The preferred specimen for most examinations is the first urine voided in the morning. This specimen will be the most concentrated; the volume and concentration usually varies during the day. The patient may be instructed to collect a **clean-catch** urine sample or a **mid-stream** urine sample.

### Mid-Stream Urine Specimen

If the urine specimen is to be used for a routine urinalysis, a mid-stream sample may be used. A mid-stream sample is one in which the patient collects the urine only in the middle of voiding.

### Clean-Catch Urine Specimen

A clean-catch urine sample must be collected for bacteriological examinations or if it is likely that the specimen would be contaminated with vaginal discharge or menstrual blood. To collect a clean-catch sample the patient first cleanses the urethral opening and the surrounding tissues. After the area has been cleansed the patient then collects a mid-stream sample.

## PROCEDURE FOR COLLECTING A CLEAN-CATCH URINE SAMPLE

A clean-catch urine specimen is necessary if it is to be tested for the presence of bacteria. Most hospitals and doctors' offices use a kit containing towelettes and a sterile disposable urine container. Male and female patients should be instructed to carefully collect the desired urine specimen.

### Instructions to the Male

The male patient should retract the foreskin on the penis (if not circumcised) using a towelette. A second towelette should be used to cleanse the urethral opening with a single stroke directed from the tip of the penis toward the ring of the glans. The towelette should then be discarded and the cleansing procedure repeated using two more towelettes. The patient should begin to void into the toilet. The urine stream should be interrupted to collect the urine into the supplied container. Only the middle portion of the urine flow should be included in the sample. After the specimen has been collected, the container should be closed. The patient should avoid touching the inside of both the container and the lid. The information on the label should then be completed and attached to the specimen container.

### Instructions to the Female

The female patient should position herself comfortably on the toilet seat and should swing one knee to the side as far as possible. She should spread the outer vulval folds (labia majora) using a towelette and the inner side of one inner fold (labium minor) should be wiped with a towelette using a single stroke from front to back. The towelette should then be discarded and a second towelette used to repeat the procedure on the opposite side. A third towelette is used to cleanse the urethral opening with a single front-to-back stroke. The patient should then begin to void into the toilet. The urine stream should be interrupted to collect the urine in a container. Only the middle portion of the urine flow should be included in the sample. Touching only the outside of the container and lid, the container should then be closed. The information on the label should be completed and attached to the container.

## PROCEDURE FOR COLLECTING A MID-STREAM URINE SAMPLE

For a routine chemical and microscopic analysis of urine, it is not necessary to have a clean-catch specimen. The sample preferred is the first morning sample of urine. However, a urine sample taken randomly during the day may be used. The cleansing procedures above are not necessary, but the urine should be collected mid-stream.

## SOURCES OF CONTAMINATION

Urine collection procedures must be followed correctly. If they are not, the urine specimen may become contaminated with epithelial cells, blood cells, microorganisms, or excessive mucus. Another source of contamination may be due to the collection container itself, which must be clean and dry. Precleaned or sterile disposable containers, made of either plastic or plastic-coated paper, are widely used. However, if reusable containers are used, they must be thoroughly washed and dried first. If bacteriological tests are ordered, a sterile container must be used. An unsterile container may be contaminated with bacteria or debris and may cause confusion when the microscopic exam is performed.

## HANDLING AND PRESERVING SPECIMENS

The way a urine specimen is handled after collection can affect the results of many of the tests. A urine specimen should be examined within one hour of voiding. If this is not possible, the urine may be refrigerated at 4–6° Celsius for up to eight hours. Urine which cannot be refrigerated or which has to be transported from home to laboratory over a long distance can have a preservative added to it. The lab personnel usually add the preservative after collection if the lab is shipping. The lab may give the patient a container with preservative added for the patient to take home and collect a specimen (i.e., 24-hour urine).

When a urine sample is allowed to sit at room temperature, any bacteria present will multiply rapidly. When this occurs, the specimen will have an unpleasant, ammonia-like odor. A delay before testing can also increase the decomposition of *casts* and the cellular components of the sample. The addition of a preservative will retard the growth of bacteria and slow the destruction of other urine components. The preservative must be carefully chosen to prevent interference with the tests which have been ordered. Some commonly used preservatives are toluene, formalin, and thymol. No preservative of any kind should be added to a urine which is to be used for bacteriological studies.

**Table 5-1.** Normal 24-hour Urine Volumes

| Age | Volume (ml/24 hours) |
|---|---|
| Newborn | 20–350 |
| One year | 300–600 |
| Ten years | 750–1500 |
| Adult | 750–2000 |

## URINE VOLUME

When a routine urinalysis is performed, the volume of the specimen is usually not recorded. However, there are certain quantitative tests which are performed on urine collected in a 24-hour period. The volume of these samples should be measured carefully and recorded. Graduated cylinders should be used when measuring these samples.

The urinary volume depends on various factors: the fluid intake, the fluid lost in exhalation and perspiration, and the status of renal and cardiac functions of the person. Excessive production of urine is called **polyuria.** The term **nocturia** refers to excessive urination at night. **Oliguria** is insufficient production of urine. The absence of urine production is **anuria.**

The normal volume of urine produced every 24 hours varies according to the age of the individual (Table 5–1). Infants and children produce smaller volumes than adults. The normal 24-hour urine volume for newborns is between 20 and 350 ml. At the age of one year 300–600 ml is normal for twenty-four hours. For ten-year-olds the volume may range from 750–1500 ml in twenty-four hours. The normal adult volume is 750–2000 ml in twenty-four hours, with 1500 ml being average.

## *LESSON REVIEW*

1. How can improper collection affect urinalysis test results?
2. Why is the first morning specimen preferred?

3. When would a preservative be necessary?
4. Name three common preservatives.
5. What is the major disadvantage of using a preservative?
6. Is the urine volume recorded for routine urinalysis?
7. What is the normal 24-hour volume of urine for each age group?
8. What three factors influence urine volume?
9. How is a clean-catch urine sample collected?
10. When is a clean-catch urine specimen required?
11. What is a mid-stream urine specimen?
12. What are the sources of contamination of a urine specimen?
13. Define anuria, clean-catch urine, mid-stream urine, nocturia, oliguria, and polyuria.

## *STUDENT ACTIVITIES*

1. Re-read the information on collection and preservation of urine.
2. Review the glossary terms.
3. Explain collection and preservation of urine specimens to the instructor.
4. Design patient instruction cards for the collection of clean-catch urine specimens (male and female).
5. Practice giving instructions for obtaining clean-catch urine samples (male and female) as outlined on the Student Performance Guides.

# Student Performance Guide

NAME ______________________

DATE ______________________

## LESSON 5–1 COLLECTION AND PRESERVATION OF URINE: MALE PATIENT

### Instructions

1. Practice instructing male patients in the proper method of urine collection.
2. Explain the procedures for collecting and preserving urine samples satisfactorily for the instructor. All steps must be completed as listed on the instructor's Performance Check Sheet.
3. Complete a written examination successfully.

### Materials and Equipment

- hand disinfectant
- clean, graduated containers and lids (disposable or reusable)
- towelettes
- labels
- hot, sudsy water to clean nondisposable containers
- marking pen
- biohazard container

## Procedure

S = Satisfactory
U = Unsatisfactory

| You must: | S | U | Comments |
|---|---|---|---|
| 1. Wash hands with hand disinfectant | | | |
| 2. Assemble equipment and materials | | | |
| 3. Clean urine bottle by soaking in hot sudsy water and rinsing three times (if using reusable container). Allow the bottle to drip dry | | | |
| 4. Explain to patient the procedure for collecting a clean-catch urine:<br>a. Collect the first urine passed in the morning | | | |
| b. Retract foreskin (if not circumcised) with towelette | | | |
| c. Use one of the towelettes to clean the urethral opening using a single stroke directed from the tip of the penis toward the ring of the glans | | | |
| d. Discard towelette | | | |
| e. Repeat the cleansing procedure with two more towelettes | | | |
| f. Void into the toilet and continue to void but interrupt the stream to collect the urine into the specimen container. Only the middle portion of the urine flow should be included in the sample. Do not touch the inside of the container or the inside of the lid | | | |
| g. Close the container and wash hands | | | |
| 5. Obtain specimen from patient, complete the information on the label (patient number, name, date, time of collection), and attach it to the specimen container | | | |
| 6. Wash hands with hand disinfectant | | | |

Comments:

Student/Instructor:

Date: ______________________ Instructor: ______________________

# Student Performance Guide

NAME ______________________

DATE ______________________

## LESSON 5–1 COLLECTION AND PRESERVATION OF URINE: FEMALE PATIENT

### Instructions

1. Practice instructing female patients in the proper method of urine collection.
2. Explain the procedures for collecting and preserving urine samples satisfactorily for the instructor. All steps must be completed as listed on the instructor's Performance Check Sheet.
3. Complete a written examination successfully.

### Materials and Equipment

- hand disinfectant
- clean, graduated containers and lids (disposable or reusable)
- towelettes
- labels
- hot, sudsy water to clean nondisposable containers
- marking pen
- biohazard container

| **Procedure** | | | S = Satisfactory<br>U = Unsatisfactory |
|---|---|---|---|
| **You must:** | **S** | **U** | **Comments** |
| 1. Wash hands with hand disinfectant | | | |
| 2. Assemble equipment and materials | | | |
| 3. Clean urine bottle by soaking in hot sudsy water and rinsing three times (if using reusable containers). Allow the bottle to drip dry | | | |
| 4. Explain to patient the procedure for collecting a clean-catch urine:<br>a. Collect the first urine passed in the morning | | | |
| b. Sit comfortably on the toilet seat, and swing one knee to the side as far as possible | | | |
| c. Spread the outer folds around the urethral opening using a towelette. Wipe the inner side of the fold with a single stroke from front to back using another towelette, and then discard the towelette | | | |
| d. Use a second towelette and repeat step c on the opposite side of the urethral opening | | | |
| e. Use a third towelette and cleanse the urethral opening with a single front-to-back stroke | | | |
| f. Void into the toilet and continue to void, but interrupt the stream to collect the urine in the container. Only the middle portion of the urine flow should be included in the sample. Do not touch the inside of the container or the inside of the lid | | | |
| g. Close the container and wash hands | | | |
| 5. Obtain specimen from patient, complete the information on the label (patient number, name, date, time of collection), and attach it to the specimen container | | | |
| 6. Wash hands with hand disinfectant | | | |

Comments:

Student/Instructor:

Date: ______________________ Instructor: ______________________

# LESSON 5–2

## Physical Examination of Urine

### LESSON OBJECTIVES

After studying this lesson, you should be able to:

- Perform a physical examination of urine.
- List three causes of abnormal odor of urine.
- Explain why normal urine has a yellow color.
- List three abnormal colors of urine and give a cause for each.
- List two conditions that may affect transparency of urine.
- Explain what determines the specific gravity of urine.
- Demonstrate the proper use of the urinometer and refractometer.
- Define glossary terms.

### GLOSSARY

**hematuria** / presence of red blood cells in urine

**ketones** / substances produced during increased metabolism of fat; sometimes called ketone bodies

**myoglobin** / protein found in muscle tissue

**porphyrins** / a group of pigments which are intermediates in the production of hemoglobin

**specific gravity** / ratio of weight of a given volume of a solution to the weight of the same volume of water; a measurement of density

**urochrome** / yellow pigment which gives color to urine

## INTRODUCTION

A routine urinalysis consists of physical, chemical, and microscopic examinations of urine. The physical examination of urine can provide useful information to the physician and should be the first part of the urinalysis performed.

The physical examination of urine includes observing the odor, color, transparency, and specific gravity. The physical examination is the easiest part of a routine urinalysis, and can be performed at the time the urine is being prepared for other procedures.

Changes in physical characteristics of urine can provide significant clues to renal or metabolic disease. However, variations in odor, color, and transparency do not always reflect pathologic changes. Sometimes, these variations are caused by the handling of the specimen (i.e., temperature of storage). For accurate evaluation of physical characteristics of urine, the sample should be examined immediately after voiding.

## ODOR OF URINE

Normal freshly-voided urine has a characteristic aromatic and not unpleasant odor. Changes in odor of urine may be due to disease, the presence of bacteria, or diet.

The odor of the urine of an uncontrolled diabetic is described as fruity. This is because of the presence of **ketones,** products of fat metabolism. If urine is allowed to stand, bacteria may break down urea to form ammonia; the resulting odor is similar to ammonia. A freshly-voided sample of urine which has a foul, pungent odor suggests the presence of bacteria due to urinary tract infection.

Foods such as garlic and asparagus can also produce an abnormal odor. Although odor may be striking in certain diseases, it is not a reliable enough characteristic to use alone in detecting disease.

## COLOR OF URINE

The normal color of urine is yellow; however, variations in color may be caused by diet, medication, and disease (Table 5–2). The urine color can sometimes provide a clue for the diagnosis of certain diseases.

***Yellow urine.*** The pigment that produces the normal yellow to amber color of urine is **urochrome.** As the urine concentration varies, so will the intensity of the color. Dilute urine samples are pale while the more concentrated urine samples are darker.

**Table 5-2.** Table of Urine Colors and Causes

| Color | Cause |
|---|---|
| Pale yellow to amber | Normal |
| Red, red-brown | Red cells, hemoglobin, myoglobin |
| Wine-red | Porphyrins |
| Brown-black | Melanin, hemoglobin in acidic urine |
| Yellow-brown, green-brown | Bilirubin, bile pigments |

***Red urine.*** The abnormal color seen most frequently is red or red-brown urine. This may be due to **hematuria**—the presence of red blood cells—or to the presence of hemoglobin or **myoglobin. Porphyrins** may cause the urine to be red or wine-red.

***Brown/black urine.*** Hemoglobin will become brown in acidic urine that has been standing. Melanin will also cause urine to become dark or black on standing.

***Yellow-brown or green-brown urine.*** Bilirubin or bile pigments often cause urine to become yellow-brown or green-brown. These urines have a yellow-green foam when shaken. Urine specimens containing bilirubin should be handled with caution to avoid possible exposure of lab personnel to the hepatitis agent.

## TRANSPARENCY OF URINE

Fresh urine is normally clear immediately after voiding. As the urine reaches room temperature, or after refrigeration, it may become cloudy. Depending on the pH of the urine, this cloudiness may be due to urates or phosphates. Mucus or white blood cells in the urine also can cause a cloudy appearance; red blood cells in urine give it a cloudy-red appearance. Fat causes urine to appear opales-

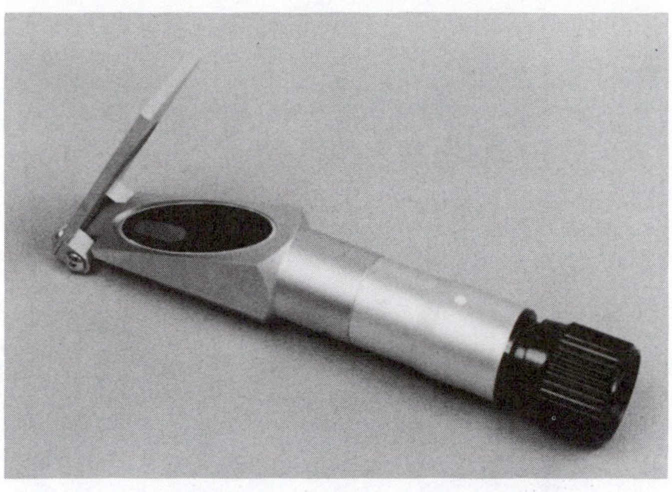

**Figure 5-1.** Refractometer (*Photo by John Estridge*)

cent. Bacteria cause turbidity in urine when present in high numbers.

It is essential that the sample be well-mixed while observing the urine for transparency. The cause of cloudiness will usually be evident during the microscopic examination.

## SPECIFIC GRAVITY

The **specific gravity** of a solution is the ratio of the weight of a given volume of the solution (urine) to the weight of an equal volume of water. The specific gravity of urine indicates the concentration of solids such as urea, phosphates, chlorides, proteins, and sugars which are dissolved in the urine.

The ability of the kidneys to concentrate is reflected by the specific gravity of the urine produced. Urine samples of small volume usually are more concentrated than those of large volume. Dehydration may cause urine to be highly concentrated.

The normal specific gravity of urine ranges from 1.005–1.030, with most samples falling between 1.010 and 1.025. Specific gravity is measured with a refractometer (Figure 5–1) or a urinometer (Figure 5–2).

To use the refractometer, one drop of well-mixed urine is put into the instrument and the value is read directly off a scale viewed through the ocular. The refractometer must be calibrated daily with distilled water (which has a specific gravity of 1.000).

The urinometer method requires a larger volume of urine (about 40–50 ml). The urinometer, which is a float with a calibrated stem, is placed into the sample with a slight spinning motion. The value is read at the meniscus of the urine. The float will rise higher in a concentrated urine and will sink lower in a dilute sample. The urinometer should also be calibrated daily with distilled water.

## PERFORMING A PHYSICAL EXAMINATION OF URINE

To perform a physical examination of urine, a fresh urine specimen must be obtained. The urine should

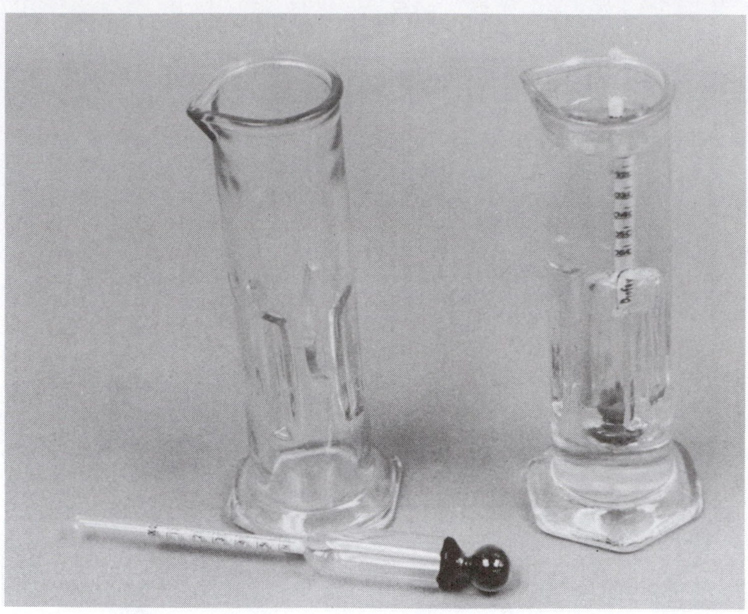

**Figure 5-2.** Urinometer (*Photo by John Estridge*)

**Table 5-3.** Physical Characteristics of Normal Urine

| Characteristic | Normal |
|---|---|
| Transparency | Clear |
| Color | Straw to amber |
| Specific gravity | 1.005–1.030 |

be observed for odor, color, and transparency after it is well mixed (by gentle swirling). The specific gravity of the urine should then be measured using a refractometer or urinometer. These observations and measurements should be recorded and the urine should be retained for chemical and microscopic examinations. The normal values for the physical characteristics of urine are shown in Table 5–3.

### *Precautions*

■ The urine should be gently, but thoroughly, mixed before making physical observations.
■ Wipe up any urine spills with disinfectant.
■ Test urinometer and refractometer daily with distilled water to check reliability.

## *LESSON REVIEW*

1. What does the physical examination of urine include?
2. What are some of the abnormal odors of urine and the causes?
3. What gives urine its normal color?
4. What is the significance of variations in urine color and what are causes of variations?

5. What is the normal transparency of urine?
6. What are some causes of cloudy urine?
7. What is the normal specific gravity of urine?
8. What kidney function is reflected by the specific gravity of urine? urines?
9. Define hematuria, ketones, myoglobin, porphyrins, specific gravity, and urochrome.

## *STUDENT ACTIVITIES*

1. Re-read the information on physical examination of urine.
2. Review the glossary terms.
3. Compare the specific gravities of the lighter-colored urines with those of the darker-colored urines.
4. Divide a urine sample. Put one part in the refrigerator; place the other part on the counter at room temperature. Observe each for transparency changes and odor changes at the end of one hour, two hours, or more.
5. Practice performing physical examinations of several urine samples as outlined on the Student Performance Guide, using the worksheet.

# Student Performance Guide

NAME ______________________

DATE ______________________

## LESSON 5–2 PHYSICAL EXAMINATION OF URINE

### Instructions

1. Practice the procedure for performing a physical examination of urine.
2. Demonstrate the procedure for a physical examination of urine satisfactorily for the instructor. All steps must be completed as listed on the instructor's Performance Check Sheet.
3. Complete a written examination successfully.

### Materials and Equipment

- hand disinfectant
- conical test tube, glass or clear plastic
- test tube rack
- fresh urine sample
- dropping pipet
- refractometer
- urinometer
- distilled water
- urinalysis report form
- soft tissue or soft paper towels
- surface disinfectant
- biohazard container

*Note:* Consult manufacturer's directions before performing the test.

| **Procedure** | | | S = Satisfactory<br>U = Unsatisfactory |
|---|---|---|---|
| **You must:** | **S** | **U** | **Comments** |
| 1. Wash hands with hand disinfectant | | | |
| 2. Assemble equipment and materials | | | |
| 3. Obtain a fresh urine specimen | | | |
| 4. Mix the urine gently by swirling and pour approximately 5 ml into a test tube | | | |
| 5. Observe and record the color of the urine (straw, yellow, red, etc.) | | | |
| 6. Record the odor of the urine | | | |
| 7. Observe and record the transparency of the urine (clear, slightly cloudy, turbid) | | | |
| 8. Measure the specific gravity by using both the refractometer and urinometer:<br>A. Refractometer<br>(1) Place one drop of distilled water on the glass plate of the refractometer and close gently | | | |
| (2) Look through ocular and read the specific gravity from the scale. For water the specific gravity should read 1.000. (If it does not, calibrate with the screwdriver provided with the refractometer) | | | |
| (3) Wipe the water from the glass plate, place one drop of urine on the plate and close gently | | | |
| (4) Look through the ocular, read the specific gravity from the scale and record | | | |
| (5) Clean the glass plate with water and dry with a soft tissue | | | |
| B. Urinometer<br>(1) Pour 40–50 ml of urine into the glass cylinder (approximately three-fourths full) | | | |
| (2) Insert urinometer with spinning motion, gently | | | |
| (3) Read the specific gravity from the scale on the stem of the urinometer as it stops spinning, and record | | | |
| (4) Rinse equipment and repeat B1–B3 with distilled water (specific gravity of water should be 1.000) | | | |

| You must: | S | U | Comments |
|---|---|---|---|
| 9. Discard urine sample properly | | | |
| 10. Clean equipment and return to proper storage | | | |
| 11. Clean work area with disinfectant | | | |
| 12. Wash hands with hand disinfectant | | | |
| Comments: | | | |
| Student/Instructor: | | | |

Date: ______________________ Instructor: ______________________

# Worksheet

NAME ______________________________ DATE ______________

SPECIMEN NO. ______________

## LESSON 5–2 PHYSICAL EXAMINATION OF URINE

Physical Examination

Volume (ml): ______________________ (only report if 24-hour urine)

| | Normal Values |
|---|---|
| Transparency: _____ clear | clear |
| _____ hazy (slightly cloudy) | |
| _____ cloudy (turbid) | |
| Color: ______________________ | straw to amber |
| Specific gravity: ______________________ | 1.005–1.030 |

# LESSON 5-3

## Chemical Examination of Urine

### LESSON OBJECTIVES

After studying this lesson, you should be able to:

- Name six routine chemical tests performed on urine and explain each.
- Demonstrate how to use and interpret a reagent strip.
- List a condition that will cause an abnormal result in each of the six chemical tests routinely performed on urine.
- Demonstrate how to perform four confirmatory chemical tests on urine.
- Discuss the precautions that must be observed in chemical testing of urine.
- Define the glossary terms.

### GLOSSARY

**bilirubin** / the yellow pigment in bile; a breakdown product of hemoglobin

**glomerular** / pertaining to the glomerulus; the filtering unit of the kidney

**glycosuria** / glucose in the urine; glucosuria

**ketonuria** / ketones in the urine

**pH** / a measure of the hydrogen ion (H+) concentration of a substance

**proteinuria** / protein in the urine, usually albumin

**urobilinogen** / a derivative of bilirubin formed by the action of intestinal bacteria

### INTRODUCTION

Tests can be performed on urine samples to detect the presence of certain compounds or chemicals. These tests are usually considered to be a part of a routine urinalysis. When performed correctly, these tests can provide valuable information to the physician. In some situations, the urine chemical test results can be critical to the diagnosis.

## METHODS OF CHEMICAL ANALYSIS

Reagent strips are the most widely used technique of detecting chemicals in urine and are available in a variety of types (Figure 5–3). A reagent strip is a firm plastic strip to which pads containing chemical reactants are attached. Most reagent strips contain reagent areas that test pH, protein, glucose, ketone, bilirubin, and blood. (Some strips may test for **urobilinogen** and bacteria.) The presence (or absence) of these chemicals in the urine provides information on the status of carbohydrate metabolism, kidney and liver function, and acid-base balance of the patient.

Reagent strips are designed to be used only once and discarded. Exact directions for the use of the strips are included in each package. These instructions must be followed precisely for accurate results. A color comparison chart is also included, usually on the label of the reagent strip container. Positive results may be checked by confirmatory tests which will be discussed later. The performance of the strips should be checked by testing strips with urine controls (positive and negative) which may be purchased or made. (See Preparation of Reagents, Appendix K, page 403.)

## PERFORMING THE CHEMICAL TESTS BY REAGENT STRIP

The urine should be tested within one hour of urine collection. If tests cannot be performed within this

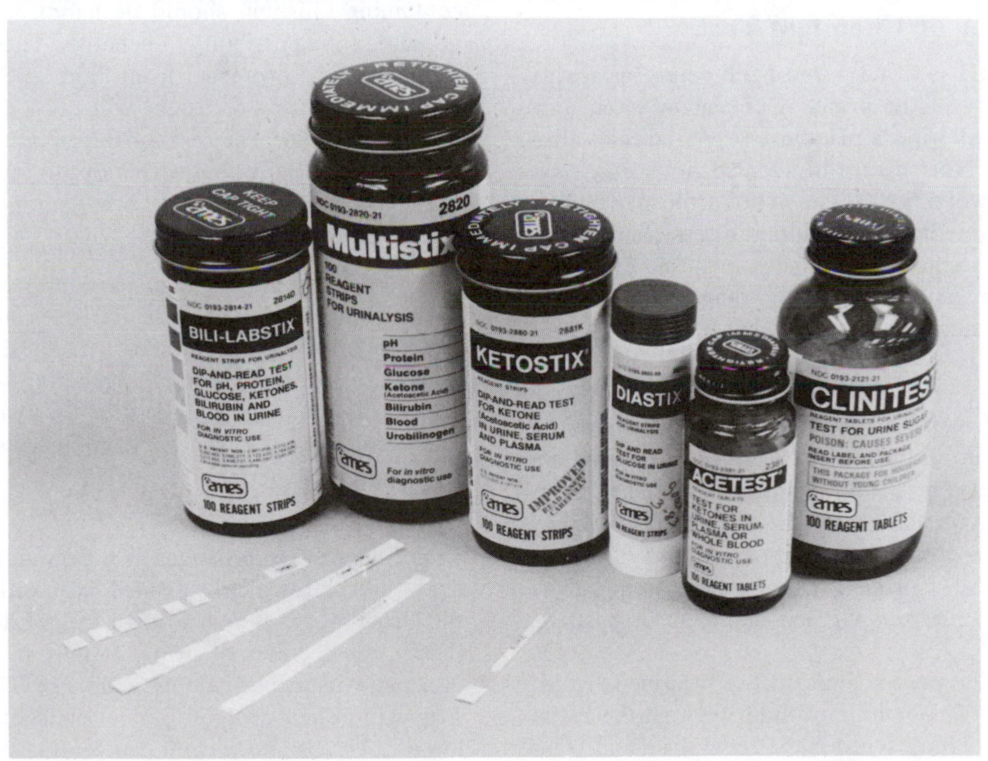


**Figure 5-3.** Various types of reagent strips used for urine testing (*Photo by John Estridge*)

time, the specimen may be refrigerated for up to eight hours. Refrigerated specimens should be allowed to return to room temperature prior to testing.

Chemical testing is performed by dipping a reagent strip into a fresh urine. The color changes on the reagent pads should be visually compared to the color chart after the appropriate time period (Color Plate No. 16). Although in most labs reagent strips are visually interpreted by the technician, there are instruments which can detect the color changes electronically. When such instruments are used, the moistened reagent strip is inserted into the instrument and the results are displayed on a lighted panel. Using such an instrument eliminates technician error due to differences in timing or interpretation of colors.

## Principles of Chemical Tests

*pH.* The **pH** is a measure of the degree of acidity or alkalinity of the urine. A pH below seven indicates an acid urine; a pH above seven indicates alkaline urine. Normal, freshly-voided urine may have a pH range of 5.5–8.0. The pH of urine may change with diet, medications, kidney disease, and metabolic diseases such as diabetes mellitus. Colors on the pH reagent pad usually range from yellow-orange for acid pH to green-blue when pH is alkaline.

*Protein.* Protein in the urine is called **proteinuria.** This is an important indicator of renal disease, but can be caused by conditions other than renal disorders. At a constant pH, the development of any green color on the protein reagent pad is due to the presence of protein. Colors range from yellow for negative to yellow-green or green for positive.

*Glucose.* The presence of glucose in urine is called **glycosuria.** This condition indicates that the blood glucose level has exceeded the renal threshold. This condition may occur in diabetes mellitus. The reagent strip is specific for glucose and uses the enzymes glucose oxidase and peroxidase, which react with glucose to form colors ranging from green (low concentration) to brown (high concentration).

*Ketone.* When the body metabolizes fats incompletely, ketones are excreted in the urine, a condition called **ketonuria.** The ketone test is based on the development of colors ranging from light pink to maroon when ketones react with nitroprusside. Ketonuria may be present in diabetes and starvation or fasting. Since ketones will evaporate at room temperature, urine should be tightly covered and refrigerated if not tested promptly.

*Bilirubin.* **Bilirubin,** a breakdown product of hemoglobin, may be an indication of liver disease, hepatitis or bile duct obstruction. Samples suspected of containing bilirubin should be handled cautiously because of the possibility of hepatitis. These samples should also be protected from light until testing is completed, since direct light will cause decomposition of bilirubin. The test for bilirubin is based on the coupling of bilirubin with a dye to form a color.

*Blood.* Presence of blood in the urine may indicate infection or trauma of the urinary tract or bleeding in the kidneys. Hemoglobin and red cells may be detected by the formation of a color due to the enzyme peroxidase (in red cells) reacting with orthotolidine, a chemical which is in the reagent pad. The resulting color ranges from orange through green to dark blue.

*Urobilinogen.* **Urobilinogen** is a degradation product of bilirubin which is formed by intestinal bacteria. Urobilinogen is normally 0.1 to 1.0 Ehrlich units (E.U.) per deciliter of urine. It may be increased in hepatic disease or hemolytic disease. The reagent strip will detect urobilinogen in concentrations as low as 0.1 E.U. The reagent pad contains a chemical which reacts with urobilinogen to form a brown-orange color.

**Table 5-4.** Normal Values for Urine Chemical Tests

| Substance Tested | Normal Value |
|---|---|
| pH | 5.5–8 |
| protein | negative to trace |
| glucose | negative |
| ketone | negative |
| bilirubin | negative |
| blood | negative |
| urobilinogen | 0.1–1.0 E.U./dl |
| bacteria (nitrite) | negative |

## Normal Values

Normal urine, when tested with a reagent strip, is negative for glucose, ketone, bilirubin, bacteria, and blood. Normal urine may be negative or contain a trace of protein. Normal, freshly-voided urine usually has a pH of 5.5–8 (Table 5–4). Positive results should be confirmed according to laboratory policy. Some laboratories retest with a reagent strip; others use confirmatory tests.

## CONFIRMATORY TESTS

Sometimes it may be necessary to measure chemicals in urine other than by the reagent strip method. The other methods are called confirmatory tests because the most common use is to confirm a positive (or negative) result obtained using the reagent strip. Confirmatory tests are more time consuming and require more reagents and equipment than the reagent strip method. Four most commonly used confirmatory tests are those for protein, reducing sugars, ketone, and bilirubin.

***Protein.*** Most simple tests for urine protein involve treating the urine with an acid to cause the protein to precipitate and therefore become visible. The amount of precipitate formed is roughly proportional to the concentration of protein present. Acids that are commonly used are acetic, nitric, and sulfosalicylic acids.

***Reducing sugars.*** A copper reduction test such as Clinitest® is the most common test performed to detect reducing sugars such as lactose and galactose. These sugars may be present in the urine of infants. The test is based on the reduction of copper ions in the Clinitest® tablet by substances such as glucose, galactose, or lactose. Therefore, the test is not specific for glucose. If a reducing sugar is present in the urine, the color changes from blue to green and then orange depending on the amount of sugar present. Since the Clinitest® is not specific for glucose and a number of substances such as penicillin, salicylates, and reducing sugars may cause positive results, Clinitest® results should not be used as the sole basis for adjusting insulin dosage.

***Ketone.*** The Acetest® is a test for ketones and is available in tablet form. The test is based on the same principle as that found in the reagent strip. If ketones are present in urine, a drop of urine added to the tablet will produce a purple color. A strip such as Ketostix® or Ketodiastix® may also be used to confirm presence of ketones.

***Bilirubin.*** The Ictotest® is a specific test for bilirubin and is four times as sensitive as the reagent strip method. The test is composed of a tablet and absorbent mat. A few drops of urine are placed on the mat, the tablet is placed over the moist area, and water is dropped on the tablet. If bilirubin is present, a purple color will develop on the mat within thirty seconds.

### *Precautions*

- Reagent strips should be tested with positive controls on each day of use to be sure that strips are working properly.

- Failure to observe color changes at the appropriate time intervals may cause inaccurate results.
- Reagents and reagent strips must be stored properly to retain reactivity.
- Observe color changes and color charts under good lighting.
- Proper collection and storage of urine is necessary to insure preservation of components such as bilirubin and ketones.
- Use care in performing the Clinitest procedure because of the heat that is generated and the caustic nature of the reagents.
- Do not allow the reagent pads of the reagent strips to touch the fingers or other surfaces.
- Wipe up any spills promptly with surface disinfectant.

## *LESSON REVIEW*

1. What are the six chemical tests routinely performed on urine?
2. Explain briefly how a reagent strip is used.
3. What type of urine specimen is preferred for chemical testing?
4. Name three confirmatory tests performed on urine.
5. Name a condition that may cause an increase of the following chemicals in urine: protein, ketones, glucose, and bilirubin.
6. Name a method of measuring urine protein other than by the reagent strip method.
7. Name a test that may be performed to detect a reducing sugar other than glucose.
8. List two precautions that must be observed to insure accurate results in chemical testing of urine.
9. Define bilirubin, glomerular, glycosuria, ketonuria, pH, proteinuria, and urobilinogen.

## *STUDENT ACTIVITIES*

1. Re-read the information on chemical examination of urine.
2. Review the glossary terms.
3. Practice performing chemical examinations on several urine samples as outlined on the Student Performance Guide, using the worksheet.
4. Compare the results of the physical examination of a sample with the chemical examination results. Are they as expected? If protein is present in a sample, is specific gravity high? If blood is positive on a reagent strip, was it detected in the physical examination?

# Student Performance Guide

NAME ______________________________

DATE ______________________________

## LESSON 5–3 CHEMICAL EXAMINATION OF URINE

### Instructions

1. Practice the procedure for performing a chemical examination of urine.
2. Demonstrate the procedure for a chemical examination of urine satisfactorily for the instructor. All steps must be completed as listed on the instructor's Performance Check Sheet.
3. Complete a written examination successfully.

### Materials and Equipment

- hand disinfectant
- fresh urine samples
- urine control solutions (positive and negative)
- reagent strips with comparative chart
- stopwatch or timer
- conical graduated centrifuge tubes
- forceps
- centrifuge
- test tubes, 13 × 100 mm and 16 × 125 mm
- dropping pipets
- distilled water
- 20% sulfosalicylic acid
- Clinitest® tablets
- Acetest® tablets
- Ictotest® tablets and absorbent pads
- test tube racks
- worksheet
- urinalysis report forms
- surface disinfectant
- biohazard container

*Note:* Consult package inserts for specific instructions before performing tests

| **Procedure** | | | S = Satisfactory<br>U = Unsatisfactory |
|---|---|---|---|
| **You must:** | **S** | **U** | **Comments** |
| 1. Wash hands with hand disinfectant | | | |
| 2. Assemble equipment and materials | | | |
| 3. Obtain urine sample (or control) | | | |
| 4. Perform reagent strip test:<br>a. Dip reagent strip into urine sample, moistening all pads | | | |
| b. Remove strip from urine immediately and tap to remove excess urine | | | |
| c. Observe reagent pads and compare colors to color chart at appropriate time intervals | | | |
| d. Record results on urinalysis report form | | | |
| e. Discard reagent strip | | | |
| 5. Perform sulfosalicylic acid test for protein (usually performed only if protein is positive by reagent strip method):<br>a. Centrifuge five ml of urine to clear the urine if it is cloudy | | | |
| b. Place four ml of clear urine into a 13 × 100 mm test tube. | | | |
| c. Add three drops of 20% sulfosalicylic acid | | | |
| d. Mix thoroughly and estimate the amount of turbidity | | | |
| e. Record results on urinalysis form as negative, trace, 1+, 2+, 3+, or 4+ | | | |
| 6. Perform Clinitest® for reducing substances:<br>a. Place 16 × 125 mm test tube into a test tube rack | | | |
| b. Place five drops of urine into the test tube | | | |
| c. Place ten drops of distilled water into the test tube | | | |
| d. Drop a Clinitest® reagent tablet into the urine-water mixture (use forceps, the Clinitest® tablet will burn fingers) | | | |
| e. Observe color while allowing tablet to effervesce or boil until boiling stops and without touching the test tube with fingers | | | |
| f. Wait fifteen seconds, shake test tube gently using forceps and compare color to color chart (tube will be hot and opening should be pointed away from the face) | | | |
| g. Record results on urinalysis report form as negative, ¼%, ½%, ¾%, 1%, or 2% or more | | | |

| You must: | S | U | Comments |
|---|---|---|---|
| 7. Perform Acetest® for ketones<br>a. Place an Acetest® tablet on a clean piece of white paper or filter paper<br>b. Place one drop of urine on top of the tablet<br>c. Compare color of tablet to color chart after thirty seconds<br>d. Record results on urinalysis report form as negative or positive | | | |
| 8. Perform Ictotest® for bilirubin<br>a. Place five drops of urine on an Ictotest® mat (if bilirubin is present, it will be absorbed onto the mat surface)<br>b. Place an Ictotest® reagent tablet on the moistened area of the mat<br>c. Let two drops of water flow onto the tablet<br>*Note:* When elevated amounts of bilirubin are present in the urine specimen, a blue to purple color forms on the mat within thirty seconds. The rapidity of the formation of the color and the intensity of the color are proportional to the amount of bilirubin in the urine (a pink or red color is a negative test)<br>d. Record results on urinalysis report form as negative or positive | | | |
| 9. Dispose of urine specimen properly | | | |
| 10. Dispose of test tube contents properly | | | |
| 11. Clean equipment and return to proper storage | | | |
| 12. Clean work area with surface disinfectant | | | |
| 13. Wash hands with hand disinfectant | | | |

Comments:

Student/Instructor:

Date: ______________________ Instructor: ______________________

# Worksheet

NAME ______________________________ DATE ____________

SPECIMEN NO. ____________

## LESSON 5–3 CHEMICAL EXAMINATION OF URINE

Chemical Examination

A. Multistix

| | | Normal Values |
|---|---|---|
| pH | ____________ | 5.5–8.0 |
| protein | ____________ | negative, trace |
| glucose | ____________ | negative |
| ketone | ____________ | negative |
| bilirubin | ____________ | negative |
| blood | ____________ | negative |
| urobilinogen | ____________ | 0.1–1.0 E.U./dl urine |

Confirmatory Test Results (circle results)

B. Protein (sulfosalicylic acid): __________ negative trace 1+ 2+ 3+ 4+

Reducing substances (Clinitest®): ______ negative ¼% ½% ¾% 1% 2% or more

Ketones (Acetest®): ________________ negative positive

Bilirubin (Ictotest®): ______________ negative positive

# LESSON 5–4

## Identification of Urine Sediment

### LESSON OBJECTIVES

After studying this lesson, you should be able to:

- Write a definition of urine sediment.
- Name four types of cells that may be seen in urine sediment.
- Name three types of casts that may appear in urine sediment.
- Explain how casts are formed.
- Name and draw eight crystals which may be seen in urine sediment.
- List the precautions that should be observed when identifying components of urine sediment.
- Identify components of urine sediment using the microscope.
- Define the glossary terms.

### GLOSSARY

**amorphous** / without shape
**cast** / mold; in urinalysis, a protein matrix formed in the tubules that becomes washed into urine
**hyaline** / transparent, pale
**sediment** / solid substances which settle to the bottom of a liquid
**supernatant** / clear liquid remaining at the top after centrifugation or settling of precipitate

## INTRODUCTION

Examining urine sediment is part of a routine urinalysis. It may provide beneficial information in evaluating the course and progress of renal disease as well as detecting the presence of infection. The urine must be freshly voided and examined as soon as possible to prevent deterioration of sediment components. Sediment is obtained by centrifugation of 10–15 ml of urine. The **supernatant** urine is carefully poured off and the sediment remaining in the tube is resuspended, placed on a slide, and examined microscopically.

## COMPONENTS OF URINE SEDIMENT

The term urine **sediment** usually refers to cells, casts, crystals, and amorphous deposits. These components of urine sediment may be identified microscopically and are usually observed unstained. (See Color Plates 17–24 for examples of some components of urine sediment.)

### Cells in Urine Sediment

***Blood Cells.*** Normal urine may contain a few blood cells. Blood cells are best identified using the high power (45X) objective.

- Erythrocytes (red blood cells)—Erythrocytes usually look like pale, light-refractive disks when viewed under high power (Figure 5–4 and Color Plates 17, 18, 19, and 21). They have no nuclei. The presence of large numbers of red cells in urine is called *hematuria* and is an abnormal condition indicating disease or trauma.
- Leukocytes (white blood cells)—A few leukocytes may be present in normal urine (Figure 5–5). The type usually present is the segmented neutrophil. Leukocytes in urine may be increased in urinary tract infections. Leukocytes are slightly larger than erythrocytes, may appear granular and have a visible nucleus (Color Plates 17, 18, and 21).

***Epithelial Cells.*** Epithelial cells are constantly being sloughed off from the lining of the urinary tract. The epithelial cells appear large and flat, with a distinct nucleus and much cytoplasm. These cells may be identified using the high power (45X) objective. The most commonly seen cell is the squamous epithelial cell (Figure 5–6); less commonly seen are the smaller bladder and renal tubular cells (Figure 5–7). The latter may indicate renal disease

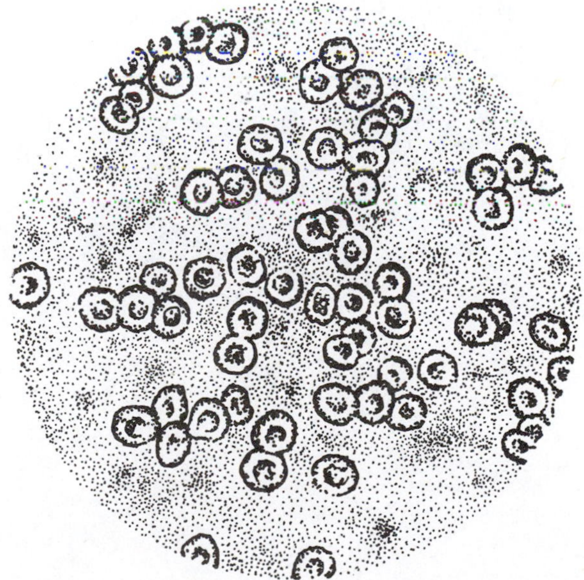

**Figure 5-4.** Erythrocytes in urine sediment

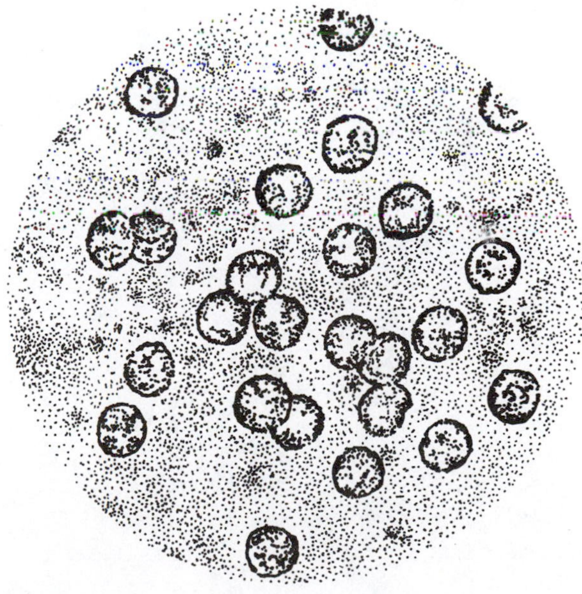

**Figure 5-5.** Leukocytes in urine sediment

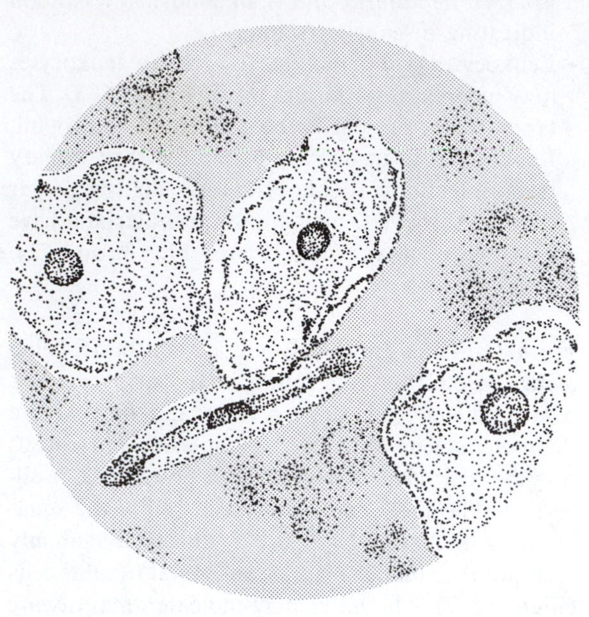

Figure 5-6. Squamous epithelial cells

if they are present in large numbers (Color Plates 17–19).

*Microorganisms.* Microorganisms should not be present in properly collected, fresh, normal urine. The presence of large numbers of microorganisms indicates infection. Microorganisms are observed using the high power (45X) objective (Figure 5–8).

- Bacteria—Bacteria may appear as tiny round or rod-shaped objects. The rod-shaped bacteria are usually more noticeable because the round ones may closely resemble amorphous material.
- Yeast—Yeast cells may be present in urine sediment. They are smaller than erythrocytes but may appear similar to them. Yeasts are ovoid and may be observed budding or in chains (Figure 5–9). To distinguish between yeasts and red cells, add one drop of dilute acetic acid to the urine sediment; red cells will lyse and yeast will not. The most common yeast found is *Candida albicans.*

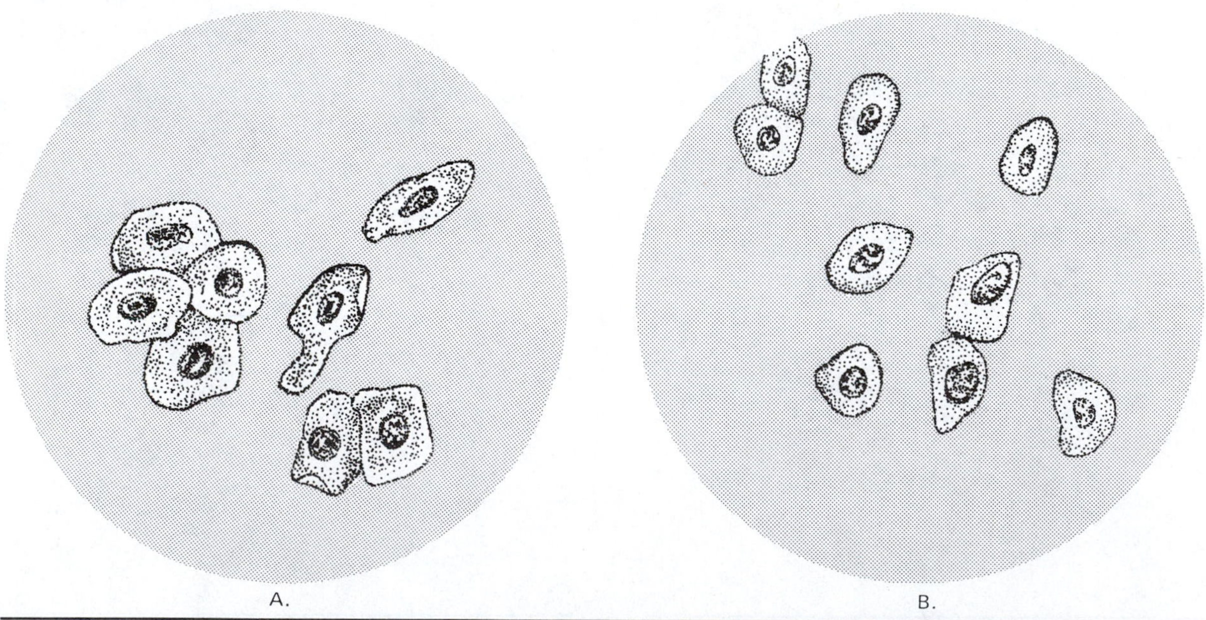


Figure 5-7. Bladder and renal tubular epithelial cells: A) bladder epithelial cells and B) renal epithelial cells

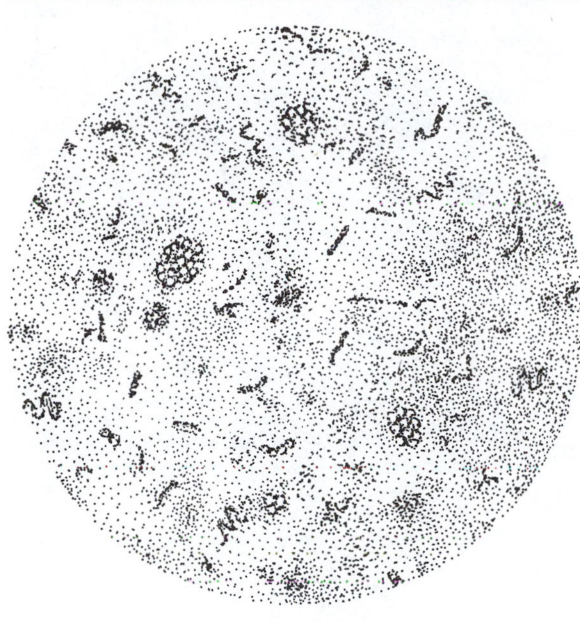

**Figure 5-8.** Bacteria in urine sediment

- Protozoa—*Trichomonas vaginalis* is the most frequently seen parasite in urine. It is a flagellated protozoan that may infect the urinary tract and is usually recognized in urine sediment because of the movement of flagellae (Figure 5-10).
- Spermatozoa—Spermatozoa may occasionally be observed in urine samples. They are easily recognized and have spherical heads and long thin tails. Spermatozoa should only be reported when they are identified in urine samples of males (Figure 5-11).

## Casts in Urine Sediment

**Casts** are formed when protein accumulates and precipitates in the kidney tubules and is washed into the urine. The presence of casts in urine, other than an occasional **hyaline** cast, may indicate renal disease. Casts are cylindrical with rounded or flat ends and are classified according to the substances observed in them (Figure 5-12). Some casts may trap cells or debris as they are formed and appear

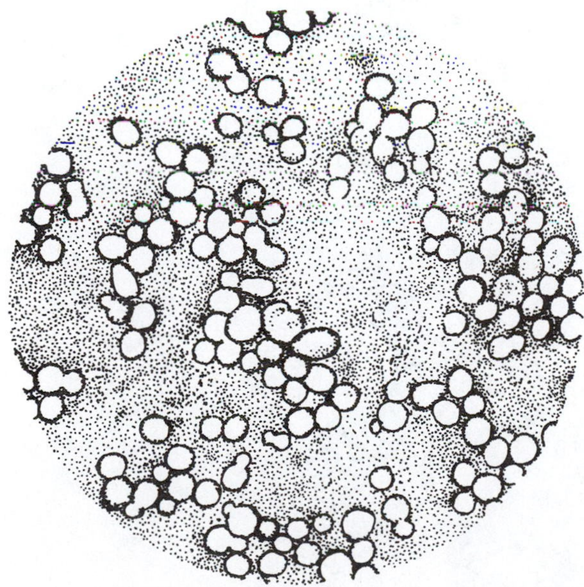

**Figure 5-9.** Yeasts in urine sediment

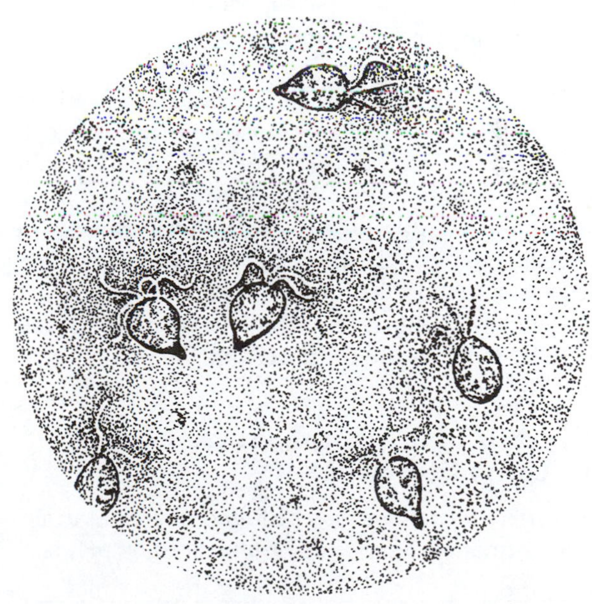

**Figure 5-10.** Protozoa in urine sediment

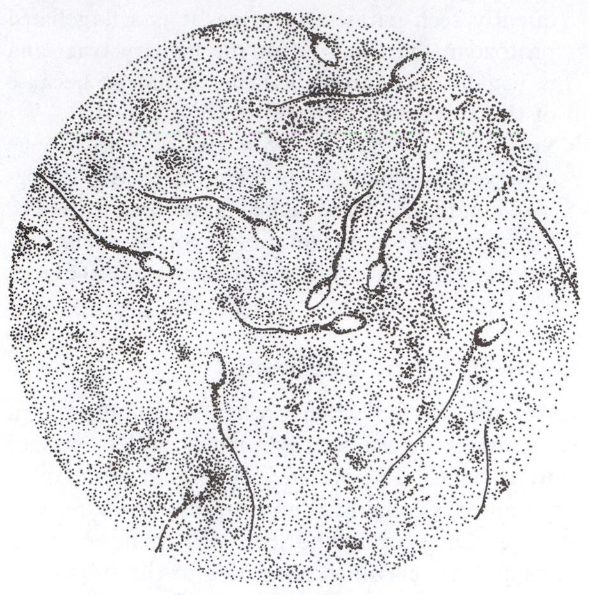

**Figure 5-11.** Spermatozoa in urine sediment

cellular or granular. Casts are viewed using the low power objective (10X) and low light.

- Hyaline—Hyaline casts are occasionally found in normal urine. They are transparent colorless cylinders and are best seen by reducing the light on the microscope (Color Plate 20).
- Granular—A granular cast contains remnants of disintegrated cells which appear as fine or coarse granules embedded in the protein.
- Cellular—Cellular casts may contain epithelial cells, red cells, or white cells in the protein.

## Crystals and Amorphous Deposits in Urine Sediment

A variety of crystals may be found in normal urine. The formation of crystals is influenced by pH, spe-

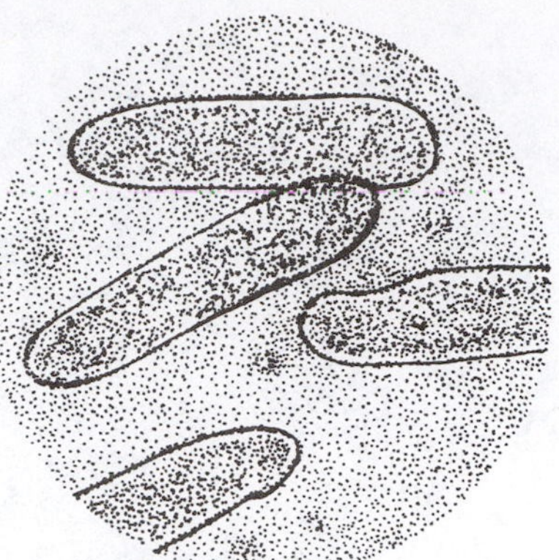

A. HYALINE

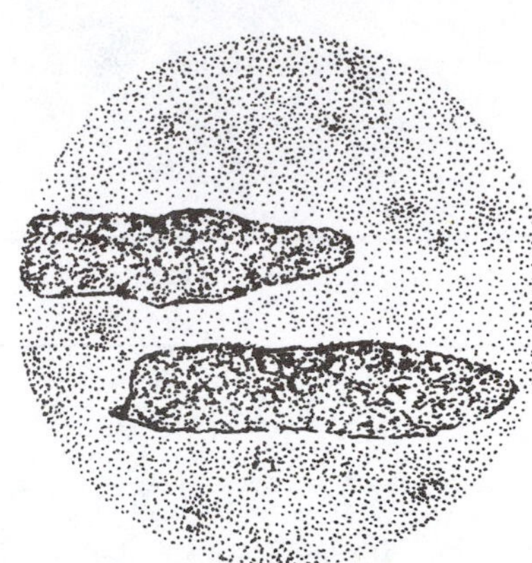

B. GRANULAR

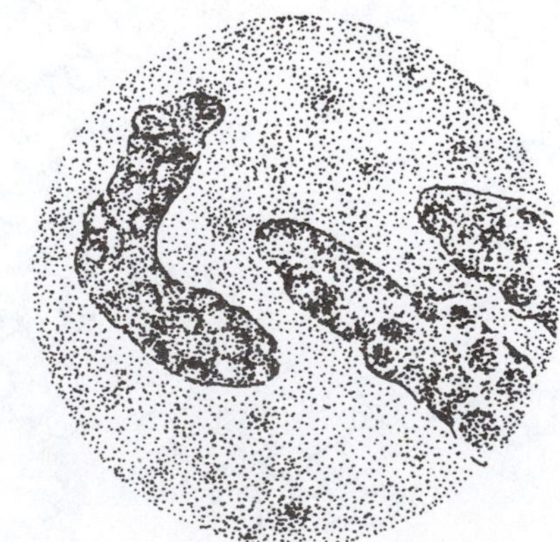

C. CELLULAR

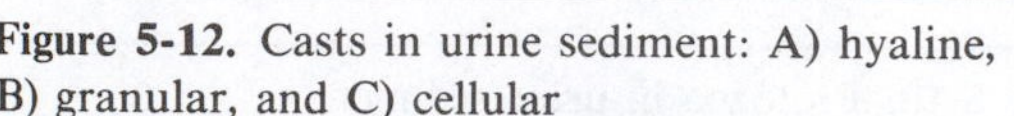

**Figure 5-12.** Casts in urine sediment: A) hyaline, B) granular, and C) cellular

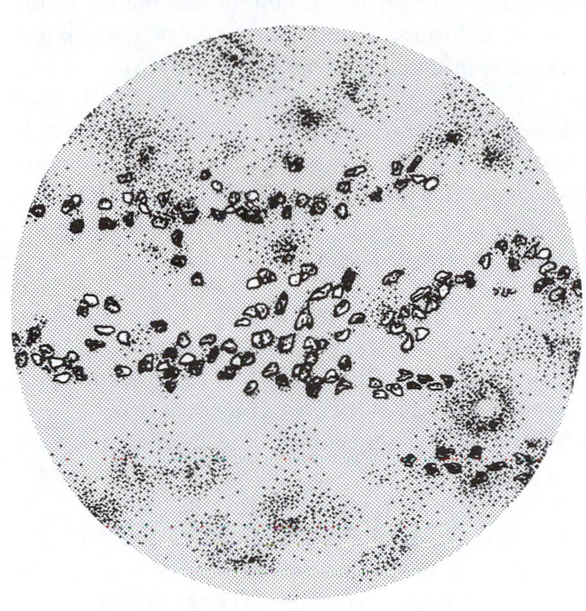

**Figure 5-13.** Amorphous urates in urine sediment

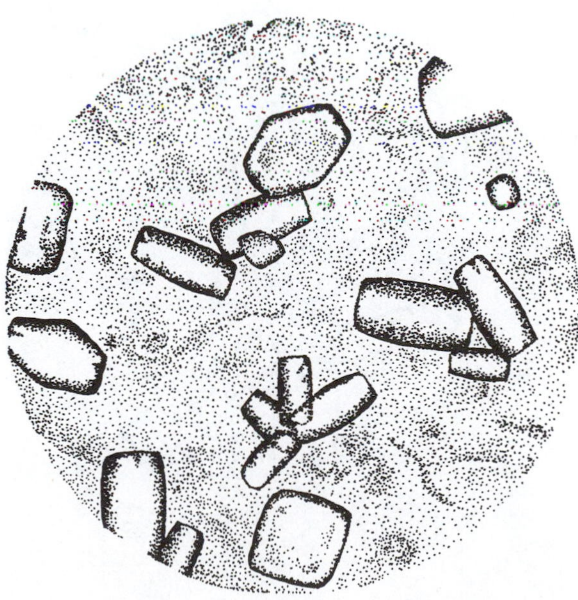

**Figure 5-14.** Uric acid crystals in urine sediment

cific gravity, and temperature of the urine. Although most urine crystals have no clinical significance, there are some rare crystals which appear in urine because of certain metabolic disorders. Therefore, it is important to be able to recognize both normal and abnormal crystals. Crystals, when seen, should be identified and reported.

*Normal Crystals in Acid Urine.* The normal crystals most commonly seen in acid urine are **amorphous** urates, uric acid, and calcium oxalate.

- Amorphous urates—The amorphous urates may appear in urine as fine granules with no specific shape. Sediment may appear pink in the urine container but, under the microscope, will appear yellowish (Figure 5–13).
- Uric acid—Uric acid may appear as yellow-brown crystals which may have a variety of shapes: irregular, rhombic, clusters, or rosettes (Figure 5–14).
- Calcium oxalate—Calcium oxalate forms colorless octahedral crystals which are refractile. They may look like "envelopes," having an X intersecting the crystal, and may vary in size (Figure 5–15).

*Normal Crystals in Alkaline Urine.* The normal crystals most commonly seen in alkaline urine are amorphous phosphates, triple phosphate, and calcium carbonate.

- Amorphous phosphates—Phosphates may appear as colorless amorphous granular masses in urine sediment. Amorphous phosphates are soluble in 10% acetic acid (Figure 5–16).
- Triple phosphate—Ammonium magnesium phosphate (triple phosphate) may form colorless, highly refractile prisms having three to six sides. The crystals are often described as having a coffin-lid appearance (Figure 5–17).

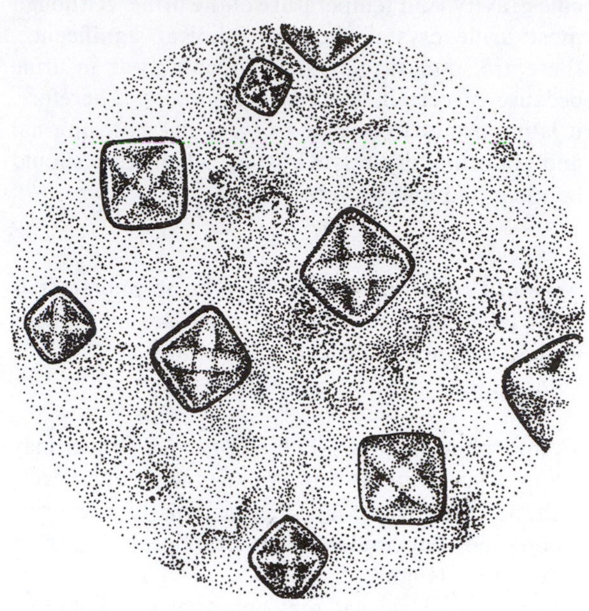

Figure 5-15. Calcium oxalate crystals in urine sediment

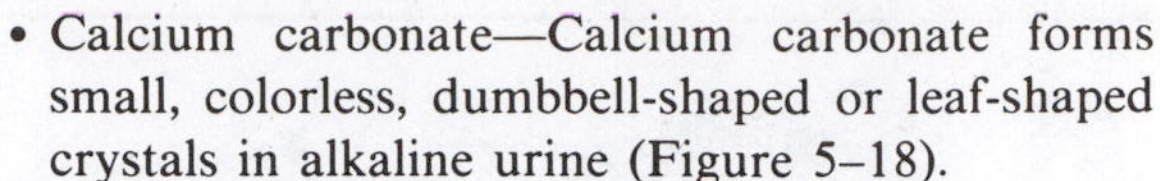

- Calcium carbonate—Calcium carbonate forms small, colorless, dumbbell-shaped or leaf-shaped crystals in alkaline urine (Figure 5–18).

***Abnormal Crystals in Urine.*** Abnormal crystals may be seen in the urine of patients with metabolic disease or after administration of drugs such as sulfonamides. Some rare crystals are cystine, tyrosine, leucine, cholesterol, and sulfonamide.

- Cystine—Cystine may form colorless, refractile, flat hexagonal crystals, usually having unequal sides. Presence of these crystals in urine indicates disease such as *cystinuria* (Figure 5–19).
- Tyrosine—Tyrosine forms fine needles arranged in sheaves. Presence of these crystals indicates liver disease or damage (Figure 5–20).
- Leucine—Leucine crystals appear as oily spheres which may be yellow-brown in color and are refractive. Presence of these crystals in urine is an indication of liver disease or damage (Figure 5–21).

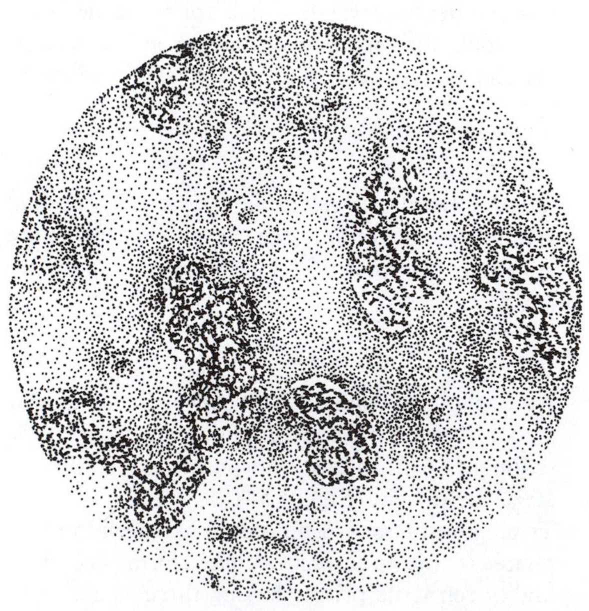

Figure 5-16. Amorphous phosphates in urine sediment

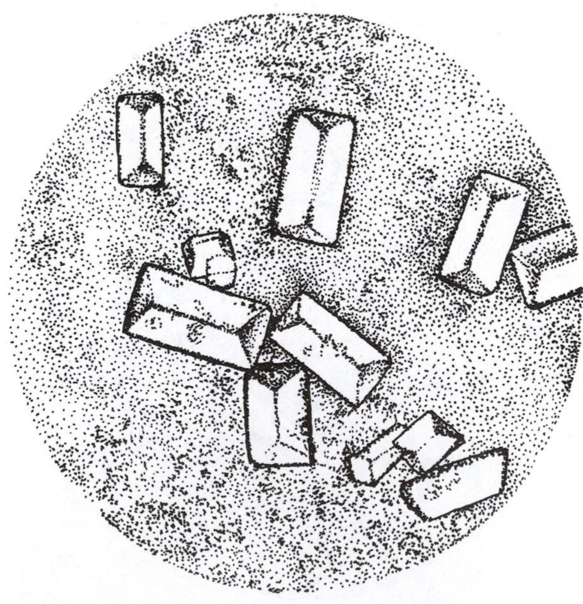

Figure 5-17. Triple phosphate crystals in urine sediment

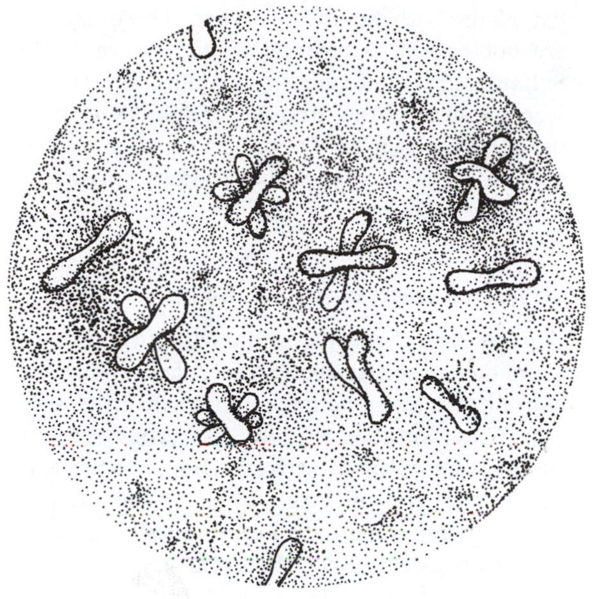

**Figure 5-18.** Calcium carbonate crystals in urine sediment

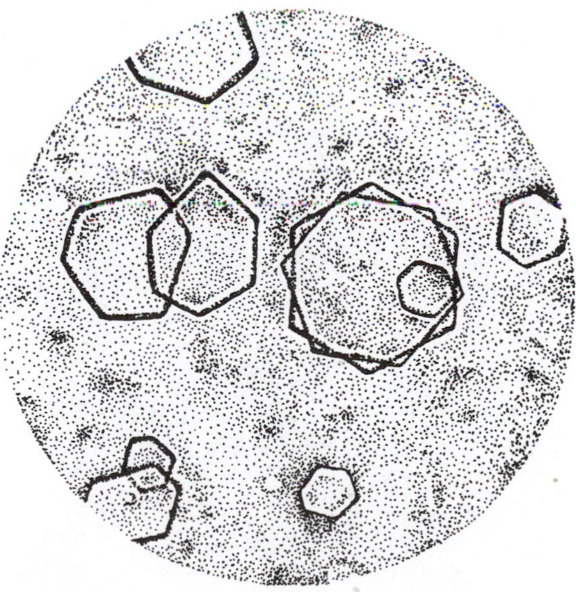

**Figure 5-19.** Cystine crystals in urine sediment

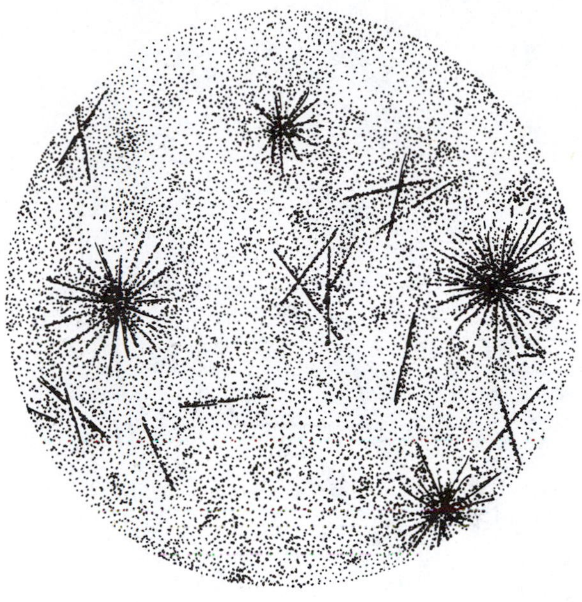

**Figure 5-20.** Tyrosine crystals in urine sediment

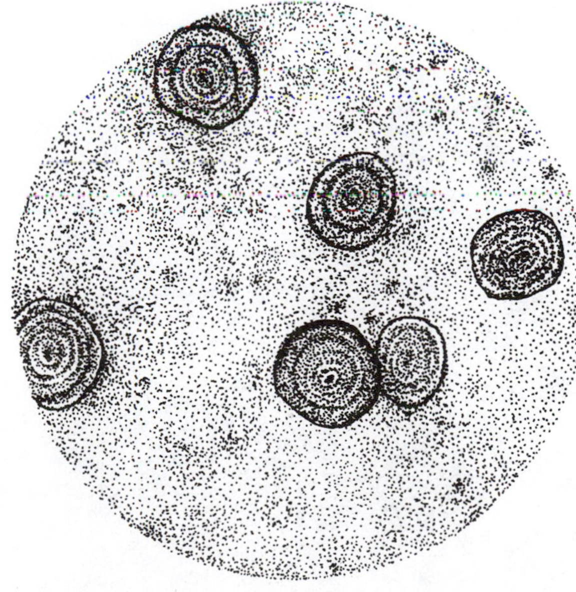

**Figure 5-21.** Leucine crystals in urine sediment

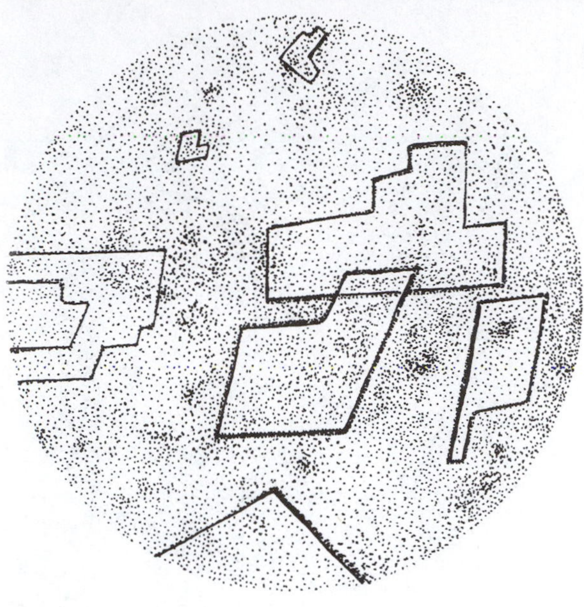

**Figure 5-22.** Cholesterol crystals in urine sediment

- Cholesterol—Cholesterol crystals are colorless, flat plates with notched corners. These crystals are not present in normal urine (Figure 5–22).
- Sulfonamide—Sulfonamide crystals are rarely seen because of the increased solubility of sulfa drugs currently used. Crystals, when seen, appear as bundles of needles with striations (Figure 5–23).

## Other Substances in Urine

Mucus threads (from the urinary tract lining) and contaminants such as fibers, hair, talc granules and oil droplets may sometimes appear in urine sediment. These substances must be recognized and should not be confused with substances in the sediment that are clinically significant. Mucus threads, when seen, are reported (Figure 5–24); contaminants or artifacts are not (Figure 5–25).

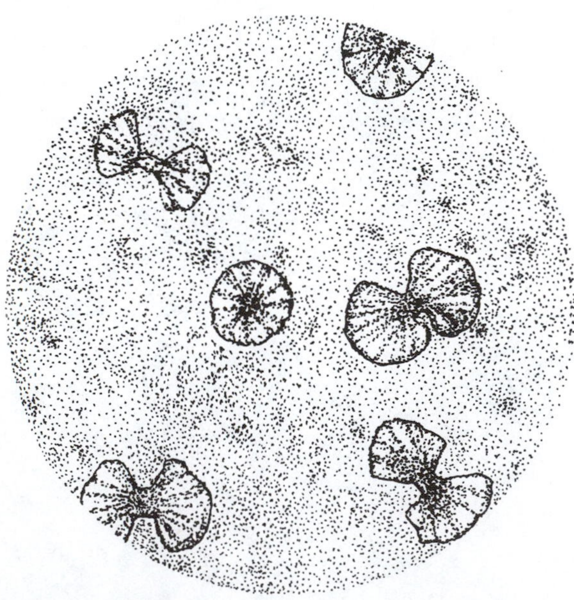

**Figure 5-23.** Sulfonamide crystals in urine sediment

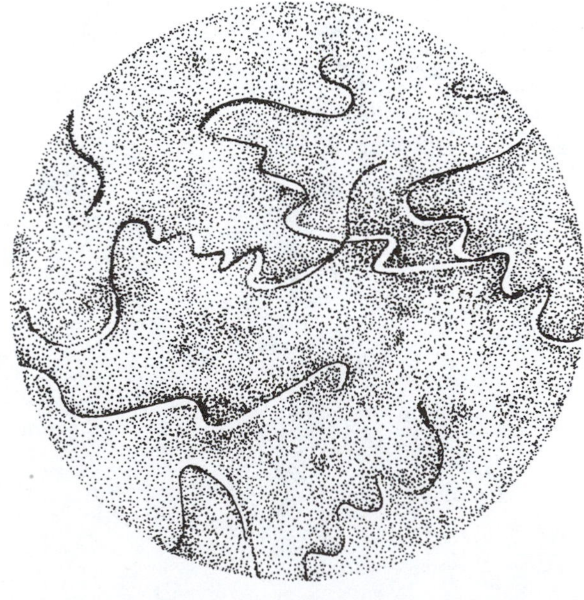

**Figure 5-24.** Mucus threads in urine sediment

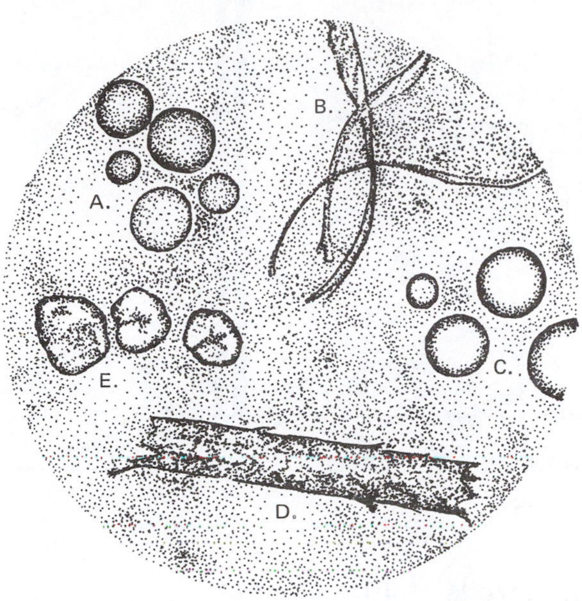


**Figure 5-25.** Common artifacts in urine sediment: A) air bubbles, B) fibers, C) oil droplets, D) hair, and E) starch granules

### *Precautions*

■ Urine samples should be handled with care and spills should be wiped with a surface disinfectant. If urine comes in contact with skin, wash the area with a hand disinfectant.

■ Urine sediment must be observed using reduced light on the microscope.

## *LESSON REVIEW*

1. Is identification of urine sediment a part of a routine urinalysis?
2. What is the significance of blood cells in urine sediment?
3. Name four types of cells that may be seen in urine sediment.
4. Should microorganisms be found in fresh, properly collected normal urine?
5. Explain how casts are formed.
6. What are three types of casts that may appear in urine sediment?
7. What are eight crystals which may be seen in urine sediment? Describe the appearance of each.
8. Define amorphous, cast, hyaline, sediment, and supernatant.

## *STUDENT ACTIVITIES*

1. Re-read the information on identification of urine sediment.
2. Review the glossary terms.
3. Practice microscopic identification of the components of one or more urine sediments as outlined on the Student Performance Guide. Compare your responses with those obtained by the instructor or fellow students.
4. Use unlabeled illustrations provided by the instructor to identify the components of urine sediment.

# Student Performance Guide

NAME ______________________

DATE ______________________

## LESSON 5–4 IDENTIFICATION OF URINE SEDIMENT

### Instructions

1. Practice identification of urine sediment.
2. Identify components of urine sediment microscopically or by visual aids satisfactorily for the instructor. All steps must be completed as listed on the instructor's Performance Check Sheet.
3. Complete a written examination successfully.

### Materials and Equipment

- hand disinfectant
- urine sediments
- microscope
- glass slides
- coverglasses
- visuals depicting various components of sediment
- surface disinfectant
- biohazard container

### Procedure

S = Satisfactory
U = Unsatisfactory

| You must: | S | U | Comments |
|---|---|---|---|
| 1. Wash hands with hand disinfectant | | | |
| 2. Assemble equipment and materials | | | |
| 3. Obtain a sample of urine sediment | | | |

| You must: | S | U | Comments |
|---|---|---|---|
| 4. Pour one drop of resuspended urine sediment onto a clean glass slide | | | |
| 5. Place coverglass over drop of urine | | | |
| 6. Place slide on microscope stage securely | | | |
| 7. Focus microscope using low power (10X) | | | |
| 8. Scan slide using reduced light on microscope | | | |
| 9. Observe and identify casts if present | | | |
| 10. Rotate high power (45X) objective into position | | | |
| 11. Scan slides and identify any blood cells, bacteria, yeasts, or epithelial cells which may be present | | | |
| 12. Identify any crystals or amorphous deposits present | | | |
| 13. Identify components of sediment not seen on slide from unlabeled illustrations | | | |
| 14. Discard sediment properly and discard slide in biohazard container | | | |
| 15. Repeat steps 3–14 using another urine sediment | | | |
| 16. Clean and return equipment to proper storage | | | |
| 17. Clean work area with surface disinfectant | | | |
| 18. Wash hands with hand disinfectant | | | |

Comments:

Student/Instructor:

Date: ______________________ Instructor: ______________________

# LESSON 5–5

## Microscopic Examination of Urine Sediment

### LESSON OBJECTIVES

After studying this lesson, you should be able to:

- Discuss briefly the proper specimen to use for microscopic examination of urine.
- Name a cause of deterioration of cellular elements in a urine sample.
- Describe how to prepare urine sediment from a urine specimen.
- List the normal values for erythrocytes, leukocytes, casts, and bacteria in urine.
- List the precautions to be observed when microscopically examining urine.
- Prepare a slide for examining urine sediment.
- Perform a microscopic examination of urine sediment and report the results.

### INTRODUCTION

The microscopic examination of urine is the third part of the routine urinalysis. A microscopic examination of urine sediment provides helpful information in evaluating the course and progression of renal disease. The examination also helps to diagnose some infections and metabolic diseases.

Early morning specimens are preferred for routine urinalysis because the specimen is usually more concentrated. If the urine is too dilute, red blood cells, white blood cells, and epithelial cells may lyse and the amount and types of urine sediment seen may be misleading. The urine should be examined as soon as possible to prevent cellular deterioration. The specimen should be a mid-stream or clean-catch specimen to avoid contamination of the specimen with epithelial cells.

### OBTAINING THE URINE SEDIMENT

To obtain the sediment, 10 to 15 ml of urine should be poured into a clean, graduated conical centrifuge tube. The tube should be centrifuged at a standard speed (usually 1500 to 2000 rpm) for five minutes. The supernatant urine is then carefully poured off (except for 0.5–1.0 ml). The sediment remaining in the tube is resuspended by gently shaking the tube.

## PERFORMING THE MICROSCOPIC EXAMINATION

A drop of resuspended sediment is poured directly onto a clean microscope slide and covered with a coverslip. The slide is first examined with the low power objective (10X) and low light to locate elements that are present in low numbers, such as casts. Ten to fifteen low power fields (LPF) are scanned and the number of casts per LPF is counted and recorded.

The high power objective (45X) is used to identify erythrocytes, leukocytes, epithelial cells, yeasts, bacteria, and crystals (ten to fifteen high power fields should be scanned). The diaphragm of the microscope should be adjusted during the scanning to obtain the proper amount of light. The number of erythrocytes, leukocytes, and epithelial cells per high power field (HPF) are counted, averaged, and recorded. Table 5–5 lists the normal values for urine sediment.

## METHOD OF COUNTING CELLS AND MAGNIFICATION

The method of counting cells and the magnification used may differ among laboratories. Therefore, the method used should always be that of the laboratory where the test is being performed. The counts for RBC, WBC, and epithelial cells represent an average of the number of cells seen in each of the 10 high power fields (HPF) scanned. The results may be reported as 0, rare, occasional or as a range such as 2–4 or 4–6.

The count for casts represents an average of the number of casts seen in each of the 10 low power fields (LPF) scanned. Casts should be categorized as hyaline, granular, or cellular. The method of reporting casts is like that for cells.

Microorganisms such as yeasts (budding) and protozoa such as *Trichomonas* should be reported if seen. Bacteria are usually only reported if large numbers are seen in a fresh urine sample that has been properly collected.

Mucus threads and crystals should be reported if seen, and crystals should be identified. Mucus and bacteria are usually reported as negative, 1+, 2+, 3+, and 4+. Spermatozoa are only reported in males.

**Table 5-5.** Normal Values for Components of Urine Sediment

| Component | Normal Value |
|---|---|
| RBC/HPF | rare |
| WBC/HPF | 0–4 |
| epith/HPF | occasional (may be higher in females) |
| casts/LPF | occasional hyaline |
| bacteria | negative |
| mucus | negative to 2+ |
| crystals | only crystals such as cystine, leucine, tyrosine, and cholesterol are considered clinically significant |

### *Precautions*

- The light level on the microscope should be reduced. The fine adjustment should be used, especially to see casts.
- Red blood cells and yeasts appear very similar. Yeasts usually cannot be positively identified unless budding is observed.
- All spills should be wiped up promptly with surface disinfectant.

## *LESSON REVIEW*

1. What kind of urine (concentrated, diluted) is the best specimen to use when identifying urine sediment? Why?
2. Under what power of magnification should a slide of urine sediment be initially examined?
3. What are the major components of urine sediment that are usually encountered?
4. How is urine sediment reported?
5. What centrifuge speed is commonly used to prepare the urine sample?
6. What volume of sample is centrifuged?
7. List the normal values for RBC, WBC, casts, and bacteria.
8. Explain the procedure for performing a microscopic examination of urine sediment.

## *STUDENT ACTIVITIES*

1. Re-read the information on microscopic examination of urine sediment.
2. Practice performing a microscopic examination of one or more urine sediments as outlined on the Student Performance Guide using the worksheet.
3. Compare the results of the microscopic examination of urine with those obtained by fellow students or the instructor.
4. Draw three components of urine sediment which were observed. Is the presence of each normal or abnormal?

# Student Performance Guide

NAME ______________________

DATE ______________________

## LESSON 5–5 MICROSCOPIC EXAMINATION OF URINE SEDIMENT

### Instructions

1. Practice the procedure for preparing and examining urine sediment.
2. Demonstrate the procedure for preparing and examining urine sediment satisfactorily for the instructor. All steps must be completed as listed on the instructor's Performance Check Sheet.
3. Complete a written examination successfully.

### Materials and Equipment

- hand disinfectant
- fresh urine sample
- conical graduated centrifuge tubes
- centrifuge
- microscope
- glass slides
- coverglasses
- worksheet (urinalysis report form)
- surface disinfectant
- biohazard container

**Procedure**

S = Satisfactory
U = Unsatisfactory

| You must: | S | U | Comments |
|---|---|---|---|
| 1. Wash hands with hand disinfectant | | | |
| 2. Assemble equipment and materials | | | |
| 3. Obtain a urine sample | | | |
| 4. Pour 10 to 15 ml of well-mixed urine into a clean conical centrifuge tube | | | |
| 5. Place filled tube in centrifuge, insert balance tube, and close lid (centrifuge must be balanced) | | | |
| 6. Centrifuge at 1500 to 2000 rpm for five minutes | | | |
| 7. Remove tube from centrifuge after rotor stops spinning | | | |
| 8. Pour off supernatant urine, leaving 0.5–1 ml of urine in tube | | | |
| 9. Resuspend urine sediment by shaking the tube | | | |
| 10. Pour one drop of resuspended urine onto a clean glass slide | | | |
| 11. Place coverslip over drop of urine | | | |
| 12. Place slide on microscope stage and focus using low power (10X) and low light | | | |
| 13. Scan ten to fifteen low power fields, count the number of casts per field, and record the average | | | |
| 14. Identify the type(s) of casts present and record | | | |
| 15. Rotate the high power objective (45X) into position | | | |
| 16. Scan ten to fifteen fields on high power | | | |
| 17. Count the number of RBC, WBC, and epithelial cells per high power field and record the average for each | | | |
| 18. Observe the sample for the presence of microorganisms, crystals, or mucus and record if present. If crystals are present, identify type | | | |

| You must: | S | U | Comments |
|---|---|---|---|
| 19. Complete the urinalysis report form | | | |
| 20. Discard sample appropriately | | | |
| 21. Clean and return equipment to proper storage | | | |
| 22. Clean work area with surface disinfectant | | | |
| 23. Wash hands with hand disinfectant | | | |
| Comments: | | | |
| Student/Instructor: | | | |

Date: ______________________ Instructor: ______________________________

# Worksheet

NAME ______________________ DATE ____________

SPECIMEN NO. ____________

## LESSON 5–5 MICROSCOPIC EXAMINATION OF URINE

| Microscopic Examination | | Normal Values |
|---|---|---|
| WBCs: | ____________ /HPF | 0–4 |
| RBCs: | ____________ /HPF | rare |
| Epithelial cells: | ____________ /HPF | occasional (higher in females) |
| Casts: | ____________ /LPF | occasional, hyaline |
| Type: | ____________ | |
| Yeasts: | negative 1+ 2+ 3+ 4+ | negative |
| Bacteria: | negative 1+ 2+ 3+ 4+ | negative |
| Mucus: | negative 1+ 2+ 3+ 4+ | negative–2+ |

Other: ______________________________

Crystals: ______ none seen

______ present

(type) ________

Amorphous deposits: ______ none seen

______ present

# UNIT 6

# Introduction To Bacteriology

## UNIT OBJECTIVES

After studying this unit, you should be able to:

- Identify three basic bacterial shapes and two Gram stain reactions.
- Prepare a bacterial smear.
- Perform a Gram stain.
- Transfer bacteria from one medium to another.
- Collect bacterial specimens from the throat and the urine.
- Culture bacteria from the throat and the urine onto appropriate growth media.

## OVERVIEW

The main objective of bacteriological procedures is to identify the organisms responsible for illness so that the physician can properly treat the patient. These procedures may be performed in physicians' offices or in the microbiology department of the medical laboratory.

Identifying bacteria involves consideration of their morphology, their Gram stain reactions, and the results of certain biochemical reactions. The morphology and the Gram stain reaction of an organism can be disclosed by preparing a bacterial smear and performing a Gram stain. The procedures for performing these are presented in Lessons 6–1, 6–2, and 6–3.

To further identify the bacteria, laboratory personnel must grow the bacteria on appropriate growth media. The procedures for the actual collection of the specimens from the patient, the transfer to proper growth media, and the selection of media are presented in Lessons 6–4, 6–5, and 6–6.

Although the strains of organisms utilized in these lessons are not considered highly pathogenic, safety precautions are still of utmost importance. All bacterial specimens should be handled as though capable of causing disease. Principles of aseptic technique must always be observed. A laboratory coat should be worn while performing these procedures to prevent bacterial stains from being splashed on clothing. A laboratory coat also prevents contamination of the worker with the bacteria.

It is equally important that a good surface disinfectant be used to wipe benchtops before and after each laboratory session and anytime an accidental spill of culture material occurs. Washing the hands often with a hand disinfectant before and after handling any specimens is also essential.

# LESSON 6–1

## Identification of Stained Bacteria

### LESSON OBJECTIVES

After studying this lesson, you should be able to:
- Identify gram-positive bacteria on a smear.
- Identify gram-negative bacteria on a smear.
- Identify the coccus form of bacteria.
- Identify the bacillus form of bacteria.
- Identify the spiral form of bacteria.
- Define the glossary terms.

### GLOSSARY

**bacillus** (pl. bacilli) / a rod-shaped bacterium
**bacteria** / a group of one-celled microorganisms; germs
**bacterial morphology** / the form or structure of bacteria; color, shape and size
**coccus** (pl. cocci) / spherical or oval-shaped bacterium
**colony** / a circumscribed mass of bacteria growing in or upon a solid or semi-solid medium; assumed to have grown from a single organism
**gram negative** / refers to bacteria which are decolorized in the Gram stain; pink-red in color after being counterstained
**gram positive** / refers to bacteria which retain the crystal violet dye in the Gram stain; purple-blue in color
**Gram stain** / a stain which differentiates bacteria according to the chemical composition of their cell walls
**spirochete** / a slender, spiral microorganism

## INTRODUCTION

Many diseases are caused by microorganisms known as **bacteria.** The three basic forms of bacteria are round (oval), rod-shaped, and spiral. The round or oval form is known as a **coccus** (Figure 6–1). Round bacteria which occur predominantly in pairs are

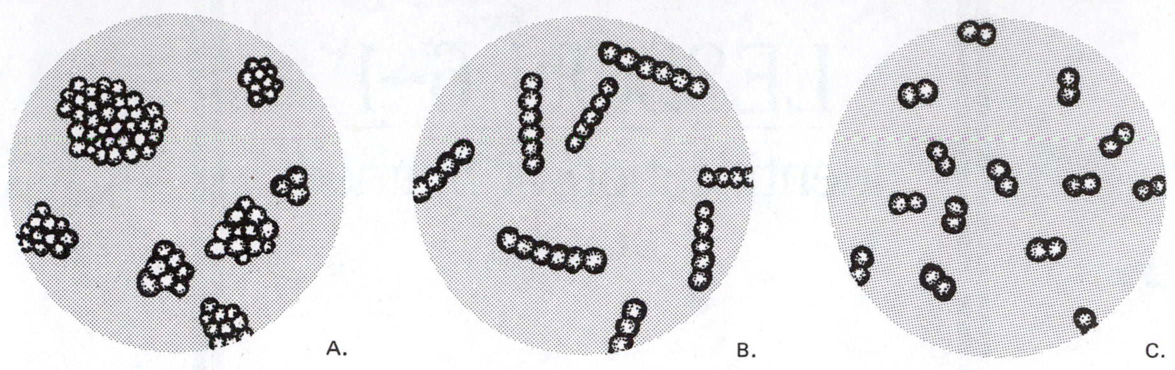


**Figure 6-1.** Microscopic appearance of round bacteria. A) round bacteria (cocci) in clusters, B) round bacteria (cocci) in chains, and C) diplococci

called *diplococci.* The rod-shaped form of bacteria is known as a **bacillus** (Figure 6–2) and the spiral one as a **spirochete** (Figure 6–3).

Most bacteria are very small and must be viewed using the oil immersion (100X) objective of the microscope. The sizes of bacteria are usually in the range of 0.1–2.0 micrometers in width and not more than five micrometers long.

Even bacteria which have color usually do not appear to be colored because they are so small. Only when many bacteria of one type are together in a **colony** is the color visible. A colony is a group of bacteria which grew from a single organism.

Since the small size of bacteria makes it difficult to see them with the microscope, stains are applied to the bacteria to make them more visible. The bacterial stain most often used is the Gram stain.

## THE GRAM STAIN

The **Gram stain** is a procedure which stains bacteria differentially according to the composition of their cell walls. The Gram stain is performed on a thin smear of the organisms to be studied. The smear is passed through a Bunsen burner flame two or three times to fix the smear to the glass slide. Crystal violet, Gram's iodine, a decolorizer, and a safranin counterstain are then applied, in sequence, to the smear.

After the stain has dried, the smear is ready for microscopic observation. The slide is placed on the microscope stage and the stained area is found with the low power (10X) objective. A drop of immersion oil is placed on the smear and the oil immersion objective (100X) is used to view the organisms. The bacteria which retain the crystal violet and appear blue-purple are called **gram positive.** The bacteria which stain red-pink with safranin are called **gram negative.**

The Gram stain can be used to give the physician information which is helpful in diagnosing and treating infections. By staining the specimen taken directly from a wound, for example, the presence or absence of bacteria in the wound can be verified. If bacteria are present, the stain will identify them as gram negative or gram positive. This information can then be used to choose the proper nutrients on which to grow the bacteria for further study. The Gram stain also helps in the choice of antibiotic treatment since gram negatives and gram positives are, in general, susceptible to different antibiotics.

## APPEARANCE OF STAINED BACTERIA

The round bacteria, the cocci, will appear similar to those shown in Figure 6–1. The most common

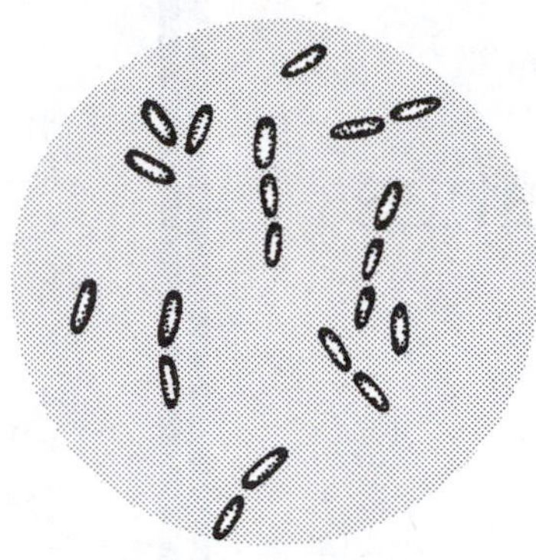

**Figure 6-2.** Microscopic appearance of rod-shaped bacteria

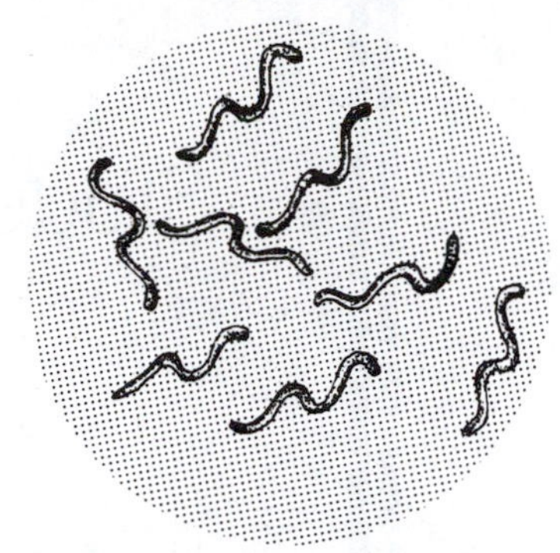

**Figure 6-3.** Microscopic appearance of spiral bacteria

cocci are *Staphylococcus* and *Streptococcus.* The *Staphylococcus* will appear singly or in grape-like clusters. Since *Staphylococci* are gram positive, they will stain dark blue (see Color Plate 25). *Streptococci* are also gram positive and appear either singly or in a bead-like chain. *Neisseria gonorrhoeae,* the causative agent of gonorrhea, is a diplococcus which is gram negative (see Color Plate 27).

The rod-shaped bacteria may be either gram positive or gram negative. A common gram-negative rod is *Escherichia coli* which is found in the intestinal tract (Figure 6–2 and Color Plate 26).

The spiral forms of bacteria usually stain gram negatively and appear as twisted rods, having from less than one turn to many turns (Figure 6–3). One bacteria with a spiral form is *Campylobacter fetus,* which can cause a variety of serious conditions in humans.

The **bacterial morphology** observed with the microscope is essential information which is used to aid in identifying bacteria. However, other characteristics such as biochemical reactions, antibiotic susceptibility, and growth on certain media must also be utilized to make the final identification of the bacteria.

## *LESSON REVIEW*

1. What is another name for the round bacteria?
2. What is the size range of most bacteria?
3. What is the best way to observe bacterial morphology?
4. The rod-shaped bacteria are known by what other name?
5. How many turns are in most spiral bacteria?
6. What is a Gram stain?
7. What cell characteristic makes a bacterium gram positive or gram negative?
8. Define bacillus, bacteria, bacterial morphology, coccus, colony, gram negative, gram positive, Gram stain, and spirochete.

## *STUDENT ACTIVITIES*

1. Re-read the information on the identification of stained bacteria.
2. Review the glossary terms.
3. Practice identifying the three morphological forms and two gram stain reactions of bacteria as outlined on the Student Performance Guide.

# Student Performance Guide

NAME ____________________

DATE ____________________

## LESSON 6–1 IDENTIFICATION OF STAINED BACTERIA

### Instructions

1. Practice identifying the three forms of bacteria and their Gram stain reactions.
2. Demonstrate the identification of stained bacteria satisfactorily for the instructor. All steps must be completed as listed on the instructor's Performance Check Sheet.
3. Complete a written examination successfully.

### Materials and Equipment

- hand disinfectant
- microscope
- immersion oil
- lens paper
- soft laboratory tissue
- prepared Gram-stained bacterial slides: coccus, bacillus, spirochete
- surface disinfectant

## Procedure

S = Satisfactory
U = Unsatisfactory

| You must: | S | U | Comments |
|---|---|---|---|
| 1. Wash hands with hand disinfectant | | | |
| 2. Assemble equipment and materials | | | |
| 3. Select one of the prepared slides and secure it on the microscope stage | | | |
| 4. Locate a stained area of the smear using the low power (10X) objective | | | |
| 5. Place a drop of immersion oil on the area to be viewed | | | |
| 6. Rotate the oil immersion lens into place carefully | | | |
| 7. Identify the type of bacteria (coccus, bacillus, spirochete) by shape | | | |
| 8. Identify the Gram stain reaction by the color | | | |
| 9. Repeat steps 3–8 until all three shapes have been identified and both Gram stain reactions have been observed | | | |
| 10. Wipe the oil off the slides gently with laboratory tissue | | | |
| 11. Clean equipment and return to proper storage | | | |
| 12. Clean work area with disinfectant | | | |
| 13. Wash hands with hand disinfectant | | | |

Comments:

Student/Instructor:

Date: ______________________ Instructor: ______________________

# LESSON 6-2

## Preparation of a Bacteriological Smear

### LESSON OBJECTIVES

After studying this lesson, you should be able to:

- Demonstrate aseptic technique.
- Prepare a smear directly from a swab.
- Prepare a smear of *Staphylococcus aureus* from tubed media.
- Prepare a smear of *Escherichia coli* from an agar plate.
- Heat-fix a bacteriological smear.
- List the precautions to be observed in the preparation of a bacteriological smear.
- Define the glossary terms.

### GLOSSARY

**aseptic techniques** / techniques used to maintain sterility or to prevent contamination

**culture** / to cultivate bacteria in a nutrient medium; a mass of growing bacteria

**flame** / sterilization of certain materials used in bacteriology by heating or passing through a flame

**inoculating loop** / a nichrome or platinum wire fashioned into a loop on one end and having a handle on the other end; used to transfer bacterial growth

**medium** / a nutritive substance, either solid or liquid, in or upon which microorganisms are grown for study

## INTRODUCTION

Preparing a bacteriological smear is a relatively simple process which can be performed quickly. The smear can be prepared directly from the specimen such as a throat swab, or from a colony of bacterial growth on a medium. Since the specimen contains live organisms, workers in the bacteriology laboratory must avoid contamination of themselves, the environment, and the specimen by using **aseptic techniques.**

## ASEPTIC TECHNIQUES

Many procedures and safety rules fall under the category of aseptic techniques. Such procedures include 1) flaming the loop before and after each use, 2) flaming the mouths of tubes before and after entering the tube (after opening and before closing the tube), and 3) placing all contaminated objects in containers of disinfectant or biohazard containers until disposal. Safety rules that follow the principles of aseptic techniques include:

- wearing a laboratory coat or apron to protect the clothing from contamination
- keeping work area clean with a surface disinfectant
- wiping up all spills promptly with disinfectant
- washing hands with hand disinfectant after every procedure
- disposing of all specimens and culture materials by incineration or autoclaving.

## THE DIRECT SMEAR

The direct smear is prepared from the swab which was used to obtain the sample. Such a smear could be from a throat culture or wound culture. If the material is also to be transferred to a medium to grow, the slide used must be sterile and free of debris. This is to prevent the transfer of organisms on an unsterile slide onto the swab and consequently onto the medium when it is inoculated.

To prepare the smear, the swab is gently rolled across the surface of the slide (Figure 6-4) leaving a thin film of the culture material on the slide. When the film has completely air dried, it is ready to be heat-fixed. This is done by holding the slide by one end with a spring-type clothespin or forceps and passing the smear area through the Bunsen burner flame two or three times (Figure 6-5). When performed correctly, the slide will not be hot enough to burn the fingers. Heat-fixing is necessary to make the organism adhere to the slide throughout the staining process. If the smear is fixed before it is air dried or if it is exposed to extreme heat, the morphology of the organisms will be affected or the slide may break. After the slide has been heat-fixed, it is ready to be stained.

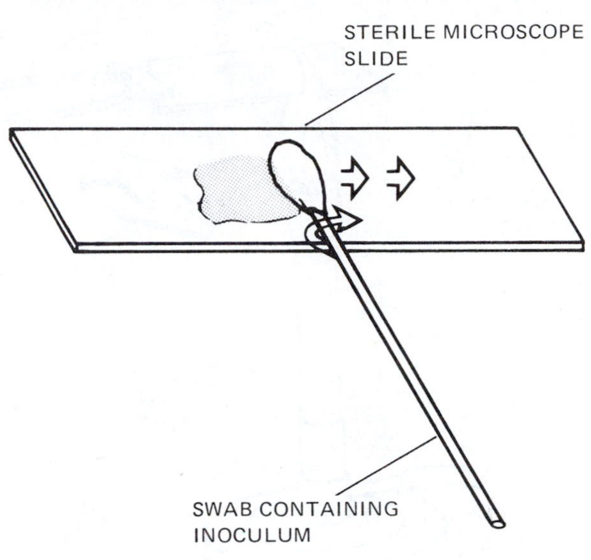


**Figure 6-4.** Preparation of a direct smear from a swab

## A SMEAR FROM BACTERIA GROWING ON MEDIA

It is also relatively simple to prepare a smear using organisms which are already growing on **media.** If the bacterial **culture** is contained on tube media, the principles of aseptic technique must be followed. Using aseptic techniques helps to avoid introducing contaminants into the tube or allowing the organisms to escape from the tube into the environment.

In order to remove a portion of the bacterial growth, the tube should be held in the left hand and the **inoculating loop** in the right hand. The loop is sterilized by heating in the Bunsen burner flame until red hot (Figure 6-6). Spattering of the culture material can be avoided by gradually placing the loop into the cool part of the flame then into

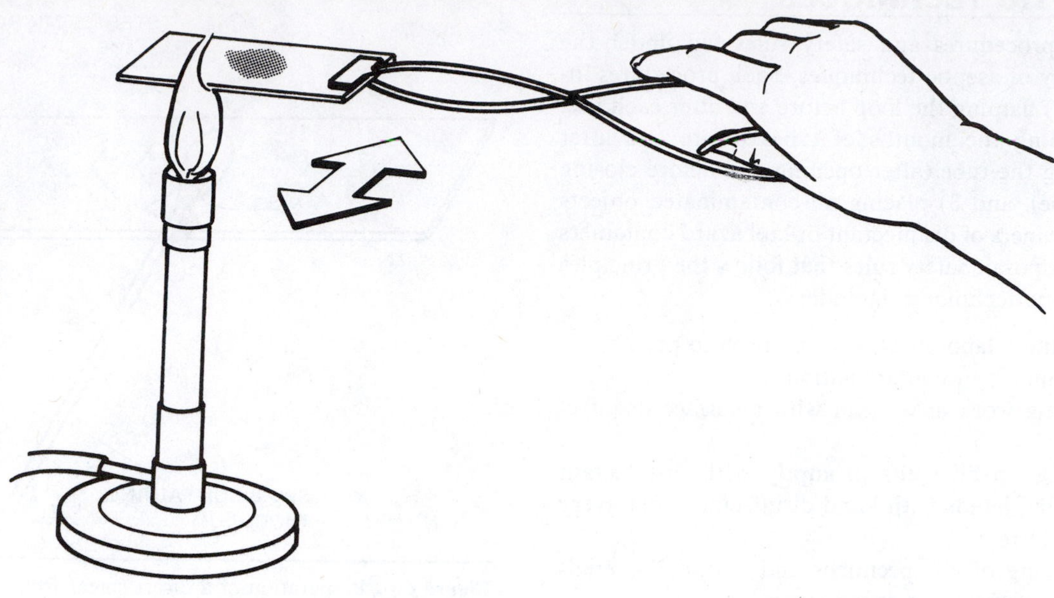

**Figure 6-5.** Heat-fixing a bacteriological smear

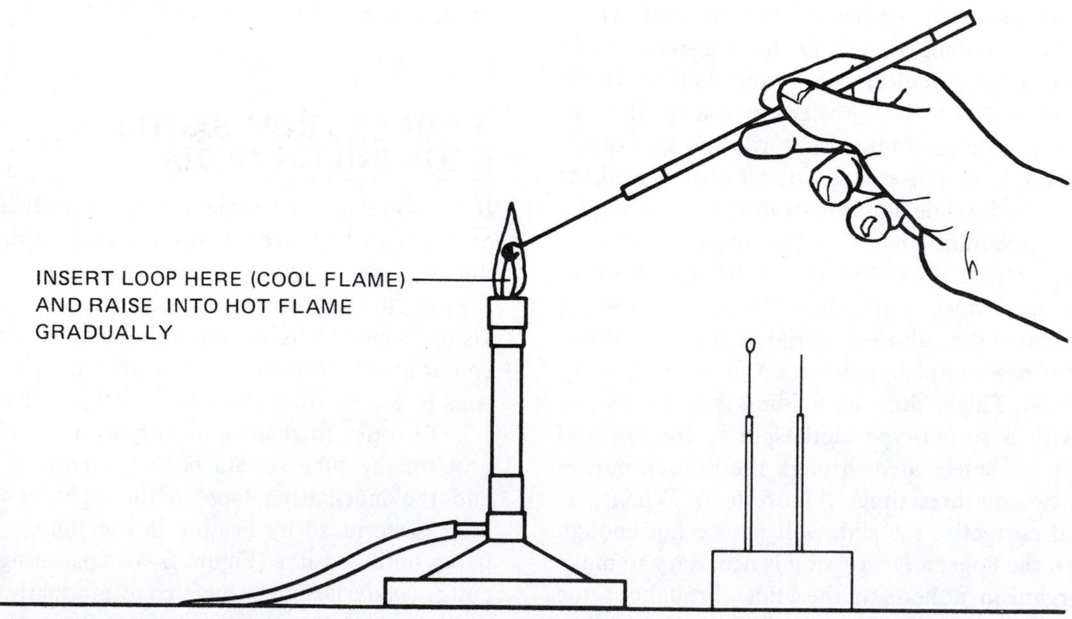


**Figure 6-6.** Sterilizing the inoculating loop

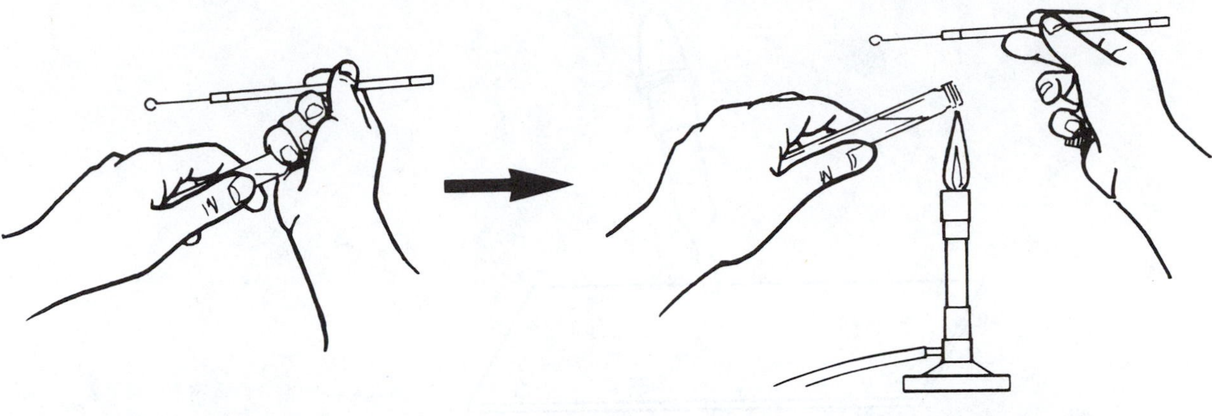

**Figure 6-7.** Flaming a culture tube

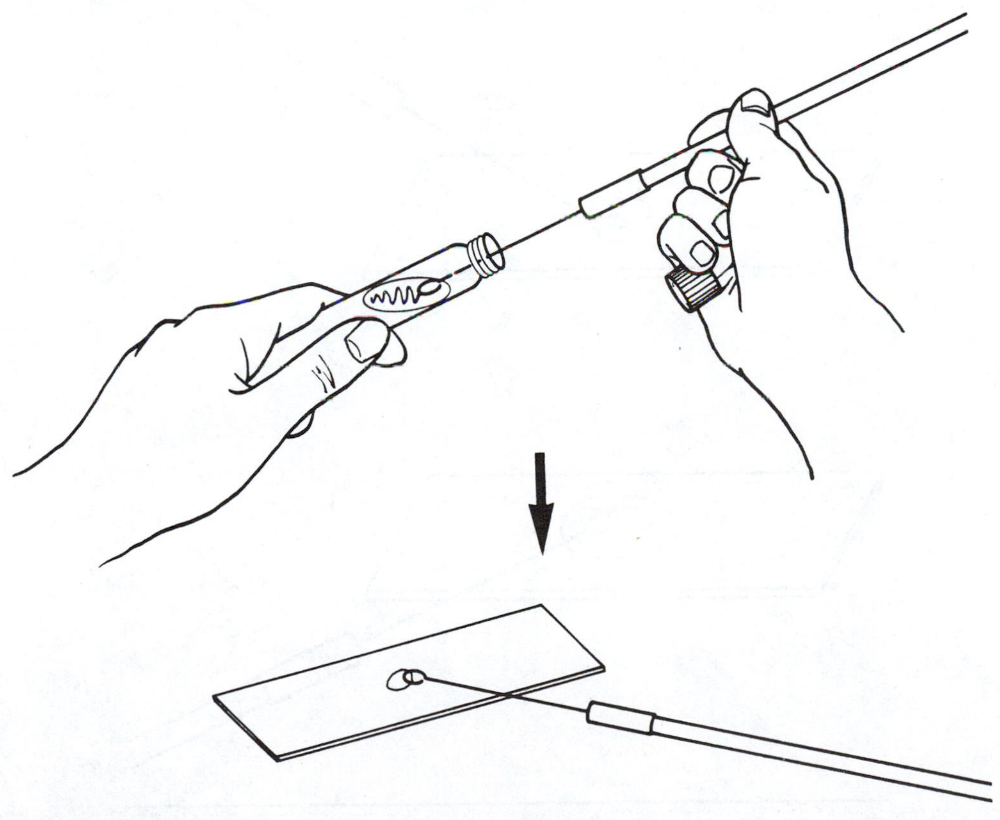

**Figure 6-8.** Transferring bacteria from a culture tube to a slide

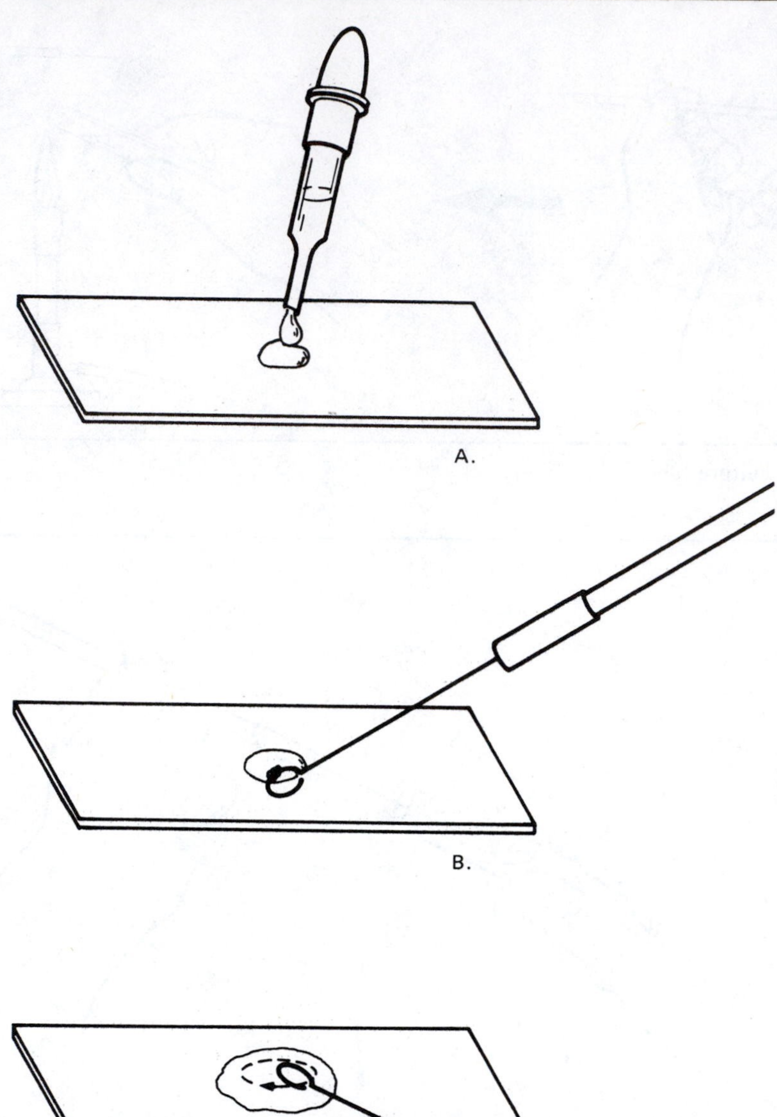


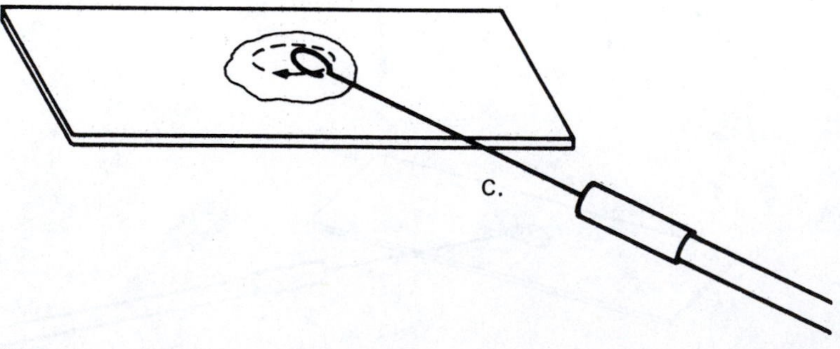


**Figure 6-9.** Making a bacterial smear using the inoculating loop

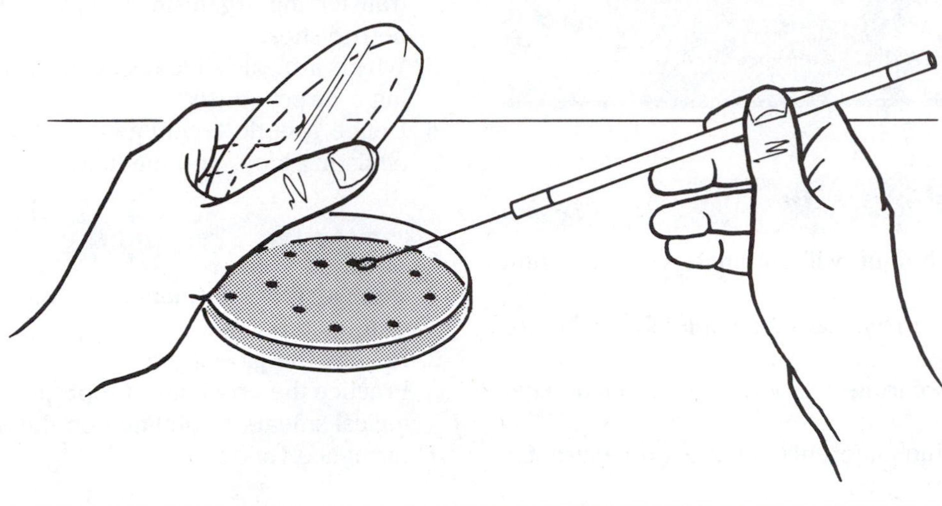

**Figure 6-10.** Removing bacteria from an agar plate using the inoculating loop

the hot part. The loop is allowed to cool briefly and the cap is removed from the tube using the fourth and fifth fingers of the right hand. Immediately the mouth of the tube is **flamed** by passing it briefly through the burner flame (Figure 6–7). The cooled loop is then used to remove a pin-point sized portion of the growth and place it onto a glass slide which has already had two loopfuls of distilled water placed on the surface (Figure 6–8). The water and the bacteria are mixed together and spread out to an area approximately the size of a nickel (Figure 6–9). The mouth of the tube is again flamed briefly, the cap is replaced on the tube, and the tube is placed into a test tube rack. The inoculating loop is flamed again and replaced in its special holder. The slide is allowed to dry and then is heat-fixed. A smear which is of proper thickness will be almost invisible when completely dried.

The procedure used to make a smear from organisms growing on a medium in a petri dish is similar. However, the petri dish is not flamed; the lid is lifted just enough to allow the entrance of the cooled sterilized loop (Figure 6–10). The smear is then prepared as explained above.

### *Precautions*

- The Bunsen burner must be situated so that laboratory supplies, hair, or articles of clothing will not catch fire.
- The prepared smear must be very thin; if it is too thick it will not stain or decolorize properly.
- After sterilization, the inoculating loop must be cooled in the air briefly before it is touched to the organisms.
- The inoculating loop should be held only by the handle, and must be replaced in its special holder when not in use.
- The inoculating loop must always be sterilized after transfer of bacteria and before it is stored in its holder.
- For the greatest margin of safety, all organisms must be handled as if they are capable of causing disease.
- To avoid morphological changes in the organisms or breakage of the slide, the smear must be completely dry before heat-fixing.

■ Wash hands with hand disinfectant before and after handling any specimen.

## *LESSON REVIEW*

1. What technique will eliminate contamination problems?
2. Why must the smear be completely dry before heat-fixing?
3. Why is wearing a laboratory apron or coat helpful?
4. Explain the difference in the procedure for transferring organisms from tubed media and petri dishes.
5. Why is a sterile slide necessary when performing a direct smear?
6. Define aseptic techniques, culture, flame, inoculating loop, and medium.

## *STUDENT ACTIVITIES*

1. Re-read the information on the preparation of a bacterial smear.
2. Review the glossary terms.
3. Practice the procedure for preparing bacteriological smears as outlined on the Student Performance Guide.

# Student Performance Guide

NAME ____________________

DATE ____________________

## LESSON 6–2 PREPARATION OF A BACTERIOLOGICAL SMEAR

### Instructions

1. Practice preparing bacteriological smears using organisms on swabs and organisms growing on tube media and in petri dishes.
2. Demonstrate the procedure for preparing bacteriological smears from the three sources satisfactorily for the instructor. All steps must be completed as listed on the instructor's Performance Check Sheet.
3. Complete a written examination successfully.

### Materials and Equipment

- hand disinfectant
- educational strain (less pathogenic strain used specifically for teaching, and that is available through catalogs) of *Escherichia coli* growing in a culture tube or petri dish
- educational strain of *Staphylococcus aureus* growing in a culture tube or petri dish
- microscope slides
- inoculating needle or loop
- diamond or carbide-tip etching pencil
- Bunsen burner
- holder for inoculating loop
- container of water
- test tube rack
- matches or flint-type lighter
- forceps, or spring-type clothespins
- swabs inoculated with organisms and stored in sterile, capped tubes
- surface disinfectant
- biohazard container

| **Procedure** | | | S = Satisfactory<br>U = Unsatisfactory |
|---|---|---|---|
| **You must:** | **S** | **U** | **Comments** |
| 1. Wash hands with hand disinfectant | | | |
| 2. Assemble equipment and materials | | | |
| 3. Light a Bunsen burner and place it in a safe, accessible area | | | |
| 4. Prepare one smear from each source listed below:<br>A. From a swab:<br>(1) Obtain a microscope slide and a swab which has been inoculated with organisms | | | |
| (2) Remove the swab from its container being careful not to touch the tip | | | |
| (3) Touch the swab to the surface of the slide and apply a film of culture material to the slide by gently rolling the swab on the surface. The size of the area should be a circle approximately ¾ in.–1 in. diameter | | | |
| (4) Return the swab to its container | | | |
| (5) Allow the smear to air dry completely | | | |
| (6) Hold the end of the slide with a clothespin or forceps and pass the smear quickly through the Bunsen flame two to three times to heat-fix. Do not heat the slide excessively; the slide should not be hot enough to burn the fingers when touched. | | | |
| (7) Allow the slide to cool | | | |
| (8) Label the slide using a diamond or carbide-tip etching pencil | | | |
| (9) Keep the slide for staining in Lesson 6–3 | | | |
| B. From the tubed medium:<br>(1) Obtain a microscope slide and culture of *Escherichia coli* growing in a culture tube | | | |
| (2) Hold the culture tube in the left hand and the inoculating loop in the right hand | | | |
| (3) Flame the inoculating needle or loop until red hot and cool briefly in the air. | | | |
| (4) Use the loop to transfer two drops of distilled water to the center of the slide | | | |
| (5) Flame the loop again | | | |

| You must: | S | U | Comments |
|---|---|---|---|
| (6) Remove the cap from the tube with the little finger of the right hand and flame the mouth of the tube | | | |
| (7) Transfer a portion of the bacterial growth to the slide | | | |
| (8) Flame tube briefly, replace the cap on the tube and set the tube in the test tube rack | | | |
| (9) Mix the water and bacterial material together using the loop and spread out to an area approximately the size of a nickel | | | |
| (10) Sterilize the loop and replace it into the holder. *Note:* Avoid spattering the culture material | | | |
| (11) Allow the smear to air dry and then heat-fix as in steps A (6) to A (9) above | | | |
| C. From a petri dish:<br>(1) Obtain a microscope slide and a petri dish culture of *Staphylococcus aureus* | | | |
| (2) Flame the inoculating loop or needle until red hot and allow to air cool briefly | | | |
| (3) Transfer two drops of water to the center of a glass slide | | | |
| (4) Flame the loop again | | | |
| (5) Lift the lid of the petri dish just enough to allow entrance of the inoculating loop or needle | | | |
| (6) Touch the sterile loop to a bacterial colony and transfer a portion of the colony to the water on the glass side | | | |
| (7) Close the petri dish | | | |
| (8) Use the loop to mix the bacteria and water together and spread them into an area about the size of a nickel | | | |
| (9) Sterilize the loop and place in holder. *Note:* Avoid spattering the culture material | | | |
| (10) Allow the smear to dry and heat-fix the slide as in steps A (6) to A (9) | | | |
| 5. Turn off the Bunsen burner | | | |
| 6. Store slides for staining | | | |
| 7. Return materials to proper storage | | | |
| 8. Clean and return equipment to proper storage | | | |

| You must: | S | U | Comments |
|---|---|---|---|
| 9. Clean work area with surface disinfectant | | | |
| 10. Wash hands with hand disinfectant | | | |
| Comments:<br><br>Student/Instructor: | | | |

Date: ______________________ Instructor: ______________________

# LESSON 6–3

## The Gram Stain

## LESSON OBJECTIVES

After studying this lesson, you should be able to:

- Perform the Gram stain procedure.
- Observe gram-positive cocci on the *Staphylococcus aureus* smear.
- Observe gram-negative rods on the *Escherichia coli* smear.
- List precautions to be observed when performing the Gram stain.
- Define the glossary terms.

## GLOSSARY

**bibulous paper** / a special absorbent paper which is used to dry slides
**counterstain** / a dye which adds a contrasting color
**mordant** / a substance which fixes a dye or stain to an object

## INTRODUCTION

The Gram stain is a procedure which is performed routinely in bacteriology laboratories. Most bacterial cells are so small and possess so little color that they are difficult to observe microscopically unless a stain is applied. The Gram stain is the most common staining technique used for bacteria. The Gram stain is performed on a bacteriological smear which has been previously heat-fixed and allowed to cool.

The staining procedure consists of applying a sequence of dye, mordant, decolorizer, and **counterstain** to a bacterial smear. The dyes are taken up differentially according to the chemical composition of the cell walls of the organisms present.

## PERFORMING THE GRAM STAIN

The heat-fixed bacteriological smear should be supported over a pan, beaker, or sink during the staining procedure. The support may be provided by parallel metal or glass rods (Figure 6–11). However, there are also various staining racks manufactured and these should be used if available.

To perform the Gram stain, the smear is placed on the supporting rods and a dye called crystal violet is poured onto the slide (Figure 6–11). After the manufacturer's recommended time has passed (usually one minute), the slide is rinsed by gently pouring tap water onto it. Gram's iodine, which is a mordant, is then added to the slide. A **mordant** is a substance which causes a dye to adhere to the object

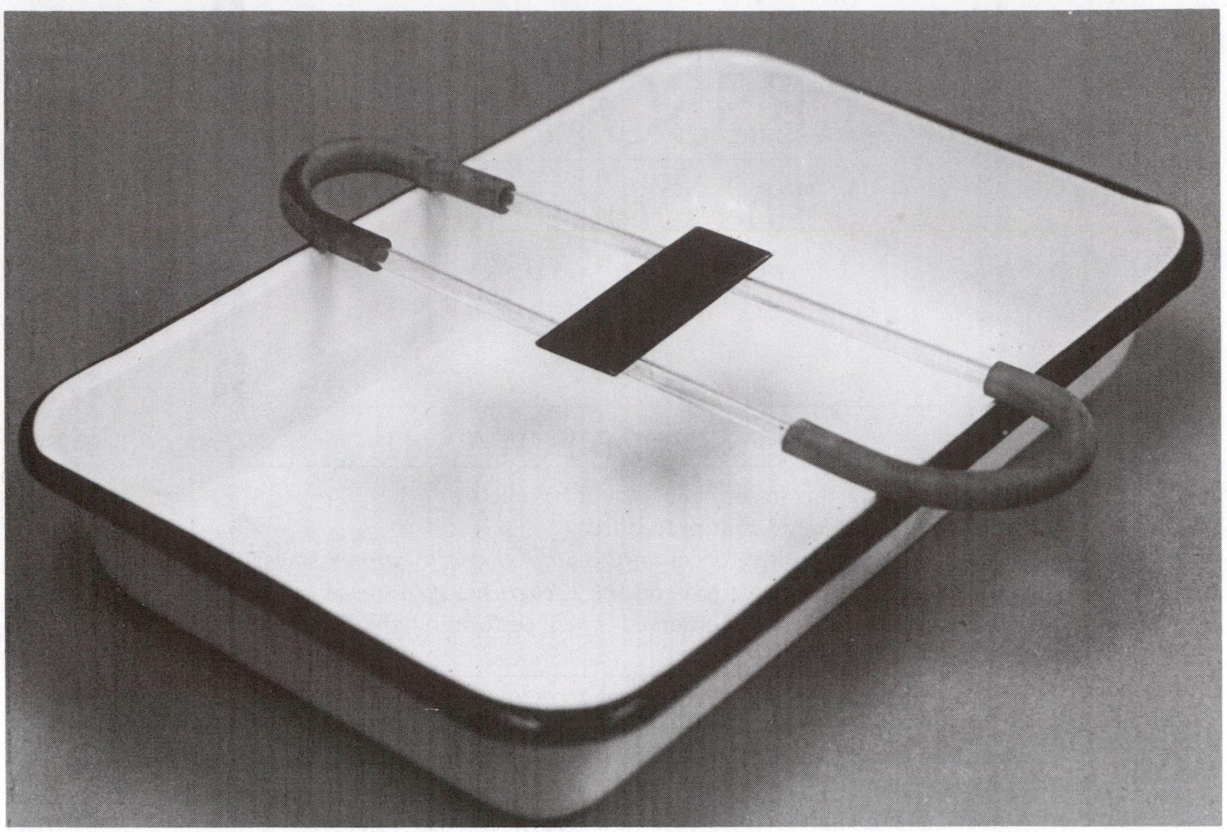

**Figure 6-11.** Slide staining rack (*Photo by John Estridge*)

being stained. When the Gram's iodine has been on the slide for the required time (usually one minute), the slide is again rinsed with water. A decolorizer, such as alcohol, is added to the slide briefly (three to five seconds) or until no more purple runs off the smear. The slide is again rinsed with water.

At this point in the staining process the gram-positive organisms will be purple-blue because their cell wall composition allows retention of the dye (Table 6–1). The gram-negative organisms will appear colorless because their cell-wall composition allows removal of the dye along with some of the cell wall constituents (Table 6–1). Prolonged decolorization can remove the dye even from the gram-positive cells. After the decolorizing procedure is finished, the slide is flooded with a red dye called safranin for approximately one minute. The safranin will have no effect on the gram-positive cells but the now colorless gram-negative cells will be stained red-pink (Table 6–1). The slides are washed by pouring distilled water on them and blotting gently with a special absorbent paper called **bibulous paper.** When the slides are completely dry, they are ready to be observed microscopically.

**Table 6-1.** Steps of Gram Stain Procedure

| | Procedure | Result |
|---|---|---|
| STEP 1 | Primary stain: Apply crystal violet stain (purple) ↓ Rinse slide | All bacteria stain purple |
| STEP 2 | Mordant: Apply Gram's iodine ↓ Rinse slide | All bacteria remain purple |
| STEP 3 | Decolorize: Apply alcohol ↓ Rinse slide | Purple stain is removed from gram-negative cells |
| STEP 4 | Counterstain: Apply safranin stain (red) ↓ Rinse slide and dry | Gram-negative cells appear pink-red; gram-positive cells appear purple |

## OBSERVING THE STAINED BACTERIOLOGICAL SMEAR

The stained smear should be observed using the oil immersion (100X) objective after the stained area has been located using the low power (10X) objective. Gram-negative organisms will appear pink-red and gram-positive organisms will appear blue-purple. *Staphylococcus aureus* is a gram-positive coccus and *Escherichia coli* is a gram-negative bacillus.

### *Precautions*

■ The staining apparatus should be arranged so that the stains will not spill onto countertops.
■ A lab coat or apron should be worn to prevent splashing of stain onto clothing.
■ The manufacturer's directions for the staining procedure must be followed carefully; the times may be different for each lot of reagents.
■ Decolorization, in particular, should be performed with care to avoid false gram negatives.

### *LESSON REVIEW*

1. What is the first stain applied to the smear?
2. What is the purpose of the Gram's iodine?
3. What is the purpose of adding the alcohol?
4. Which bacteria are stained by the safranin?
5. How are the slides dried in order to view them microscopically?

6. Describe the appearance of the *Staphylococcus aureus* smear.
7. Describe the appearance of the *Escherichia coli* smear.
8. Define bibulous paper, counterstain, and mordant.

## *STUDENT ACTIVITIES*

1. Re-read the information on the Gram stain.
2. Review the glossary terms.
3. Practice performing the Gram stain as outlined on the Student Performance Guide.

# Student Performance Guide

NAME ________________________________

DATE ________________________________

## LESSON 6–3 THE GRAM STAIN

### Instructions

1. Practice performing the Gram stain procedure using smears of a gram-negative and gram-positive culture (or smears prepared in Lesson 6–2).
2. Demonstrate the procedure for the Gram stain satisfactorily for the instructor. All steps must be completed as listed on the instructor's Performance Check Sheet.
3. Complete a written examination successfully.

### Materials and Equipment

- hand disinfectant
- Gram stain kit or individual Gram stain reagents (in plastic squeeze bottles)
- unstained smears—gram-positive cocci (*Staphylococcus aureus*) or smears prepared in Lesson 6–2
- unstained smears—gram-negative rods (*Escherichia coli*) or smears prepared in Lesson 6–2
- staining rack
- forceps or springtype wooden clothespins
- pasteur pipet with rubber bulb
- paper towels or soft laboratory tissue
- bibulous paper
- microscope
- immersion oil
- lens paper
- surface disinfectant
- biohazard container

*Note:* Follow manufacturer's instructions for specific staining times.

## Procedure

S = Satisfactory
U = Unsatisfactory

| You must: | S | U | Comments |
|---|---|---|---|
| 1. Wash hands with hand disinfectant | | | |
| 2. Assemble equipment and materials | | | |
| 3. Place slide to be stained on the staining rack with smear side up | | | |
| 4. Flood the slide with crystal violet for the manufacturer's recommended time (approximately one minute) | | | |
| 5. Rinse the stain off the slide by pouring water gently from a beaker, a small diameter laboratory hose, or a plastic squeeze bottle | | | |
| 6. Tilt the slide to remove excess water | | | |
| 7. Flood the slide with Gram's iodine | | | |
| 8. Leave the Gram's iodine on the slide for the recommended time (one minute) | | | |
| 9. Rinse the slide gently with water | | | |
| 10. Tilt the slide to remove excess water | | | |
| 11. Add 95% ethyl alcohol decolorizer by the drop onto the slide using a pasteur pipet with bulb or plastic squeeze bottle | | | |
| 12. Tilt the slide immediately; a purple color should run off the slide | | | |
| 13. Decolorize quickly two to three times (steps 11–12) or until no purple color runs off the slide. *Note:* Do not decolorize longer than three to five seconds or gram positives will appear gram negative | | | |
| 14. Rinse the slide immediately with a gentle stream of tap water to remove the decolorizer | | | |
| 15. Counterstain the smear by adding the safranin dye for the recommended time (one minute) | | | |
| 16. Rinse the slide gently with tap water | | | |

| You must | S | U | Comments |
|---|---|---|---|
| 17. Tilt the slide to remove excess water | | | |
| 18. Wipe the back of the slide with paper towel or soft tissue to remove water and dye | | | |
| 19. Place the smear between two sheets of bibulous paper and gently blot dry, or allow slide to air dry by standing the slide on end | | | |
| 20. Place the dry smear on the microscope stage | | | |
| 21. Use the low power (10X) objective to locate the stained area | | | |
| 22. Place a drop of immersion oil on the stained area | | | |
| 23. Rotate the oil immersion objective into place carefully | | | |
| 24. Observe that the *Staphylococcus* organisms are gram-positive cocci and are arranged in clusters | | | |
| 25. Observe that the *Escherichia* organisms are gram-negative bacilli | | | |
| 26. Rotate the low power objective into position | | | |
| 27. Remove the slide from the microscope stage | | | |
| 28. Clean the oil immersion objective thoroughly | | | |
| 29. Return equipment to proper storage | | | |
| 30. Clean work area with surface disinfectant | | | |
| 31. Wash hands with hand disinfectant | | | |

Comments:

Student/Instructor:

Date: ______________________ Instructor: ______________________

# LESSON 6–4
## Inoculation of Media

## LESSON OBJECTIVES

After studying this lesson, you should be able to:

- Transfer bacteria from one medium to another.
- Streak an agar plate and an agar slant.
- Inoculate broth medium.
- Utilize aseptic technique during the transfer of bacteria.
- List the precautions to be observed in culture transfer.
- Define the glossary terms.

## GLOSSARY

**aerosol** / a suspension of fine solid or liquid particles in the air

**agar plate** / agar medium dispensed into sterile petri dishes and allowed to solidify

**agar slant** / agar medium dispensed into tubes and allowed to solidify at an angle

**broth** / liquid nutrient medium in tubes

**incubator** / temperature-controlled chamber into which inoculated media is placed so that bacterial growth will occur

**inoculation** / the introduction of organisms into media

**inoculum** / the portion of culture organisms which is being introduced into a medium

**quadrant** / one fourth; one quarter of an agar plate

## INTRODUCTION

The transfer of culture material from one medium or source to another medium is **inoculation.** The medium used may be solid or liquid and may be in either a culture tube or a petri dish. Aseptic techniques must be strictly observed to insure safety and good results.

## INOCULATION OF A TUBE OF BROTH MEDIUM

At times it may be necessary to inoculate a tube of broth medium. The organisms may be transferred from an **agar slant** or other source into the **broth.** If an agar slant is used, the procedure can be performed by holding both tubes in the left hand and

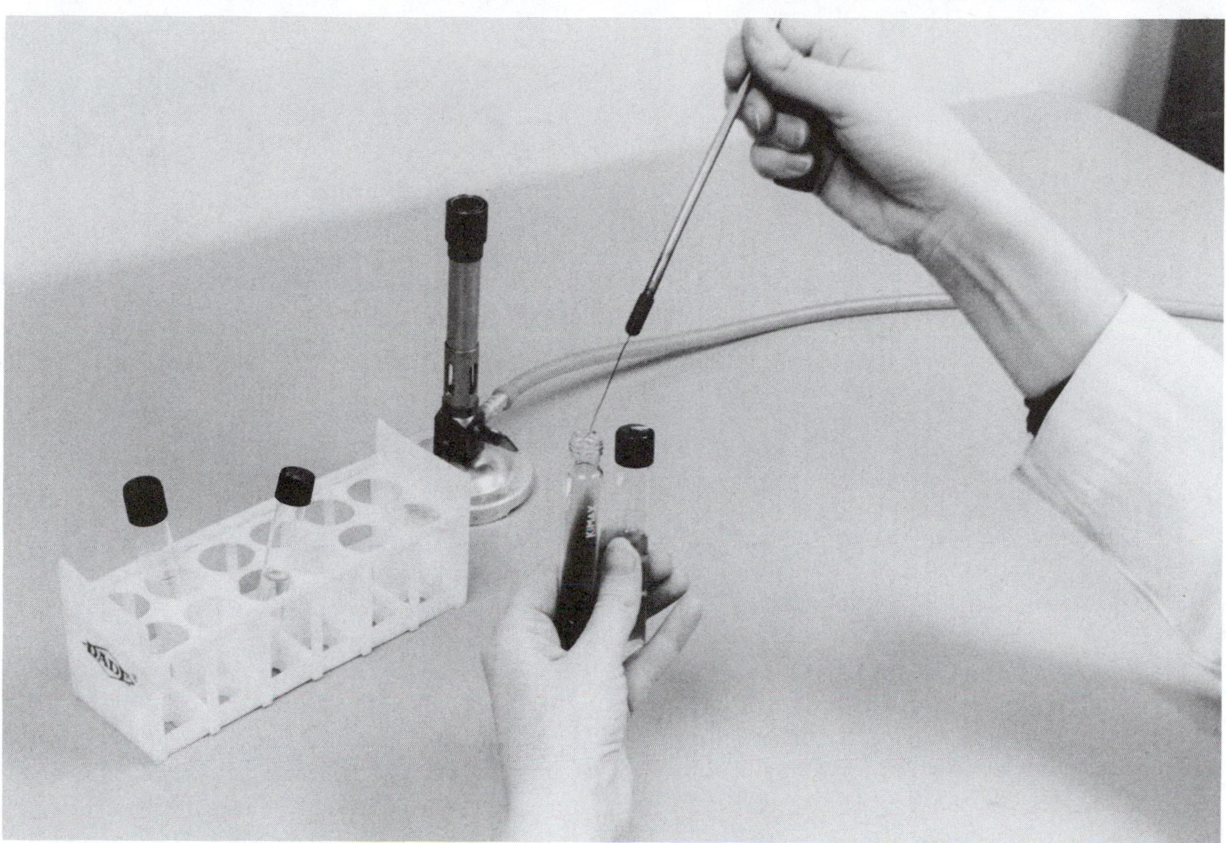

**Figure 6-12.** Transferring organisms from agar slant to broth (*Photo by John Estridge*)

the inoculating loop in the right (Figure 6–12). The loop should be flamed. The cap can then be removed from the agar tube, using the fourth and fifth fingers of the right hand (which is still holding the loop). The mouth of the tube is briefly flamed and a portion of culture picked up on the flamed and cooled loop. The loop is withdrawn, the mouth of the tube is briefly flamed, and the cap is replaced on the agar tube. The cap is then removed from the second tube (broth), the mouth of the tube is flamed briefly, and the loop is immersed into the broth, agitating it several times to disperse the **inoculum** (Figure 6–13). The loop is withdrawn, the mouth of the tube is flamed, and the cap is replaced on the broth tube. The loop is then flamed and replaced into its holder. The broth tube is placed in a test tube rack in the **incubator** set at 37°C and left overnight, or for eighteen to twenty-four hours.

This method prevents the loop or the caps from being laid on the countertop and thus prevents contamination. If these procedures are performed carelessly, the surroundings and/or personnel may become contaminated. One way contamination may occur is through the formation of aerosols. **Aerosols** are formed when a broth is shaken, a loop spatters in the flame, or something happens which causes the organisms to become airborne.

A broth can also be inoculated by using a swab. The swab which contains the inoculum is inserted into the broth and agitated to disperse the culture

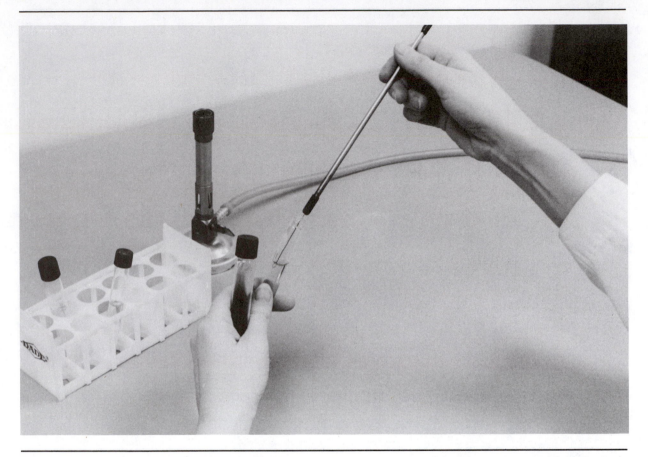

**Figure 6-13.** Inoculation of broth (*Photo by John Estridge*)

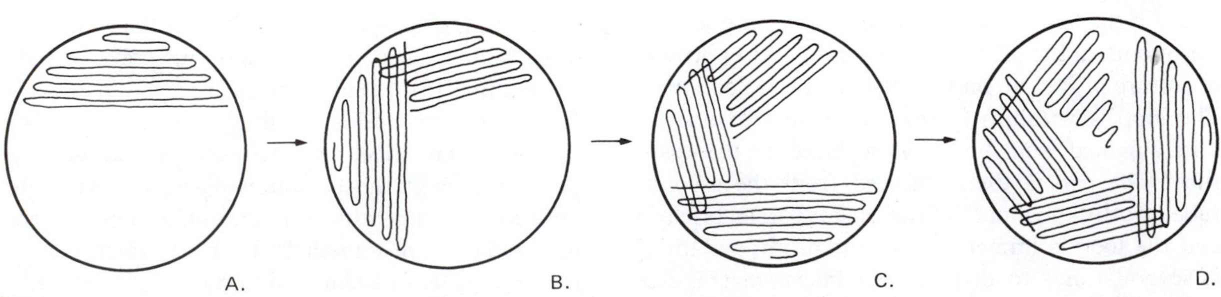


**Figure 6-14.** Streaking an agar plate in four quadrants

material. The tip is then pressed against the inner surface of the tube to express any remaining material. The swab is then withdrawn from the tube. The tube is then flamed and capped as in the procedure utilizing the loop. The swab should be placed in a biohazard container or a container of disinfectant for disposal.

## INNOCULATION OF AN AGAR PLATE

The transfer of organisms from an agar slant onto an **agar plate** is performed in a similar manner. The tube is held in the left hand, the loop in the right hand and the cap of the tube is removed with the fingers of the right hand. The loop and the mouth of the tube are then flamed. When the organisms have been removed from the tube with the loop, the mouth of the tube is flamed and the cap is replaced. The tube is set in the test tube rack. The left hand is then free to lift the lid on the agar plate (petri dish). To avoid contamination or formation of aerosols, the lid is lifted only about two and one-half inches—just enough to allow entrance of the loop. The inoculum is spread with the loop by streaking it across one **quadrant** of the agar surface (Figure 6–14). The loop is then flamed and cooled. The petri dish is turned one quarter turn and the inoculum is spread into the second quadrant with the loop crossing the first quadrant two or three times. The loop is again flamed and cooled and the inoculum is spread into the third quadrant by entering the second quadrant with the loop two or three times (Figure 6–14). When streaking the organism from the third quadrant into the fourth, the loop should enter the previously-streaked third quadrant only two or three times.

Because the loop is flamed between the streaking of each quadrant, the number of organisms introduced into each quadrant is fewer than the number in the one before. When a plate is streaked in this manner, the final quadrant should contain only a few organisms. This technique is called streaking for isolated colonies and is illustrated in Figure 6–14.

After streaking, the plate is labeled on the bottom. It is then placed overnight (eighteen to twenty-four hours) in the incubator set at 37°C to allow for growth of the organisms. Agar plates are incubated upside down to prevent condensate (which forms on the lid) from dropping onto the agar surface. If the plate was streaked properly, quadrant four should contain only a few isolated colonies of the organism after the overnight incubation period.

## INOCULATION OF AN AGAR SLANT

Organisms may also be transferred onto an agar slant in a culture tube to allow growth. Aseptic techniques are used, including flaming the mouth of the tube and the loop. When the cap has been removed, the inoculum can be introduced into the tube by a swab or loop. A swab can be used in the same manner as a loop with the inoculum being spread in a zig-zag manner from the far end of the slant toward the opening of the tube. Alternately, the swab may be used to introduce the inoculum onto the slant and the loop is then used to spread the inoculum (Figure 6–15). The mouth of the tube is again flamed briefly and the cap is replaced on the tube. The loop is flamed, cooled, and replaced in its holder. The slant is then placed in a test tube rack in the 37°C incubator overnight.

Each laboratory will have its particular way of performing these basic procedures. However, every method must contain good aseptic techniques. If aseptic measures are not followed, bacteria in the air or even from the skin will be introduced and will grow along with the inoculum. Perfection of the streaking method will result in scattered isolated pure colonies of bacteria which can be picked up and transferred for further studies.

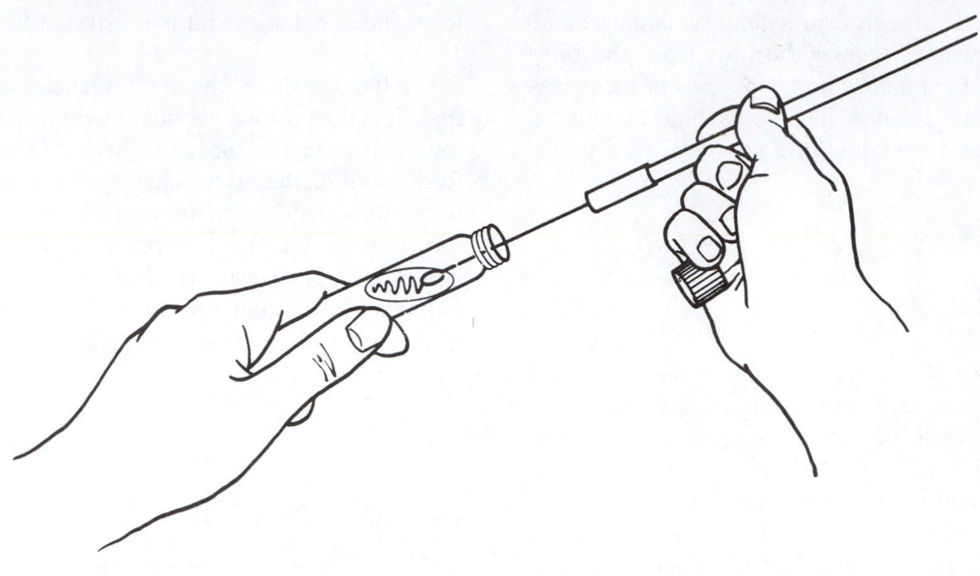

**Figure 6-15.** Inoculation of an agar slant

### *Precautions*

■ Aseptic techniques must be observed at all times.

■ The loop should be checked periodically to be sure it has a smooth surface. A misshaped loop may tear the agar surface when streaking the inoculum.

■ The loop must be cooled after flaming; a hot loop will kill the organisms, damage agar surfaces, and cause aerosols to form.

■ The loop must be replaced into its special holder between uses.

## *LESSON REVIEW*

1. What is an inoculum?
2. What is an aerosol?
3. How can aerosol formation be avoided?
4. How is an agar plate streaked to produce isolated colonies?
5. Why are isolated colonies needed?
6. How is the number of organisms reduced from quadrant to quadrant?
7. What kind of pattern is used to inoculate an agar slant?
8. Why is aseptic technique important?
9. Explain the procedure for transferring organisms from a culture tube onto a plate.
10. Define aerosol, agar plate, agar slant, broth, incubator, inoculation, inoculum, and quadrant.

## *STUDENT ACTIVITIES*

1. Re-read the information on the inoculation of media.
2. Review the glossary terms.
3. Practice the procedures for transferring organisms to broths, agar slants, and petri dishes as outlined on the Student Performance Guide.

# Student Performance Guide

NAME ____________________

DATE ____________________

## LESSON 6–4
## INOCULATION OF MEDIA

### Instructions

1. Practice inoculating broth, agar slant, and petri dish media.
2. Demonstrate the procedure for inoculating broth, agar, and petri dish media satisfactorily for the instructor. All steps must be completed as listed on the instructor's Performance Check Sheet.
3. Complete a written examination successfully.

### Materials and Equipment

- hand disinfectant
- inoculating loop or needle
- Bunsen burner
- matches or flint-type lighter
- agar slants (tryptose or comparable agar)
- agar plates (tryptose or comparable agar)
- broth tubes (tryptose or comparable)
- sterile swabs
- educational strains of *Staphylococcus aureus* or *Escherichia coli*
- test tube racks
- incubator (37°C)
- surface disinfectant
- biohazard container

**Procedure**

S = Satisfactory
U = Unsatisfactory

| You must: | S | U | Comments |
|---|---|---|---|
| 1. Wash hands with hand disinfectant | | | |
| 2. Assemble equipment and materials | | | |
| 3. Light the Bunsen burner | | | |
| 4. Select the culture to be transferred | | | |
| 5. Select a tube of broth, an agar slant, and an agar plate to be inoculated | | | |
| 6. Label each appropriately with the following: name of culture used, your name, and the date. Agar plates are always labeled on the bottom of the petri dish | | | |
| 7. Inoculate the agar slant:<br>a. Hold the tube containing the bacterial culture and the agar slant tube in the left hand | | | |
| b. Hold the inoculating loop in the right hand similar to a pencil | | | |
| c. Flame the loop and cool it | | | |
| d. Remove the cap from the tube containing the bacterial growth with the fifth finger of the right hand | | | |
| e. Flame the mouth of the open tube briefly | | | |
| f. Remove a portion of the bacterial growth with the loop (try to get a part of an isolated colony) | | | |
| g. Withdraw the loop from the tube, flame the mouth, replace the cap. Limit the movement of the loop through the air to avoid aerosols | | | |
| h. Remove the cap from the tube containing the agar slant and flame the mouth | | | |
| i. Inoculate the slant, starting at the far end of the slant and continuing in a zigzag motion toward the mouth of the tube | | | |
| j. Withdraw the loop, flame it, and replace it in its holder. *Note:* Avoid spattering the culture material | | | |
| k. Flame the mouth of the tube and replace the cap on the tube (do not tighten) | | | |
| l. Place the slant in a test tube rack | | | |

| You must: | S | U | Comments |
|---|---|---|---|
| 8. Inoculate the broth:<br>a. Repeat steps 7 (A) through 7 (G), substituting the broth in place of the agar slant. Observe aseptic technique | | | |
| b. Remove the cap from the broth tube | | | |
| c. Insert the loop containing the bacterial growth beneath the surface of the broth and agitate to disperse the organisms throughout the broth | | | |
| d. Withdraw the loop, flame it, and replace it in holder. *Note:* Avoid spattering culture material | | | |
| e. Flame the mouth of the tube briefly and replace the cap on the broth tube (do not tighten) | | | |
| f. Place broth in a test tube rack | | | |
| 9. Inoculate the agar plate:<br>a. Place the petri dish containing the agar plate on the counter | | | |
| b. Hold the tube containing the bacterial growth in the left hand and the inoculating loop in the right hand | | | |
| c. Flame the loop and allow to cool | | | |
| d. Remove the cap from the tube, briefly flame the mouth of the tube, and use the loop to obtain a portion of a colony of the bacterial culture | | | |
| e. Withdraw the loop, flame the mouth of the tube, replace the cap onto the tube, and place tube in test tube rack | | | |
| f. Open the petri dish lid with the left hand just enough (two and one-half inches) to allow the entrance of the loop | | | |
| g. Streak one quadrant by spreading the organisms, making six to eight streaks | | | |
| h. Flame the loop and cool it | | | |
| i. Turn the petri dish one quarter turn | | | |
| j. Streak the second quadrant making six to eight streaks, entering the previously streaked quadrant two to three times | | | |
| k. Repeat steps i–j for the third quadrant | | | |
| l. Begin the streaks in the fourth quadrant as in the other quadrants; continue making the streaks, decreasing the width and increasing the distance between the streaks to form a "tornado-like" pattern | | | |

| You must: | S | U | Comments |
|---|---|---|---|
| 10. Turn off the Bunsen burner. *Note:* Never leave lighted burner unattended | | | |
| 11. Place the broth and slant tubes into a test tube rack in a 37°C incubator (leave caps slightly loosened). Place the agar plate upside down in the 37°C incubator | | | |
| 12. Clean equipment and return to proper storage | | | |
| 13. Clean work area with surface disinfectant | | | |
| 14. Wash hands with hand disinfectant | | | |
| 15. Check the broth, slant, and agar plate for bacterial growth after overnight incubation. The broth should be cloudy, indicating growth of organisms. The slant should have a zigzag formation of bacterial growth on the surface. The agar plate should have bacteria growing in all four quadrants with some isolated colonies in the third and fourth quadrants. | | | |

Comments:

Student/Instructor:

Date: ______________________ Instructor: ______________________

# LESSON 6–5

## Collection and Handling of Bacteriological Specimens

### LESSON OBJECTIVES

After studying this lesson, you should be able to:

- List the most frequently cultured sites.
- Collect a throat culture.
- Instruct a patient to collect a urine specimen for bacterial culture.
- Define the glossary terms.

### GLOSSARY

**flora** / organisms adapted for living in a specific environment

**transport medium** / a medium into which a specimen is placed to preserve it during transport to the laboratory

## INTRODUCTION

The correct collection and handling of the specimens to be used in the various bacteriological procedures is absolutely essential if the results are to be of any value in diagnosis and treatment. Improper collection may result in not obtaining the organisms responsible for the illness. An improperly handled specimen may become contaminated or may contaminate the environment. If a sample is not processed properly the organisms collected may die before they can be transferred to growth media. A variety of disposable, sterile supplies and containers are available to meet most specimen collection and transport requirements (Figure 6–16).

## MOST FREQUENTLY CULTURED SITES

Two of the most frequently cultured sites are the throat and the genito-urinary tract. The next most frequently performed cultures are of wounds, sputum, and cultures of suspected fungal infections.

Cultures of the throat are collected by using a cotton or polyester-tipped swab. Polyester swabs are preferred since some interfering substances on the cotton fibers may inhibit or kill certain organisms. The urinary tract can be tested for the presence of disease-causing organisms by sampling a clean-catch urine. The procedure for collecting samples from wounds or fungal infections depends on the

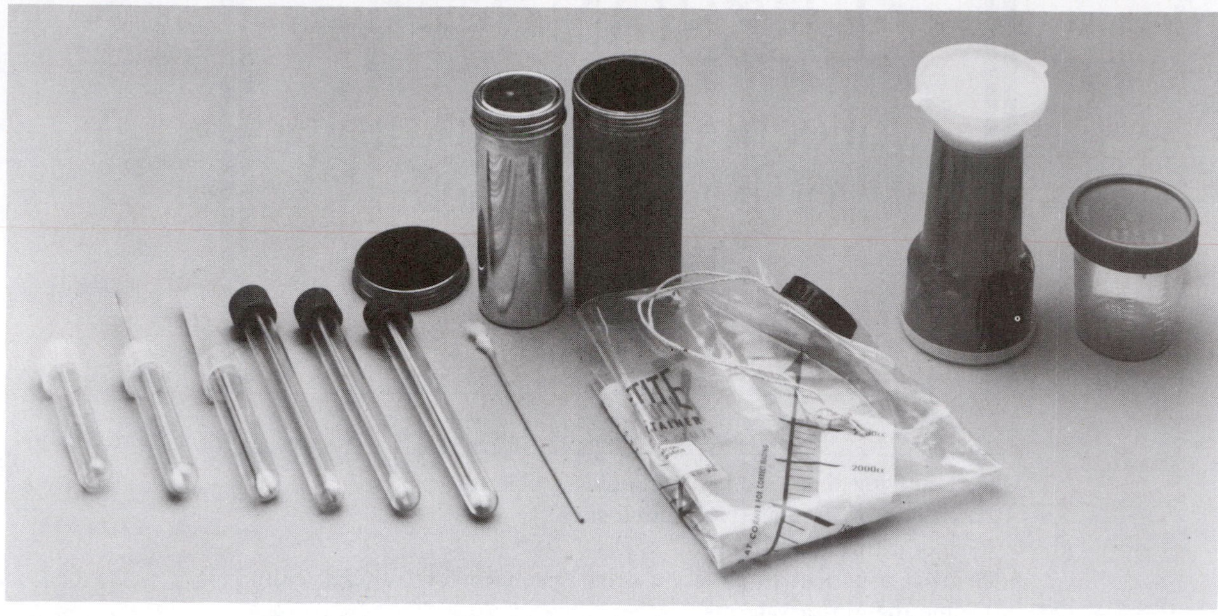

**Figure 6-16.** Examples of supplies for collection and transport of bacteriological specimens (*Photo courtesy of Becton Dickinson & Co.*)

particular situation and will not be covered in this lesson.

## COLLECTING A THROAT CULTURE

Throat cultures are collected by gently swabbing the back of the throat and the surfaces of the tonsils with a sterile swab. The mouth or tongue surfaces should not be touched. This will prevent contaminating the swab with the normal **flora** of the mouth. The procedure can be accomplished more easily if the patient's tongue is depressed and he/she makes the sound of "ah."

The throat is most often cultured when the physician suspects that the patient has a "strep throat" infection. This disease is caused by organisms called *Streptococci.* The most important group of these is called Group A *Streptococci.* It is essential to identify these organisms if present in the throat and to start antibiotic treatment. Left untreated, this infection can have serious complications such as rheumatic fever, rheumatic endocarditis, or glomerulonephritis.

## PERFORMING A URINE CULTURE

Urine samples for culture must be collected by the clean-catch method directly into sterile containers. Urine cultures are performed whenever the patient reports symptoms which indicate infection somewhere in the urinary tract. The organism which is most commonly isolated from urine is *Escherichia coli.*

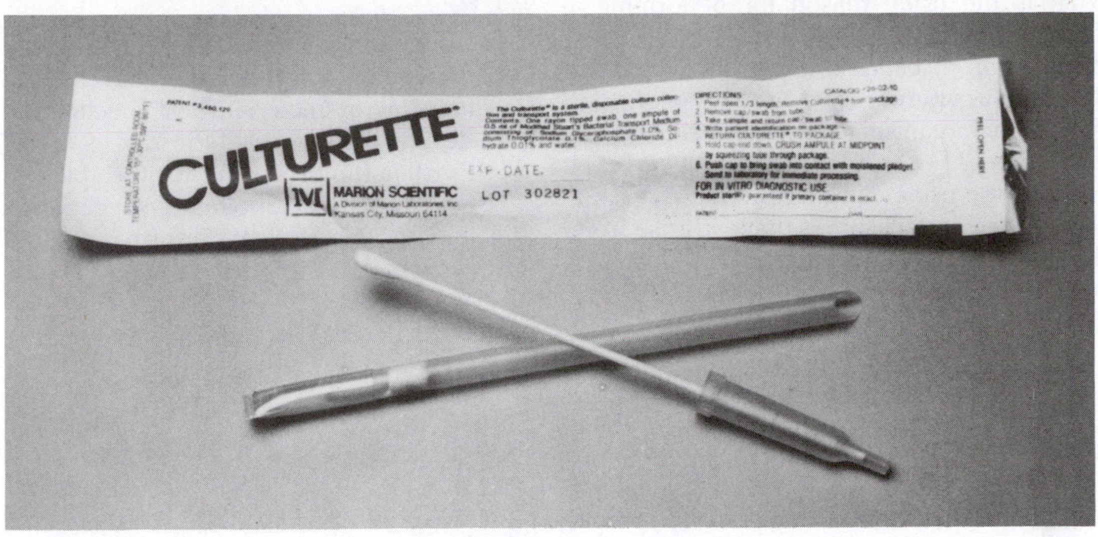


**Figure 6-17.** Culturette® system for collection and transport of bacteriological specimens (*Photo courtesy of Marion Laboratories, Inc., Marion Scientific Division*)

## HANDLING THE SPECIMEN AFTER COLLECTION

After the urine sample has been collected into a sterile container, it should have a proper label attached and then be promptly transported to the lab. It should be processed within one to two hours but may be refrigerated if necessary. No preservatives should be added since most are toxic to bacteria.

The material on the swab from the throat should be inoculated immediately onto the proper medium. However, that is not always possible and several devices have been marketed which can be used to transport samples to the laboratory. One system widely used is the Culturette® (Figure 6–17). It is a sterile swab in a plastic tube which contains an ampule of modified Stuart's **transport medium** to preserve the organism during transport to the laboratory.

### *Precautions*

■ Materials for laboratory culture should be transported to the laboratory and transferred to growth media as soon as possible.

■ Improper collection can cause the loss of the organism responsible for the illness.

■ If aseptic technique is not observed, a contaminating organism may be introduced into the culture.

## *LESSON REVIEW*

1. Why is it important to process the bacteriological specimens promptly?
2. What are the most frequently cultured sites?
3. When performing a throat culture, why is it important not to swab the mouth and tongue?

4. What is the usual reason for performing a throat culture?
5. What group of bacteria is usually looked for in a throat culture?
6. What is the organism most commonly isolated from urines?
7. When is the urine culture requested?
8. Name three complications that can arise from "strep throat."
9. Define flora and transport medium.

## *STUDENT ACTIVITIES*

1. Re-read the information on the collection and handling of bacteriological specimens.
2. Review the glossary terms.
3. Practice the procedure for the collection and handling of bacteriological specimens as outlined on the Student Performance Guide.

# Student Performance Guide

NAME ________________________

DATE ________________________

## LESSON 6–5 COLLECTION AND HANDLING OF BACTERIOLOGICAL SPECIMENS

### Instructions

1. Practice the procedure for the collection and handling of throat and urine specimens.
2. Demonstrate the procedure for collection and handling of the urine and throat specimens satisfactorily for the instructor. All steps must be completed as listed on the instructor's Performance Check Sheet.
3. Complete a written examination successfully.

### Materials and Equipment

- hand disinfectant
- sterile swabs (or Culturettes®, if available)
- sterile culture tubes with caps (for transporting swabs)
- sterile urine containers
- materials for clean-catch urine collection
- tongue depressors
- labels
- pen, pencil
- surface disinfectant
- biohazard container

**Procedure**

S = Satisfactory
U = Unsatisfactory

| You must: | S | U | Comments |
|---|---|---|---|
| 1. Wash hands with hand disinfectant | | | |
| 2. Assemble equipment and materials | | | |

| You must: | S | U | Comments |
|---|---|---|---|
| 3. Collect a throat culture: | | | |
| a. Explain the procedure to the patient | | | |
| b. Remove the swab from the package or Culturette® tube carefully to avoid contamination of the swab tip | | | |
| c. Have the patient open mouth wide | | | |
| d. Depress the patient's tongue with a tongue depressor and have the patient say "ah" | | | |
| e. Swab the back of the throat and the surfaces of the tonsils gently. Avoid touching the surfaces of the mouth and tongue | | | |
| f. Replace swab into Culturette® tube or sterile tube. When using Culturette, crush the enclosed ampule according to package instructions | | | |
| g. Label the tube with the patient's name, identification number, the date, and patient's room number if hospitalized | | | |
| h. Transport specimen to the laboratory promptly | | | |
| 4. Collect a urine specimen for culture: | | | |
| a. Explain to the patient the procedure for clean-catch urine collection (Lesson 5–1) | | | |
| b. Emphasize the necessity of avoiding contamination of the container or the specimen | | | |
| c. Label the sterile container with the patient's name, room number, and ID number (if hospitalized), and date | | | |
| d. Transport specimen to the laboratory promptly | | | |
| 5. Clean equipment and return to proper storage | | | |
| 6. Dispose of used materials in proper receptacles | | | |
| 7. Clean work area with surface disinfectant | | | |
| 8. Wash hands with hand disinfectant | | | |

Comments:

Student/Instructor:

Date: ______________________ Instructor: ______________________

# LESSON 6–6

## Transferring a Urine Culture and a Throat Culture to Growth Media

### LESSON OBJECTIVES

After studying this lesson, you should be able to:

- Transfer the throat culture onto growth media.
- Transfer the urine specimen onto growth media.
- List the different types of media and their uses.
- Define the glossary terms.

### GLOSSARY

**agar** / common name for agar-agar; a gelatinous seaweed extract which is added to bacterial media to make it semi-solid or solid

**nonselective media** / media which will support the growth of most bacteria

**pathogen** / an organism which causes disease

**primary plating medium** / the initial growth medium upon which the bacterial specimen is placed

**selective media** / media which support the growth of certain bacteria while inhibiting the growth of others

## INTRODUCTION

Once proper collection of a specimen has been accomplished, it is equally important that it be promptly transferred to an appropriate growth medium. An almost endless variety of growth media is available, and it is imperative that the medium used will promote the optimum growth of the organism.

## LIQUID, SEMI-SOLID, AND SOLID MEDIA

A growth medium may be liquid, semi-solid, or solid. One liquid medium used for general purposes is tryptic soy broth (TSB). Liquid media, including TSB, can be solidified by adding a specified amount of a gelling substance called **agar.** Semi-solid media can be prepared by the addition of a smaller amount of agar. It is usually desirable to grow bacteria on solid media in order to observe the individual colonies.

The broth with the agar added may be made into plates or slants. *Agar slants* are made by allowing the agar to solidify in tubes placed in a slanted position. For medical laboratory work, the agar is more commonly poured into sterile petri dishes and allowed to solidify. These are called *agar plates.*

### Selective and Nonselective Media

Media can be further divided into **selective** and **nonselective** types. The selective media allow the growth of certain bacteria while inhibiting the growth of others. The nonselective media are those which support the growth of most bacteria. An example of a selective medium is MacConkey's, which supports the growth of gram-negative bacteria and inhibits the growth of gram positives. Another selective medium is Thayer-Martin, which is used to grow cultures of *Neisseria gonorrhoeae.* A common nonselective medium is blood agar which is prepared by adding sheep blood to tryptic soy agar (TSA).

### Primary Plating Media

Most bacteriology departments in medical laboratories have a list of **primary plating media** which is to be used when initially growing organisms. This list is based mainly on the origin of the specimen. For example, material from a throat swab is placed on blood agar which is a good growth medium for most of the **pathogens** from the throat. Blood agar supports the growth of the *Streptococci* and also demonstrates the phenomenon of hemolysis. A green appearance of the blood agar around the colonies is called *alpha* ($\alpha$) *hemolysis.* Complete clearing of the agar around the colonies is called *beta* ($\beta$) *hemolysis.* The presence and type of hemolysis is important in the diagnosis of the *Streptococci* which are pathogenic to humans.

Urine specimens are placed onto blood agar and MacConkey's. The organism *Escherichia coli* is commonly isolated from urines. The MacConkey's will support the growth of the *Escherichia coli,* which is gram negative, and inhibit the growth of any gram positives present. The recommended list is always followed unless the requesting physician notes that an organism which requires special growth media is suspected.

## TRANSFERRING THE THROAT CULTURE

The organisms obtained from the throat swab are transferred to a blood agar plate. This is accomplished by gently rolling the swab across the surface of one quadrant of the plate (Figure 6–18). The inoculating loop is then used to streak the plate for isolated colonies as in Lesson 6–4. The plate is then incubated at 37°C overnight. It is important to produce isolated individual colonies which can be picked up with the loop and transferred for further study and identification. Group A *Streptococci* may be identified by placing an antibiotic disk, bacitracin, on a streaked area of agar and observing inhibition of bacterial growth after overnight incu-

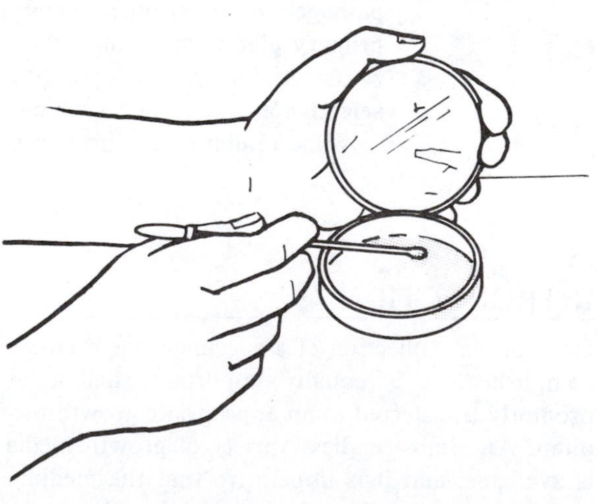

**Figure 6-18.** Transferring throat culture swab to an agar plate

bation. Growth of some streptococcus strains is enhanced by incubation in an environment of increased carbon dioxide ($CO_2$). A special $CO_2$ incubator may be used for this. Or, the culture may be placed in a candle jar—a lidded jar containing a lighted candle to convert part of the oxygen to $CO_2$. Rapid tests (fifteen to seventy minutes) for identifying the Group A *Streptococci* are now also available.

## TRANSFERRING THE URINE SPECIMEN

Urine specimens are usually transferred onto blood agar and MacConkey's agar. Special calibrated loops which have capacities of either 0.01 or 0.001 ml are used. The agar plates are inoculated by making one streak down the center of the plate, then making fifteen to twenty streaks at right angles to the first over the entire surface of the plate. Finally, a third set of streaks is made at right angles to the second set so that the plate is almost solidly streaked (Figure 6–19). The blood agar will support the growth of most bacteria. The MacConkey's agar allows the growth of gram negatives and also demonstrates the utilization of lactose which is helpful in the identification of the organism.

### Colony Count

The number of bacteria which are present in a urine sample can be estimated by counting the colonies which grow out after eighteen to twenty-four hours incubation. For example, if thirty colonies are counted and a 0.001 ml loop was used, the bacterial count is 30,000 per ml of urine. The number of colonies is multiplied by 1,000 since only 1/1000 ml of urine was cultured. An infection is usually indicated when the count is over 100,000 organisms per ml of urine (Figure 6–21).

## IDENTIFICATION OF BACTERIA

After an organism has been isolated from a culture, it may be identified by the use of any one of several identification kits, such as agglutination kits or the biochemical strip tests. These strip tests are available for the identification of some of the gram-negative and gram-positive organisms (Color Plate 30).

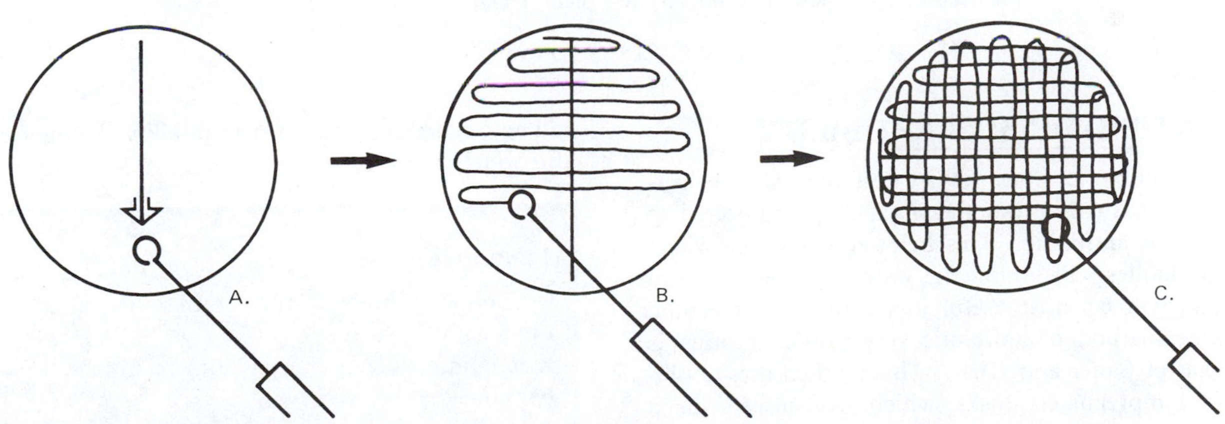


**Figure 6-19.** Streaking a urine plate. A) Make one streak down the center of the plate using a calibrated loop. B) Make several streaks at right angles to the initial streak, crossing over the original streak several times. C) Make several streaks at right angles to the second set of streaks so that the plate is almost solidly streaked

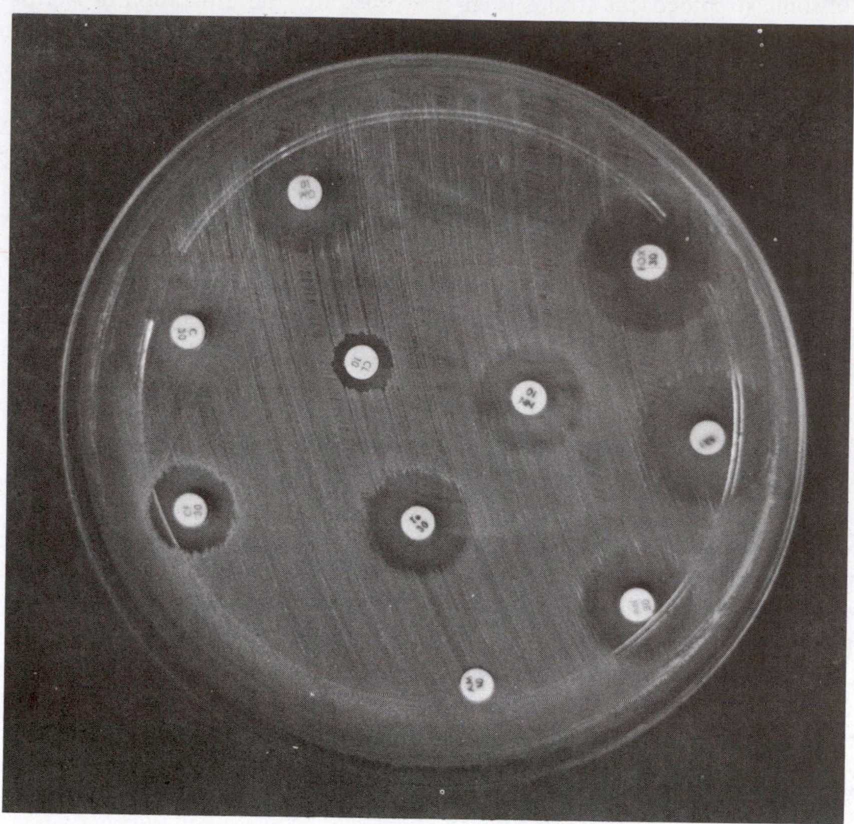

**Figure 6-20.** Antibiotic susceptibility test plate (*Photo by John Estridge*)

## ANTIBIOTIC SUSCEPTIBILITY

An antibiotic susceptibility test may also be performed. In this test, the organism is subjected to various antibiotics. This helps to determine which antibiotics will inhibit the growth of the organism and will be most useful in treating the infection. One method of antibiotic susceptibility testing is that of Bauer and Kirby. This method uses antibiotic-impregnated disks which are placed on a streaked plate. Susceptibility to a certain antibiotic is shown by inhibition of growth around that disk (Figure 6–20 and Color Plate 29). Semi-automated and automated methods of susceptibility testing are also widely used.

### *Precautions*

- Aseptic technique must be observed at all times.
- Recommended primary plating media should be utilized.
- Care should be used in streaking to avoid damaging the agar surfaces.

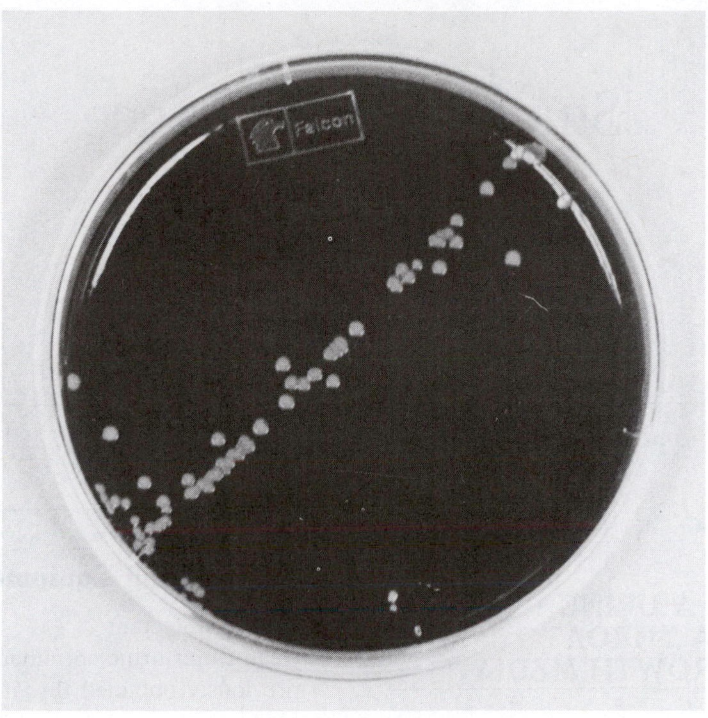


**Figure 6-21.** Isolated colonies on a blood agar plate (*Photo by John Estridge*)

## *LESSON REVIEW*

1. How is the primary plating medium chosen?
2. What is the difference between a broth medium and an agar medium?
3. What is an agar plate?
4. Material from a throat swab is usually placed on which medium?
5. Urine specimens are placed on which media?
6. If a 0.001 ml loop is used and sixty colonies are counted, what is the estimated number of bacteria per ml of urine?
7. What effect does MacConkey's have on gram-positive bacteria?
8. Why is it important to produce isolated colonies?
9. Define agar, nonselective media, pathogen, primary plating medium, selective media.

## *STUDENT ACTIVITIES*

1. Re-read the information on transferring a urine culture and throat culture to growth media.
2. Review the glossary terms.
3. Practice the procedures for transferring the throat culture and the urine specimen to growth media as outlined on the Student Performance Guide.

# Student Performance Guide

NAME ______________________

DATE ______________________

## LESSON 6–6
## TRANSFERRING A URINE CULTURE AND A THROAT CULTURE TO GROWTH MEDIA

### Instructions

1. Practice transferring the throat and urine specimens to growth media.
2. Demonstrate the procedure for transferring the throat and urine specimens to growth media satisfactorily for the instructor. All steps must be completed as listed on the instructor's Performance Check Sheet.
3. Complete a written examination successfully.

### Materials and Equipment

- hand disinfectant
- clean-catch urine specimen
- previously obtained throat cultures
- blood agar plates
- MacConkey agar plates
- inoculating loop, with holder
- special calibrated loop (0.01 or 0.001 ml)
- test tube rack
- Bunsen burner
- matches or flint-type lighter
- incubator
- wax pencil or marking pen
- surface disinfectant
- biohazard container

## Procedure

S = Satisfactory
U = Unsatisfactory

| You must: | S | U | Comments |
|---|---|---|---|
| 1. Wash hands with hand disinfectant | | | |
| 2. Assemble equipment and materials | | | |
| 3. Light the Bunsen burner | | | |
| 4. Perform the procedure for transferring the throat culture: | | | |
| a. Remove the swab from the transport tube | | | |
| b. Raise the lid of the petri dish containing blood agar high enough to allow entrance of the swab | | | |
| c. Gently roll the swab across the surface of the agar at the top of one quadrant | | | |
| d. Replace swab into tube | | | |
| e. Flame the loop and cool briefly | | | |
| f. Use the loop to streak the organisms from quadrant one into quadrant two | | | |
| g. Repeat for each quadrant, flaming the loop between quadrants, until the plate has been streaked to produce isolated colonies | | | |
| h. Replace the lid on the petri dish | | | |
| i. Flame the loop and return it to the holder | | | |
| j. Label the bottom of the agar plate properly | | | |
| 5. Perform the procedure for transferring the urine specimen to growth media: | | | |
| a. Flame the 0.001 ml calibrated loop (0.01 ml loop may be used) | | | |
| b. Insert the loop into the well-mixed urine sample | | | |
| c. Remove the loop from the urine and check to see that the loop is filled with urine | | | |
| d. Transfer the loopful of urine to the blood agar by making a single streak down the center of the plate | | | |
| e. Spread the urine over the plate by making twenty to twenty-five streaks at right angles to the original streak, crossing the original streak each time | | | |
| f. Turn the petri dish one half turn and streak twenty to twenty-five times at right angles to the first set of streaks, crossing through all of them each time | | | |
| g. Replace the lid on the petri dish | | | |
| h. Repeat steps 5a–5g using a MacConkey plate | | | |

| You must: | S | U | Comments |
|---|---|---|---|
| i. Flame the loop and return it to the holder | | | |
| j. Label the bottom of the agar plates properly | | | |
| 6. Turn off Bunsen burner | | | |
| 7. Return equipment to proper storage | | | |
| 8. Place agar plates upside down in 37°C incubator | | | |
| 9. Dispose of contaminated materials properly | | | |
| 10. Wipe the work area with surface disinfectant | | | |
| 11. Wash hands with hand disinfectant | | | |
| 12. Examine the agar plates after the overnight (eighteen to twenty-four hours) incubation. The throat culture plate should have isolated colonies in the fourth quadrant. The urine culture plates should have isolated colonies spread over the entire surface | | | |
| 13. Count the number of colonies on the urine blood agar plate | | | |
| 14. Calculate the number of organisms per ml of urine by multiplying the number of colonies by 1,000 (multiply by 100 if 0.01 ml loop is used) | | | |
| 15. Record the results | | | |
| 16. Dispose of plates as instructed by teacher | | | |
| 17. Wash hands with hand disinfectant | | | |

Comments:

Student/Instructor:

Date: ______________________ Instructor: ______________________

# References and Suggested Readings

American Association of Blood Banks. *Technical Manual of the American Association of Blood Banks.* 7th ed. Philadelphia: J. B. Lippincott, 1977.

Anderson, Shauna C. *Introductory Laboratory Exercises for Medical Technologists.* St. Louis: C. V. Mosby, 1978.

Barrett, James T. *Basic Immunology and Its Medical Applications.* 2nd ed. St. Louis: C. V. Mosby, 1980.

Bauer, John D., Ackerman, Phillip G. and Toro, Gelson. *Clinical Laboratory Methods.* 8th ed. St. Louis: C. V. Mosby, 1974.

Brock, Thomas D. and Katherine M. *Basic Microbiology with Applications.* Englewood, N.J.: Prentice-Hall, Inc., 1973.

Brown, Barbara A. *Hematology: Principles and Procedures.* Philadelphia: Lea & Febiger, 1973.

Bryant, Neville J. *An Introduction to Immunohematology.* 2nd ed. Philadelphia: W. B. Saunders, 1982.

Coltey, Roger W. *Survey of Medical Technology.* St. Louis: C. V. Mosby, 1978.

Crabtree, Koby T., and Hinsdill, Ronald D. *Fundamental Experiments In Microbiology.* Philadelphia: W. B. Saunders, 1974.

Davidsohn, Israel and Henry, John Bernard. *Clinical Diagnosis By Laboratory Methods.* 15th ed. Philadelphia: W. B. Saunders, 1974.

Diggs, L. W., Sturm, Dorothy and Bell, Ann. *The Morphology of Human Blood Cells.* 4th ed. Abbott Park, IL: Abbott Laboratories, 1984.

Dougherty, William M. *Introduction to Hematology.* 2nd ed. St. Louis: C. V. Mosby, 1976.

Finegold, Sydney M., Martin, William J. and Scott, Elvyn G. *Bailey and Scott's Diagnostic Microbiology.* 5th ed. St. Louis: C. V. Mosby, 1978.

Fischbach, Frances T. *A Manual of Laboratory Diagnostic Tests.* Philadelphia: J. B. Lippincott, 1980.

Frobisher, Martin and others. *Fundamentals of Microbiology.* 9th ed. Philadelphia: W. B. Saunders, 1974.

Kaplan, Martin and others. *Clinical Chemistry: Interpretation and Techniques.* 2nd ed. Philadelphia: Lea & Febiger, 1983.

Koneman, Elmer W. and others. *Color Atlas and Textbook of Diagnostic Microbiology.* Philadelphia: J. B. Lippincott, 1978.

Lamberg, Stanley Lawrence and Rothstein, Robert. *Laboratory Manual of Hematology and Urinalysis.* Westport, Connecticut: AVI Publishing Co., Inc., 1978.

Lindberg, David S., Britt, Mary Stevenson and Fisher, Frances W. *Williams' Introduction to the Profession of Medical Technology.* 4th ed. Philadelphia: Lea & Febiger, 1984.

Miale, John B. *Laboratory Medicine—Hematology.* 6th ed. St. Louis: C. V. Mosby, 1982.

*Modern Urine Chemistry.* 4th and 6th printing. Elkhart, Indiana: Ames Division, Miles Laboratories, Inc., 1978.

Nester, Eugene, and others. *Microbiology, Third Edition.* Philadelphia: Saunders College Publishing, 1983.

Peacock, Julia E. and Tomar, Russel H. *Manual of Laboratory Immunology.* Philadelphia: Lea & Febiger, 1980.

Pittiglio, D. Harmening. *Modern Blood Banking and Transfusion Practices.* Philadelphia: F. A. Davis Co., 1983.

Raphael, Stanley S. *Lynch's Medical Laboratory Technology.* 3rd ed. Vol. I and II. Philadelphia: W. B. Saunders, 1976.

Scimone, John. *Laboratory Manual of Clinical Bacteriology.* Westport, Connecticut: AVI Publishing Co., Inc., 1978.

Seiverd, Charles E. *Hematology for Medical Technologists.* 5th ed. Philadelphia: Lea & Febiger, 1983.

Simmons, Arthur. *Technical Hematology.* 3rd ed. Philadelphia: J. B. Lippincott, 1980.

Thomas, Clayton L. *Taber's Cyclopedic Medical Dictionary.* 14th ed. Philadelphia: F. A. Davis Company, 1981.

Tietz, Norbert W. *Fundamentals of Clinical Chemistry.* Philadelphia: W. B. Saunders Co., 1976.

Williams, Harriet B. *Laboratory Manual of Serology, Immunology and Blood Banking.* Westport, Connecticut: AVI Publishing Co., Inc., 1978.

Wintrobe, Maxwell M. *Clinical Hematology.* 6th ed. Philadelphia: Lea & Febiger, 1967.

Wittman, Karl S. and Thomas, John C. *Medical Laboratory Skills.* New York: McGraw Hill, 1977.

Woosley, Hugh A. and Cuviello, Patrick V. *Basic Medical Laboratory Subjects.* Indianapolis: Bobbs-Merrill Co., 1982.

# Glossary

**absorbance** the light absorbed (not transmitted) by a liquid containing colored molecules; designated in formulas by "A"; also called optical density (O.D.)

**acid** a substance which liberates hydrogen ions in solution; turns litmus paper red

**aerosol** a suspension of fine solid or liquid particles in the air

**agar** common name for agar-agar; a gelatinous seaweed extract which is added to bacterial media to make it semi-solid or solid

**agar plate** agar medium dispensed into sterile petri dishes and allowed to solidify

**agar slant** agar medium dispensed into tubes and allowed to solidify at an angle

**agglutination** clumping of cells or particles; in serology due to reaction of the particle with antibody

**agglutination inhibition** interference of agglutination

**aggregate** total substances making up a mass; a clustering of particles

**amorphous** without shape

**anemia** decrease below the normal red cell count or in the blood hemoglobin level

**anhydrous** containing no water

**anisocytosis** marked variation in the size of erythrocytes

**anticoagulant** agent which prevents blood coagulation

**antiserum** serum containing antibodies

**anuria** absence of urine production

**artery** a blood vessel that carries oxygenated blood from the heart to the tissues

**aseptic techniques** techniques used to maintain sterility or to prevent contamination

**aspiration** act of drawing in by suction

**autoclave** a device for sterilization by steam pressure

**bacillus** a rod-shaped bacterium (pl. bacilli)

**bacteria** a group of one-celled microorganisms; germs

**bacterial morphology** the form or structure of bacteria; color, shape, and size

**band cell** an immature neutrophil with a nonsegmented nucleus; a stab cell

**base** a substance which accepts hydrogen ions; turns litmus paper blue

**basophil** a leukocyte containing basophilic-staining granules

**basophilic** blue in color; having affinity for the basic stain

**bibulous paper** a special absorbent paper which is used to dry slides

**bilirubin** the yellow pigment in bile; a breakdown product of hemoglobin

**binocular** having two oculars or eyepieces

**blank** reagent blank; solution which contains some or all of the reagents used in the test but does not contain the substance being measured

**blood bank** place where blood is typed, tested, and stored until it is needed for transfusion

**blood group antibody** a serum protein that reacts specifically with a blood group antigen

**blood group antigen** a substance or structure on the red cell membrane which causes antibody formation and reacts with that antibody

**broth** liquid nutrient medium in tubes

**buffer** a substance which prevents changes in the pH of solutions when additional acid or base is added

**buffy coat** a light-colored layer of leukocytes and platelets which forms on the top of the red cell layer when a sample of blood is centrifuged or allowed to stand

**capillary** a minute blood vessel which connects the smallest arteries to the smallest veins

**capillary action** the action by which a fluid will enter a tube or pipet because of the attraction between the glass and liquid

**capillary tube** a glass tube of very small diameter used for laboratory procedures

**carcinogenic** having the ability to produce or cause cancer

**cast** mold; in urinalysis, a protein matrix formed in the tubules that becomes washed into the urine

**CBC** complete blood count, a commonly performed group of hematological tests

**Celsius** temperature scale having the freezing point of water at zero (0°) and the boiling point at one hundred (100°); indicated by "C"; also called Centigrade

**certified medical laboratory technician** a professional who has completed a minimum of two years of specific training in an accredited program, consisting of one year of college and one year of clinical training, and has passed a national certifying examination

**certified medical technologist** a professional who has a bachelor's degree from an accredited college or university, has completed one year of clinical training, and has passed a national certifying examination

**clean-catch urine** a urine sample collected after the urethral opening and surrounding tissues have been cleansed

**coagulation** formation of a fibrin clot which aids in stopping bleeding

**coagulation factors** proteins present in plasma which interact to form the fibrin clot

**coarse adjustment** adjusts position of microscope objectives; used to initially bring objects into focus

**coccus** spherical or oval-shaped bacterium (pl. cocci)

**colony** a circumscribed mass of bacteria growing in or upon a solid or semi-solid medium; assumed to have grown from a single organism

**condenser** apparatus located below the microscope stage which directs light into the objective

**counterstain** a dye which adds a contrasting color

**critical measurements** measurements made when accuracy of the concentration of a solution is important; measurements made using glassware which is manufactured to strict standards

**culture** to cultivate bacteria in a nutrient medium; a mass of growing bacteria

**cuvette** a small test tube used to hold liquids to be examined in the spectrophotometer; must be manufactured to certain standards for clarity and lack of distortion in the glass

**cyanmethemoglobin** a stable compound formed when hemoglobin is combined with Drabkin's reagent

**cystinuria** the presence of cystine in urine; results in the development of recurrent urinary calculi

**cytoplasm** the fluid portion of the cell outside the nucleus

**diffraction grating** a device which disperses a light beam into a spectrum

**diluting fluid** diluting solution which will not damage the cells being counted

**diplococci** round bacteria which occur predominantly in pairs

**distilled water (dist. $H_2O$)** the condensate collected when water has been boiled (distilled) to remove impurities

**Drabkin's reagent** a diluting reagent used for hemoglobin determination; contains iron, potassium, cyanide, and sodium bicarbonate

**dysfunction** impaired or abnormal function

**EDTA** ethylene diamine tetraacetic acid, commonly used anticoagulant for hematological studies

**eosin** a dye that produces a red stain

**eosinophil** an acid-staining leukocyte; numbers may increase in allergic reactions

**eosinophilic** having affinity for the acid stain; reddish in color

**erythrocyte** red blood cell, RBC, transports oxygen to the tissue and carbon dioxide ($CO_2$) to the lungs

**erythrocytosis** increase above the normal number of red cells in circulation

**eyepiece** ocular

**Fahrenheit** a temperature scale having the freezing point of water at 32° and the boiling point at 212°; indicated by "F"

**fibrin** protein filaments formed in the coagulation process resulting from the action of the enzyme, thrombin, on the plasma protein, fibrinogen

**fine adjustment** adjusts position of microscope objectives; used to sharpen focus

**fixative** preservative; chemical which prevents deterioration of cells or tissues

**flame** sterilization of certain materials used in bacteriology by heating or passing through a flame

**flora** organisms adapted for living in a specific environment

**fume hood** a device which draws contaminated air out of an area and either cleanses and recirculates it or discharges it to the outside

**galvanometer** instrument which measures electrical current

**gauge** a measure of the diameter of a needle

**globin** the portion of the hemoglobin molecule composed of protein

**glomerular** pertaining to the glomerulus; the filtering unit of the kidney

**glycosuria** glucose in the urine; glucosuria

**graduated flask** container used for estimating volumes; has 50 ml to 100 ml increment marks

**gram** basic metric unit of weight or mass

**gram negative** refers to bacteria which are decolorized in the Gram stain; pink-red in color after counterstained

**gram positive** refers to bacteria which retain the crystal violet dye in the Gram stain; purple-blue in color

**Gram stain** a stain which differentiates bacteria according to the chemical composition of their cell walls

**HCG** human chorionic gonadotropin, a hormone found in pregnant women; sometimes called uterine chorionic gonadotropin (UCG)

**hemacytometer** a heavy glass slide made to precise specifications and used to count cells microscopically; a counting chamber

**hemacytometer coverglass** a special coverglass of uniform thickness used with a hemacytometer

**hematocrit** the volume of erythrocytes packed by centrifugation in a given volume of blood and expressed as a percentage; abbreviated "crit" or "hct"

**hematology** the science concerned with the study of blood and blood forming tissues

**hematoma** the swelling of tissue around a vessel due to leakage of blood from the vessel into the tissue

**hematuria** presence of red blood cells in urine

**heme** the portion of the hemoglobin molecule containing iron

**hemoglobin** a red blood cell constituent which is composed of heme and globin and which carries oxygen; abbreviated "Hb" or Hgb"

**hemolysis** the destruction of red blood cells resulting in the liberation of hemoglobin from the cells

**hemolytic disease of the newborn (HDN)** a disease in which antibody from the mother destroys the red cells of the fetus

**hemorrhage** excessive or uncontrolled bleeding

**hemostasis** process of stopping blood flow

**heparin** an anticoagulant used in certain laboratory procedures

**heterophile antibody** antibody which is increased in infectious mononucleosis

**hyaline** transparent, pale

**hypochromia** a condition in which the red cell has a hemoglobin content below normal for its size

**hypochromic** having reduced color or hemoglobin content

**hypodermic needle** a hollow needle used for injections or for obtaining fluid specimens

**immunity** resistance to disease or infection

**immunization** process by which an antibody is produced in response to an antigen

**immunohematology** blood banking; the study of blood group antigens and antibodies

**incubator** temperature-controlled chamber into which inoculated media is placed so that bacterial growth will occur

**indices** plural of index; indexes; erythrocyte indices are values which compare a blood sample to standard values

**inflammation** a tissue reaction to injury

**inoculating loop** a nichrome or platinum wire fashioned into a loop on one end and having a handle on the other end; used to transfer bacterial growth

**inoculation** the introduction of organisms into media

**inoculum** the portion of culture organisms which is being introduced into a medium

**iris diaphragm** regulates the amount of light which strikes the object being viewed through the microscope

**isotonic solution** a solution which has the same concentration of dissolved particles as that solution with which it is compared

**ketones** substances produced during increased metabolism of fat; sometimes called ketone bodies

**ketonuria** ketones in the urine

**lancet** a sterile, sharp, pointed blade which can be used to perform a capillary puncture

**lateral** toward the side

**lens** a transparent material, curved on one or both sides, which spreads or focuses light

**lens paper** a special nonabrasive material used to clean optical lenses

**leukocyte** white blood cell, WBC, provides protection from disease

**leukocytosis** increase above the normal number of leukocytes in the blood

**leukopenia** decrease below the normal number of leukocytes in the blood

**liter** basic metric unit of volume

**lumen** the open space within a tubular organ or tissue

**lymphocyte** a small basophilic staining leukocyte having a round or oval nucleus and which is important in the immune process

**lymphocytosis** an increase above normal in the number of lymphocytes in the blood

**macrocytic** a cell which is larger than normal

**mean corpuscular hemoglobin** MCH; average red cell hemoglobin concentration; an estimate of the hemoglobin concentration in a red cell in a blood specimen; measured in picograms (pg)

**mean corpuscular hemoglobin concentration** MCHC; compares the weight of hemoglobin in a red cell to the size of the cell; reported in percentage or g/dl

**mean corpuscular volume** MCV; average red cell volume; an estimate of the volume of a red cell in a blood specimen; measured in femtoliters (fl) or cubic microns ($\mu^3$)

**median cephalic vein** a vein located in the bend of the elbow and frequently used for venipuncture

**medical technology** the health profession concerned with the performance of laboratory analyses used in the diagnosis and treatment of disease as well as in health maintenance

**medium** a nutritive substance, either solid or liquid, in or upon which microorganisms are grown for study (pl. media)

**megakaryocyte** a large bone marrow cell which releases platelets into the blood stream

**meniscus** the curved surface of a liquid in a container

**meter** basic metric unit of distance or length

**methylene blue** a dye that produces a blue stain

**microbiology** the scientific study of microorganisms such as bacteria

**microcytic** having a smaller than normal cell size

**microhematocrit** a hematocrit performed on a small sample of blood

**microhematocrit centrifuge** a machine which spins capillary tubes at a high speed to cause rapid separation of liquid from solid components

**micron** a unit of measurement, $1 \times 10^{-6}$ meter or one micrometer

**micropipet** pipet which holds a very small volume

**microscope arm** the portion of the microscope which connects the lenses to the base

**microscope base** the portion of the microscope which rests on the table and supports the instrument

**mid-stream urine** a urine sample collected in the middle of voiding

**monochromatic** consisting of one color; light which is one wavelength

**monochromator** device which allows only one color of light to reach the cuvette

**monocular** having one ocular

**monocyte** the largest of the leukocytes; usually has a convoluted nucleus

**mordant** a substance which fixes a dye or stain to an object

**morphology** study of form and structure of cells, tissues, organs

**myoglobin** protein found in muscle tissue

**neutrophil** most numerous leukocyte, neutral staining, first line of defense against infection

**nocturia** excessive urination at night

**noncritical measurement** measurement which is estimated; measurement made in containers (such as the Erlenmeyer flask) which estimate volume

**nonselective media** media which will support the growth of most bacteria

**normochromic** having normal color

**normocytic** having a normal cell size and shape

**nosepiece** revolving unit to which microscope objectives are attached

**nucleus, pl. nuclei** the central structure of a cell which contains DNA and controls cell growth and function

**objective** magnifying lens which is closest to the object being viewed with a microscope

**ocular** eyepiece of a microscope; contains a magnifying lens

**oliguria** decreased production of urine

**opalescent** reflecting an iridescent light

**pathogen** an organism which causes disease
**pathologist** a physician specially trained in the nature and cause of disease
**percent transmittance** the percentage of light which passes through a liquid sample
**petri dish** a shallow covered dish made of plastic or glass
**pH** a measure of the hydrogen ion (H+) concentration of a substance
**phlebotomist** one trained to draw blood
**phlebotomy** venipuncture; entry of a vein with a needle
**photoelectric cell** a device which detects light and converts it into electricity
**picogram** micromicrogram; $1 \times 10^{-12}$ gram
**plasma** the liquid part of the blood in which the cellular elements are suspended
**platelet** a small disk-shaped fragment of cytoplasm from a megakaryocyte which plays an important role in blood coagulation; a thrombocyte
**poikilocytosis** significant variation in the shape of erythrocytes
**polychromatic** multicolored
**polyuria** excessive production of urine
**porphyrins** a group of pigments which are intermediates in the production of hemoglobin
**prefix** modifying word or syllable(s) placed at the beginning of a word
**primary plating medium** the initial growth medium upon which the bacterial specimen is placed
**proteinuria** protein in the urine, usually albumin

**quadrant** one fourth; one quarter of an agar plate

**ratio** relationship in degree or number between two things
**reagents** substances which are used in laboratory analyses
**red cell diluting pipet** pipet used to dilute blood for a red cell count; RBC pipet
**reticulocyte** an immature erythrocyte which has retained basophilic substance in the cytoplasm
**reticulocytopenia** decrease below the normal number of reticulocytes
**reticulocytosis** an increase above the normal number of reticulocytes in the circulating blood
**reticulum** a network
**Rh (D) immune globulin** a concentrated purified solution of human anti–D used for injection; RhIG
**rouleau** a group of red cells arranged like a roll of coins (pl. rouleaux)

**Sahli pipet** a pipet with a volume of 0.02 ml, used for manual hemoglobin determinations
**saline** an isotonic solution of sodium chloride and distilled water; normal saline; physiological saline; usually made in 0.85 or 0.9% concentration for use in medical laboratory procedures
**sediment** solid substances which settle to the bottom of a liquid
**sedimentation** the process of solid particles settling at the bottom of a liquid
**selective media** media which support the growth of certain bacteria while inhibiting the growth of others
**serology** laboratory study of serum and the reactions between antigens and antibodies
**S.I. units** standardized units of measure; international units
**solute** a liquid, gas, or solid which is dissolved in a liquid to make a solution
**solvent** that liquid into which the solute is dissolved
**specific gravity** ratio of weight of a given volume of a solution to the weight of the same volume of water; a measurement of density
**spectrophotometer** an instrument which can be used to determine the concentration of a solution by measuring the light transmitted or absorbed by the solution
**spirochete** a slender, spiral microorganism
**stage** platform on which object to be viewed microscopically is placed
**standard curve** a graph which shows the relationship between the concentration of a solution and the absorbance or percent transmittance of the solution
**stem** main part of a word; root word
**suffix** modifying word or syllable(s) placed at the end of a word
**supernatant** clear liquid remaining at the top after centrifugation or settling of precipitate in a solution
**supravital stain** a stain which will color living cells or tissues
**synthesis** the combining of elements to produce a compound
**syringe** a hollow, tube-like container with a plunger, used for injecting or withdrawing fluids

**TC** to contain
**TD** to deliver
**terminology** special terms used in any specialized field

**thrombocyte** platelet
**thrombocytopenia** a decrease below the normal number of platelets in the blood
**thrombocytosis** an increase above the normal number of platelets in the blood
**tourniquet** a band used to constrict the blood flow in the vein from which blood is to be drawn
**transport medium** a medium into which a specimen is placed to preserve it during transport to the laboratory
**turbid** cloudy, not clear; used to describe urine

**urobilinogen** a derivative of bilirubin formed by the action of intestinal bacteria
**urochrome** yellow pigment which gives color to urine

**vacuole** a clear space in cytoplasm filled with fluid or air
**vasoconstriction** a contracting or narrowing of a vessel
**vein** a blood vessel that carries deoxygenated blood to the heart
**venipuncture** entry of a vein with a needle; a phlebotomy

**white cell diluting pipet** pipet used to dilute blood for white cell count; WBC pipet
**Wintrobe tube** a slender thick-walled tube marked from 0–100 mm; used in Wintrobe method of macrohematocrit and erythrocyte sedimentation rate
**working distance** distance between the microscope objective and the slide when the object is in sharp focus

# APPENDIX A
## Safety Agreement Form

Although there are many hazards present in the medical laboratory, it is possible to make the laboratory a safe working environment. Each laboratory worker must agree to observe all safety rules posted or unposted which are required by the instructor or employer. No set of rules can cover all of the hazards that may be present. However, several general rules are listed below:

1. Refrain from horseplay.
2. Avoid eating, drinking, smoking, or gum chewing.
3. Wear a laboratory jacket or coat.
4. Pin long hair away from face and neck to avoid contact with chemicals, equipment, or flames.
5. Wear closed-toe shoes.
6. Avoid wearing chains, bracelets, rings, or other loose hanging jewelry.
7. Use gloves if cuts or open sores are present on hands.
8. Clean work area before beginning laboratory procedures and at the end of each procedure.
9. Wash hands before and after laboratory procedures and at any other time necessary.
10. Wear safety glasses when working with chemicals and the autoclave.
11. Wipe up spills promptly and appropriately.
12. Avoid tasting any chemicals.
13. Follow manufacturer's instructions for operating equipment.
14. Handle equipment with care.
15. Report any broken, frayed, or exposed electrical cord.

16. Report any broken glassware or damaged equipment.
17. Store equipment properly.
18. Report any accident to the instructor immediately.
19. Allow visitors only in the nonworking area of the laboratory.
20. Handle carefully any biological specimens, including human blood and diagnostic products made from human blood.

Please initial the items listed below:
Initial

_______ I agree to follow all set rules and regulations as required by the instructor, including those listed above.

_______ I have been informed that biological specimens and blood products may possess the potential of transmitting diseases such as hepatitis and acquired immunodeficiency syndrome (AIDS).

_______ I understand that even though diagnostic products are tested for Hepatitis B surface antigen (HBsAg), no known test can offer assurance that products derived from human blood will not transmit hepatitis.

Student Name (please print) ____________________________________________

Student Signature ______________________________ Date ________________

Parent Signature (if student under 18) ______________________ Date ________________

# APPENDIX B
# Abbreviations, Prefixes, Suffixes, and Stems

## ABBREVIATIONS COMMONLY USED IN A MEDICAL LABORATORY

| | |
|---|---|
| **BP** | blood pressure |
| **BUN** | blood urea nitrogen |
| **C** | Centigrade, Celsius |
| **CBC** | complete blood count |
| **cc, ccm** | cubic centimeter |
| **cm** | centimeter |
| **CNS** | central nervous system |
| **CO** | carbon monoxide |
| **$CO_2$** | carbon dioxide |
| **CSF** | cerebral spinal fluid |
| **E.U.** | Ehrlich units |
| **F** | Fahrenheit |
| **FUO** | fever of unknown origin |
| **g, gm** | gram |
| **GI** | gastrointestinal |
| **GU** | genitourinary |
| **Hb** | hemoglobin |
| **HCl** | hydrochloric acid |
| **Hct** | hematocrit |

| | |
|---|---|
| **Hgb** | hemoglobin |
| **$H_2O$** | water |
| **HPF** | high power field |
| **IM** | infectious mononucleosis |
| **IU** | international unit |
| **IV** | intravenous |
| **l, L** | liter |
| **LPF** | low power field |
| **MCH** | mean corpuscular hemoglobin |
| **MCHC** | mean corpuscular hemoglobin concentration |
| **MCV** | mean corpuscular volume |
| **mg** | milligram |
| **MI** | myocardial infarction |
| **ml, mL** | milliliter |
| **MLT** | medical laboratory technician |
| **mm** | millimeter |
| **MT** | medical technologist |
| **NaCl** | sodium chloride, saline |
| **nm** | nanometer |
| **O.D.** | optical density |
| **pH** | a number indicating the relative acidity of a solution |
| **RBC** | red blood cell |
| **S.I.** | Le Système International d'Unités (International System of Units) |
| **sp. gr.** | specific gravity |
| **Staph** | *Staphylococcus* |
| **stat** | immediately |
| **Strep** | *Streptococcus* |
| **UA** | urinalysis |
| **WBC** | white blood cell |

## SELECTED PREFIXES COMMONLY USED IN MEDICAL TERMINOLOGY

| Prefix | Definition | Example of term |
|---|---|---|
| **a, an** | absent, deficient | anemia |
| **ab** | away from | absent |
| **ad** | toward | adrenal |
| **ambi** | both | ambidextrous |
| **aniso** | unequal | anisocytosis |
| **ante** | before | antenatal |
| **ant(i)** | against | antibiotic |
| **auto** | self | autograft |
| **baso** | blue | basophil |
| **bi** | two | binuclear |
| **bio** | life | biology |
| **brady** | slow | bradycardia |
| **circum** | around | circumnuclear |
| **co, com, con** | with, together | concentrate |
| **contra** | against | contraception |
| **de** | down, from | decay |
| **di** | two | dimorphic |
| **dia** | through | dialysis |
| **dipl** | double | diplococcus |
| **dis** | apart, away from | disease |
| **dys** | bad, difficult, improper | dysphagia |
| **e, ecto, ex** | out from | ectoparasite |
| **end(o)** | inside, within | endoparasite |
| **enter(o)** | intestine | enterotoxin |
| **epi** | upon, after | epidermis |
| **equi** | equal | equilibrium |
| **hemi** | half | hemisphere |
| **hyper** | above, excessive | hyperglycemia |
| **hypo** | under, deficient | hypoventilation |
| **infra** | beneath | infracostal |
| **inter** | among | intercostal |
| **intra** | within | intracranial |
| **iso** | equal | isotonic |
| **macr(o)** | large | macrocyte |
| **mal** | bad, abnormal | malformation |
| **medi** | middle | median |
| **mega** | huge, great | megaloblast |

| Prefix | Definition | Example of term |
|---|---|---|
| **melan** | black | melanoma |
| **meta** | after, next | metamorphosis |
| **micro** | small | microscope |
| **mon(o)** | one, single | monoxide |
| **morph** | shape | morphology |
| **necro** | dead | necropsy |
| **neo** | new | neoplasm |
| **neutro** | neutral | neutrophil |
| **olig** | few | oliguria |
| **orth** | straight, normal | orthopedic |
| **pan** | all | pandemic |
| **para** | beside | paraplegic |
| **per** | through | percolate |
| **peri** | around | pericardium |
| **phago** | to eat | phagocyte |
| **poly** | many | polyuria |
| **post** | after | post-op |
| **pre, pro** | before | prenatal |
| **pseudo** | false | pseudoappendicitis |
| **psych(o)** | mind | psychology |
| **py(o)** | pus | pyuria |
| **quad(r)** | four | quadrant |
| **retro** | backward | retroactive |
| **semi** | half | semiconscious |
| **steno** | narrow | stenosis |
| **sub** | under | subcutaneous |
| **super, supra** | above | superinfection |
| **syn** | together | synergistic |
| **tachy** | swift | tachycardia |
| **tetra** | four | tetramer |
| **therm** | heat | thermometer |
| **trans** | through | transport |
| **tri** | three | trimester |
| **uni** | one | unicellular |

## SELECTED SUFFIXES COMMONLY USED IN MEDICAL TERMINOLOGY

| Suffix | Definition | Example of term |
|---|---|---|
| **algia** | pain | neuralgia |
| **blast** | primitive, germ | erythroblast |
| **centesis** | puncture, aspiration | amniocentesis |
| **cide** | death, killer | bacteriocide |
| **ectomy** | excision, cut out | gastrectomy |
| **emesis** | vomiting | hematemesis |
| **emia** | in the or of the blood | bilirubinemia |
| **ferent** | carry | afferent |
| **genic** | origin, producing | pyogenic |
| **ia, iasis** | state, condition | iatrogenic |
| **iole** | small | bronchiole |
| **itis** | inflammation | pharyngitis |
| **lysis** | free, breaking down | hemolysis |
| **oid** | resembling, similar to | blastoid |
| **(o)logy** | study of | pathology |
| **oma** | tumor | hepatoma |
| **opathy, pathia** | disease | adenopathy |
| **osis** | state or condition, increase | leukocytosis |
| **ostomy** | create an opening | ileostomy |
| **otomy** | cut into | phlebotomy |
| **penia** | lack of | leukopenia |
| **phil** | affinity for; liking | eosinophil |
| **phyte** | plant | dermatophyte |
| **plastic, plasia** | to form or mold | hyperplasia |
| **pnea** | breathing | apnea |
| **poiesis** | to make | hemopoiesis |
| **rrhage** | excessive flow | hemorrhage |
| **rrhea** | flow | diarrhea |
| **scope, scopy** | view | arthroscope |
| **stasis** | same, standing still | hemostasis |
| **troph(y)** | nourishment | hypertrophy |

## SELECTED STEMS COMMONLY USED IN MEDICAL TERMINOLOGY

| Stem | Definition | Example of term |
|---|---|---|
| **adeno** | gland | lymphadenitis |
| **alg** | pain | analgesic |
| **arter** | artery | arteriogram |
| **arthr** | joint | arthritis |
| **audio** | hearing | auditory |
| **brachi** | arm | brachial |
| **bronch(i)** | air tube in lungs | bronchitis |
| **calc** | stone | calcify |
| **carcin** | cancer | carcinogen |
| **cardi** | heart | myocardium |
| **caud** | tail | caudate |
| **ceph(al)** | head | encephalitis |
| **chol** | bile, gall bladder | cholesterol |
| **chondr** | cartilage | chondroplasia |
| **chrom** | color | chromogen |
| **cran** | skull | craniotomy |
| **cut** | skin | subcutaneous |
| **cyan** | blue | cyanosis |
| **cyst** | bladder, bag | cystocele |
| **cyt(o)** | cell | monocyte |
| **dactyl** | finger | arachnodactyly |
| **dent, dont** | teeth | orthodontist |
| **derm** | skin | dermatitis |
| **edema** | swelling | edematous |
| **erythro** | red | erythrocyte |
| **febr** | fever | afebrile |
| **gastr(o)** | stomach | gastritis |
| **genito** | reproductive | genital |
| **gloss** | tongue | glossitis |
| **glyco** | sweet | glycosuria |
| **gran** | grain | granulocyte |
| **hem(a), haem,** | blood | hematology |
| **hepat(o)** | liver | hepatitis |
| **histo** | tissue | histology |
| **hydro** | water | hydrocephalic |
| **hystero** | uterus | hysterectomy |
| **iatro** | physician | podiatrist |

| Stem | Definition | Example of term |
|---|---|---|
| **leuk** | white | leukocyte |
| **lip** | fat | lipoma |
| **lith** | stone | cholelithiasis |
| **mening** | membrane covering brain | meningitis |
| **myel** | marrow | myelogram |
| **myo** | muscle | myositis |
| **nephro** | kidney | nephron |
| **neur** | nerve | neurectomy |
| **noct** | night | nocturia |
| **onc** | tumor | oncology |
| **oo** | egg | oogenesis |
| **ophthal** | eye | ophthalmologist |
| **os, osteo** | bone | osteosarcoma |
| **oto** | ear | otitis |
| **path** | disease | pathogen |
| **ped** | child | pediatrician |
| **phleb** | vein | phlebitis |
| **phob** | fear | phobia |
| **phot** | light | photosensitive |
| **pneum** | air | pneumonitis |
| **pod** | foot | pseudopod |
| **pulm** | lung | pulmonary |
| **ren** | kidney | adrenal |
| **rhin** | nose | rhinoplasty |
| **scler** | hard | sclerosis |
| **sep** | poison | septic |
| **soma(t)** | body | somatic |
| **sperm** | seed | spermatogenesis |
| **stoma** | mouth, opening | stomatitis |
| **therm** | temperature | thermometer |
| **thorac** | chest | thoracotomy |
| **thromb** | clot | thrombocyte |
| **tome** | knife | microtome |
| **tox** | poison | toxin |
| **ur(o), uria** | urine | hematuria |
| **vas** | vessel | intravascular |
| **ven** | vein | intravenous |

# APPENDIX C
## Table of Normal Hematological Values

| Test | Normal Range |
|---|---|
| **Hemoglobin:** | |
| Newborn | 16.0–23.0 g/dl |
| Children | 10.0–14.0 g/dl |
| Adult males | 13.5–17.5 g/dl |
| Adult females | 12.5–15.5 g/dl |
| **Microhematocrit:** | |
| Newborn | 51–60% |
| One year | 32–38% |
| Six years | 34–42% |
| Adult males | 42–52% |
| Adult females | 36–48% |
| **Leukocyte Counts:** | |
| Newborn | $9.0–30.0 \times 10^9/1$ |
| One year | $6.0–14.0 \times 10^9/1$ |
| Six years | $4.5–12.0 \times 10^9/1$ |
| Adult | $4.5–11.0 \times 10^9/1$ |
| **Erythrocyte Counts:** | |
| Adult males | $4.5 \times 6.0 \times 10^{12}/1$ |
| Adult females | $4.0 \times 5.5 \times 10^{12}/1$ |

| Test | Normal Range | |
|---|---|---|
| **Erythrocyte Indices:** | | |
| Mean Corpuscular Volume (MCV) | 80–100 fl | |
| Mean Corpuscular Hemoglobin (MCH) | 27–32 pg | |
| Mean Corpuscular Hemoglobin Concentration (MCHC) | 33–38% | |
| **Platelet Count** | $0.15–0.40 \times 10^{12}/1$ | |
| **Reticulocyte Percentages:** | | |
| | | Upper limit of Normal |
| Newborn | 2.5–6.5% | 10% |
| Adult | 0.5–1.5% | 3% |
| **Erythrocyte Sedimentation Rate (ESR),** Wintrobe method | | |
| Children | 0–13 mm/hr | |
| Adult males | 0–9 mm/hr | |
| Adult females | 0–20 mm/hr | |
| **Bleeding Time:** | | |
| Ivy method | 1–7 minutes | |
| Duke method | 1–3 minutes | |
| **Capillary Coagulation** | 2–6 minutes | |

**Differential Leukocyte Count:**

| White cell | 1 month | six-year-old | 12-year-old | adult |
|---|---|---|---|---|
| Neutrophil (seg) | 15–35% | 45–50% | 45–50% | 50–65% |
| Neutrophil (band) | 7–13% | 0–7% | 6–8% | 0–7% |
| Eosinophil | 1–3% | 1–3% | 1–3% | 1–3% |
| Basophil | 0–1% | 0–1% | 0–1% | 0–1% |
| Monocyte | 5–8% | 4–8% | 3–8% | 3–9% |
| Lymphocyte | 40–70% | 40–45% | 35–40% | 25–40% |

Platelets: An average of 5–15 platelets per oil immersion field is considered normal

# APPENDIX D
# Table of Normal Urine Values

**Urine Volume:**

| Age | Volume (ml/24 hours) |
|---|---|
| Newborn | 20–350 |
| One year | 300–600 |
| Ten years | 750–1500 |
| Adult | 750–2000 |

**Physical and Chemical Characteristics of Urine:**

| | Range | Average/Normal |
|---|---|---|
| Color | straw to amber | yellow |
| Transparency | | clear |
| Specific gravity | 1.005–1.030 | 1.015 |
| pH | 5.5–8 | 6 |
| Protein | negative-trace | negative |
| Glucose | | negative |
| Ketone | | negative |
| Bilirubin | | negative |
| Blood | | negative |
| Urobilinogen | | 0.1–1.0 EU/dl |
| Bacteria (nitrite) | | negative |

**Components of Urine Sediment:**

| | Normal |
|---|---|
| RBC/HPF | rare |
| WBC/HPF | 0–4 |
| Epith/HPF | occasional (may be higher in females) |
| Casts/LPF | occasional hyaline |
| Bacteria | negative |
| Mucus | negative to 2+ |
| Crystals | only crystals such as cystine, leucine tyrosine, and cholesterol are considered clinically significant |

# APPENDIX E
## Metric Conversions

**COMMONLY USED PREFIXES IN THE METRIC SYSTEM**

| Abbreviation | Prefix | | Meaning | Multiple of basic unit | Weight gram (g) | Length meter (m) | Volume Liter (L) |
|---|---|---|---|---|---|---|---|
| k | kilo | = | 1000 | $10^3$ | kg | km | kl |
| h | hecto | = | 100 | $10^2$ | hg* | hm* | hl* |
| da | deca | = | 10 | $10^1$ | dag* | dam* | dal* |
| d | deci | = | .1 | $10^{-1}$ | dg* | dm* | dl |
| c | centi | = | .01 | $10^{-2}$ | cg* | cm | cl* |
| m | milli | = | .001 | $10^{-3}$ | mg | mm | ml |
| $\mu$ | micro | = | .000001 | $10^{-6}$ | $\mu$g | $\mu$m | $\mu$l |
| n | nano | = | | $10^{-9}$ | ng | nm | nl* |
| p | pico | = | | $10^{-12}$ | pg | pm* | pl* |

* units not commonly used in the laboratory

## COMMON METRIC EQUIVALENTS

| | | | | | | | |
|---|---|---|---|---|---|---|---|
| **Mass:** | $10^{-3}$ kg | = | 1 gram | = | $10^3$ mg | = | $10^6$ μg |
| | $10^{-3}$ g | = | 1 mg | = | $10^3$ μg | = | $10^6$ ng |
| | $10^{-9}$ g | = | 1 ng | = | $10^3$ pg | | |
| **Volume:** | $10^{-3}$ kl | = | 1 liter | = | $10^3$ ml | = | $10^6$ μl |
| | $10^{-3}$ l | = | 1 ml | = | $10^3$ μl | = | $10^6$ nl |
| | $10^{-1}$ l | = | 1 dl | = | $10^2$ ml | | |
| **Length:** | $10^{-3}$ km | = | 1 meter | = | $10^3$ mm | = | $10^6$ μm |
| | $10^{-3}$ m | = | 1 mm | = | $10^3$ μm | = | $10^6$ nm |
| | $10^{-2}$ m | = | 1 cm | = | 10 mm | = | $10^4$ μm |
| | $10^{-3}$ mm | = | 1 nm | = | 10 Å | | |

## CONVERSION OF ENGLISH UNITS TO METRIC UNITS

| | English unit | English abbreviation | | Multiply by | To get metric unit | Metric abbreviation |
|---|---|---|---|---|---|---|
| **Distance** | 1 mile | mi | = | 1.6 | kilometers | km |
| | 1 yard | yd | = | 0.9 | meters | m |
| | 1 inch | in | = | 2.54 | centimeters | cm |
| **Mass** | 1 pound | lb | = | 0.454 | kilograms | kg |
| | 1 pound | lb | = | 454 | grams | g |
| | 1 ounce | oz | = | 28 | grams | g |
| **Volume** | 1 quart | qt | = | 0.95 | liters | l |
| | 1 fluid ounce | fl. oz. | = | 30 | milliliters | ml |
| | 1 teaspoon | tsp | = | 5 | milliliters | ml |

## CONVERSION OF METRIC UNITS TO ENGLISH UNITS

| | Metric unit | Metric abbreviation | | Multiply by | To find English unit | English abbreviation |
|---|---|---|---|---|---|---|
| **Distance** | 1 kilometer | km | = | 0.6 | miles | mi |
| | 1 meter | m | = | 3.3 | feet | ft |
| | 1 meter | m | = | 39.37 | inches | in |
| | 1 centimeter | cm | = | 0.4 | inches | in |
| | 1 millimeter | mm | = | .04 | inches | in |
| **Mass** | 1 gram | g | = | .0022 | pounds | lb |
| | 1 kilogram | kg | = | 2.2 | pounds | lb |
| **Volume** | 1 liter | l | = | 1.06 | quarts | qt |
| | 1 milliliter | ml | = | .03 | fluid ounces | fl. oz. |

## INTERNATIONAL SYSTEM OF UNITS (S.I. UNITS)

| Common Usage | SI Equivalent |
|---|---|
| micron ($\mu$) | micrometer ($\mu$m; $10^{-6}$ meter) |
| cubic micron ($\mu^3$) | femtoliter (fl; $10^{-15}$ liter) |
| micromicrogram ($\mu\mu$g) | picogram (pg; $10^{-12}$ gram) |
| microgram (mcg) | microgram ($\mu$g; $10^{-6}$ gram) |
| Angstrom (Å) | nm $\times 10^{-1}$ |
| millimicron (m$\mu$) | nanometer (nm; $10^{-9}$ meter) |
| lambda ($\lambda$) | microliter ($\mu$l; $10^{-6}$ liter) |

| Test | Old Unit | S.I. Unit |
|---|---|---|
| Cell counts | cells/mm$^3$ or cells/cumm | cells/$\mu$l or cells/liter |
| Hematocrit | % (Ex. 41%) | decimal (Ex. 0.41) |
| Hemoglobin | g/dl | g/liter |
| MCV | $\mu^3$ | fl |
| MCH | $\mu\mu$g | pg |
| MCHC | % | g/dl (or g/1) |

# APPENDIX F
## Temperature Conversions

Temperatures may be converted from Fahrenheit to Celsius (or Celsius to Fahrenheit) by using the conversion chart below.

| F | C | F | C | F | C |
|---|---|---|---|---|---|
| 23 | −5 | 101 | 38.3 | 115 | 46.1 |
| 32 | 0 | 102 | 38.9 | 116 | 46.7 |
| 70 | 21.1 | 103 | 39.4 | 117 | 47.2 |
| 75 | 23.9 | 104 | 40 | 118 | 47.8 |
| 80 | 26.7 | 105 | 40.6 | 119 | 48.3 |
| 85 | 29.4 | 106 | 41.1 | 120 | 48.9 |
| 90 | 32.2 | 107 | 41.7 | 125 | 51.7 |
| 95 | 35 | 108 | 42.2 | 130 | 54.4 |
| 96 | 35.6 | 109 | 42.8 | 135 | 57.2 |
| 97 | 36.1 | 110 | 43.3 | 140 | 60 |
| 98 | 36.7 | 111 | 43.9 | 150 | 65.6 |
| 98.6 | 37 | 112 | 44.4 | 212 | 100 |
| 99 | 37.2 | 113 | 45 | 230 | 110 |
| 100 | 37.8 | 114 | 45.6 | | |

Temperature conversions may also be performed using the formulas below:

| | |
|---|---|
| **PROBLEM:** | Convert 98.6° F (normal body temperature) to Celsius (C) degrees. |
| **FORMULA:** | $C = \frac{5}{9}(F - 32)$ |
| **SOLUTION:** | $C = \frac{5}{9}(98.6 - 32)$ |
| | $C = \frac{5}{9}(66.6)$ |
| | $C = 36.99$ or $37$ |
| **ANSWER:** | 98.6° F is equal to 37° C |

| | |
|---|---|
| **PROBLEM:** | Convert 37° C to Fahrenheit (F) degrees. |
| **FORMULA:** | $F = \frac{9}{5}(C) + 32$ |
| **SOLUTION:** | $F = \frac{9}{5}(37) + 32$ |
| | $F = 66.6 + 32$ |
| | $F = 98.6$ |
| **ANSWER:** | 37° C is equal to 98.6° F |

# APPENDIX G
## Percent Transmittance–Absorbance Conversion Chart

| % T | A | % T | A | % T | A | % T | A |
|---|---|---|---|---|---|---|---|
| 1 | 2.000 | 1.5 | 1.824 | 23 | .638 | 23.5 | .629 |
| 2 | 1.699 | 2.5 | 1.602 | 24 | .620 | 24.5 | .611 |
| 3 | 1.523 | 3.5 | 1.456 | 25 | .602 | 25.5 | .594 |
| 4 | 1.398 | 4.5 | 1.347 | 26 | .585 | 26.5 | .577 |
| 5 | 1.301 | 5.5 | 1.260 | 27 | .569 | 27.5 | .561 |
| 6 | 1.222 | 6.5 | 1.187 | 28 | .553 | 28.5 | .545 |
| 7 | 1.155 | 7.5 | 1.126 | 29 | .538 | 29.5 | .530 |
| 8 | 1.097 | 8.5 | 1.071 | 30 | .523 | 30.5 | .516 |
| 9 | 1.046 | 9.5 | 1.022 | 31 | .509 | 31.5 | .502 |
| 10 | 1.000 | 10.5 | .979 | 32 | .495 | 32.5 | .488 |
| 11 | .959 | 11.5 | .939 | 33 | .482 | 33.5 | .475 |
| 12 | .921 | 12.5 | .903 | 34 | .469 | 34.5 | .462 |
| 13 | .886 | 13.5 | .870 | 35 | .456 | 35.5 | .450 |
| 14 | .854 | 14.5 | .838 | 36 | .444 | 36.5 | .438 |
| 15 | .824 | 15.5 | .810 | 37 | .432 | 37.5 | .426 |
| 16 | .796 | 16.5 | .782 | 38 | .420 | 38.5 | .414 |
| 17 | .770 | 17.5 | .757 | 39 | .409 | 39.5 | .403 |
| 18 | .745 | 18.5 | .733 | 40 | .398 | 40.5 | .392 |
| 19 | .721 | 19.5 | .710 | 41 | .387 | 41.5 | .382 |
| 20 | .699 | 20.5 | .688 | 42 | .377 | 42.5 | .372 |
| 21 | .678 | 21.5 | .668 | 43 | .367 | 43.5 | .362 |
| 22 | .658 | 22.5 | .648 | 44 | .357 | 44.5 | .352 |

| % T | A | % T | A | % T | A | % T | A |
|---|---|---|---|---|---|---|---|
| 45 | .347 | 45.5 | .342 | 73 | .1367 | 73.5 | .1337 |
| 46 | .337 | 46.5 | .332 | 74 | .1308 | 74.5 | .1278 |
| 47 | .328 | 47.5 | .323 | 75 | .1249 | 75.5 | .1221 |
| 48 | .319 | 48.5 | .314 | 76 | .1192 | 76.5 | .1163 |
| 49 | .310 | 49.5 | .305 | 77 | .1135 | 77.5 | .1107 |
| 50 | .301 | 50.5 | .297 | 78 | .1079 | 78.5 | .1051 |
| 51 | .2924 | 51.5 | .2882 | 79 | .1024 | 79.5 | .0996 |
| 52 | .2840 | 52.5 | .2798 | 80 | .0969 | 80.5 | .0942 |
| 53 | .2756 | 53.5 | .2716 | 81 | .0915 | 81.5 | .0888 |
| 54 | .2676 | 54.5 | .2636 | 82 | .0862 | 82.5 | .0835 |
| 55 | .2596 | 55.5 | .2557 | 83 | .0809 | 83.5 | .0783 |
| 56 | .2518 | 56.5 | .2480 | 84 | .0757 | 84.5 | .0731 |
| 57 | .2441 | 57.5 | .2403 | 85 | .0706 | 85.5 | .0680 |
| 58 | .2366 | 58.5 | .2328 | 86 | .0655 | 86.5 | .0630 |
| 59 | .2291 | 59.5 | .2255 | 87 | .0605 | 87.5 | .0580 |
| 60 | .2218 | 60.5 | .2182 | 88 | .0555 | 88.5 | .0531 |
| 61 | .2147 | 61.5 | .2111 | 89 | .0505 | 89.5 | .0482 |
| 62 | .2076 | 62.5 | .2041 | 90 | .0458 | 90.5 | .0434 |
| 63 | .2007 | 63.5 | .1973 | 91 | .0410 | 91.5 | .0386 |
| 64 | .1939 | 64.5 | .1905 | 92 | .0362 | 92.5 | .0339 |
| 65 | .1871 | 65.5 | .1838 | 93 | .0315 | 93.5 | .0292 |
| 66 | .1805 | 66.5 | .1772 | 94 | .0269 | 94.5 | .0246 |
| 67 | .1739 | 67.5 | .1707 | 95 | .0223 | 95.5 | .0200 |
| 68 | .1675 | 68.5 | .1643 | 96 | .0177 | 96.5 | .0155 |
| 69 | .1612 | 69.5 | .1580 | 97 | .0132 | 97.5 | .0110 |
| 70 | .1549 | 70.5 | .1518 | 98 | .0088 | 98.5 | .0066 |
| 71 | .1487 | 71.5 | .1457 | 99 | .0044 | 99.5 | .0022 |
| 72 | .1427 | 72.5 | .1397 | 100 | .0000 | | |

# APPENDIX H
## Hematology—CBC Report Form

Date ______________________

Student ______________________

Specimen No. ______________________

| | | Normal |
|---|---|---|
| WBC/1 | __________ | $4.5 - 11.0 \times 10^9/1$ |
| RBC/1 | __________ | $4.5 - 6.0 \times 10^{12}/1$ Male<br>$4.0 - 5.5 \times 10^{12}/1$ Female |
| Hgb g/dl | __________ | 13.5 − 17.5 g/dl Male<br>12.5 − 15.5 g/dl Female |
| Hct % | __________ | 42 − 52% Male<br>36 − 48% Female |
| MCV (fl) | __________ | 80 − 100 fl |
| MCH (pg) | __________ | 27 − 32 pg |
| MCHC (%) | __________ | 33 − 38% |

| **Differential count:** | **Normal** |
|---|---|
| __% segmented neutrophils | 50–65% |
| __% lymphocytes | 25–40% |
| __% monocytes | 3–9% |
| __% eosinophils | 1–3% |
| __% basophils | 0–1% |
| __% bands | 0–7% |
| __ other | |

**RBC morphology:**

| | | |
|---|---|---|
| Cell size: | ☐ normocytic | |
| | ☐ microcytic | normocytic |
| | ☐ macrocytic | |
| Cell color: | ☐ normochromic | normochromic |
| | ☐ hypochromic | |
| Platelet | ☐ appear adequate | 5–15/ oil immersion field |
| Estimate: | ☐ appear decreased | <4/ oil immersion field |
| | ☐ appear increased | >16/ oil immersion field |

Comments: ______________________________________________

______________________________________________

# APPENDIX I
## Routine Urinalysis Report Form

**ROUTINE URINALYSIS REPORT FORM**

Date ______________________________

Student ______________________________

Specimen No. ______________________________

Instructions: Record results as indicated:

I. *Physical Examination*

| | Normal Values |
|---|---|
| Volume (ml): ______________________ | (only report if 24-hour urine) |
| Transparency: ___ clear | clear |
| ___ hazy (slightly cloudy) | |
| ___ cloudy (turbid) | |
| Color: ______________________ | straw to amber |
| Specific gravity: ______________________ | 1.005–1.030 |

II. *Chemical Examination*

A. Multistix

| | | Normal Values |
|---|---|---|
| pH | ________ | 5.5–8.0 |
| protein | ________ | negative, trace |
| glucose | ________ | negative |
| ketone | ________ | negative |
| bilirubin | ________ | negative |
| blood | ________ | negative |
| urobilinogen | ________ | 0.1 – 1.0 e.u./dl urine |

B. *Confirmatory Test Results* (circle results)

| | | |
|---|---|---|
| Protein (sulfosalicylic acid): | negative | trace 1+ 2+ 3+ 4+ |
| Reducing substances (Clinitest®): | negative | ¼% ½% ¾% 1% 2% or more |
| Ketones (Acetest®): | negative | positive |
| Bilirubin (Ictotest®): | negative | positive |

III. *Microscopic Examination*

| | | Normal Values |
|---|---|---|
| WBCs: | ________/HPF | 0–4 |
| RBCs: | ________/HPF | rare |
| Epithelial cells: | ________/HPF | occasional (higher in females) |
| Casts: | ________/LPF | Occasional, hyaline |

Type present: ________

Crystals: _____ none seen

_____ present

(type)________

Amorphous deposits: _____ none seen

_____ present

| | | Normal Values |
|---|---|---|
| Yeasts: | negative 1+ 2+ 3+ 4+ | negative |
| Bacteria: | negative 1+ 2+ 3+ 4+ | negative |
| Mucus: | negative 1+ 2+ 3+ 4+ | negative–2+ |

Other: ________________

# APPENDIX J
## Examples of Preparing Solutions and Dilutions

**Preparation of a v/v Percentage Solution**

**PROBLEM:** Prepare one liter of 2% acetic acid from concentrated (glacial) acetic acid.

**SOLUTION:**

1. A 2% solution of acetic acid contains 2 ml of concentrated acetic acid in each 100 ml of solution.
2. Therefore, one liter of 2% acetic acid contains 2 ml × 10, or 20 ml of concentrated acetic acid.
3. To prepare the solution:
   a. Fill a one-liter volumetric flask approximately half full of distilled water
   b. Add 20 ml of concentrated acetic acid and swirl to mix
   c. Fill the flask to the line with distilled water.

### Preparing a Solution Using proportions

**PROBLEM:** A buffer is made by adding 2 parts of "solution A" to 5 parts of "solution B." How much of solution A and solution B would be required to make 70 ml of the buffer?

**FORMULA:**

$$\frac{\text{Total volume required}}{\text{parts of "A"} + \text{parts of "B"}} = \text{volume of one part}$$

**SOLUTION:**

$$\frac{\text{70 ml required}}{\text{2 parts "A"} + \text{5 parts "B"}} = \text{volume of one part}$$

$$\frac{70}{7} = 10 \text{ ml} = \text{volume of one part}$$

2 parts of solution "A" $= 2 \times 10 = 20$ ml
5 parts of solution "B" $= 5 \times 10 = 50$ ml

**ANSWER:** The buffer would be made by mixing 20 ml of solution A with 50 ml of solution B to give a total volume of 70 ml.

### Using the Formula: $C_1V_1 = C_2V_2$ to Prepare a Solution

**PROBLEM:** Prepare 100 ml of a 2% solution of acetic acid using a 10% acetic acid solution.

**FORMULA:** $C_1V_1 = C_2V_2$

**where:**
$C_1$ = concentration of first solution
$C_2$ = concentration of second solution
$V_1$ = required volume of first solution
$V_2$ = required volume of second solution

**SOLUTION:**

$$(2)(100 \text{ ml}) = (10)(V_2)$$

$$200 \text{ ml} = 10\ (V_2)$$

$$\frac{200}{10} \text{ ml} = V_2$$

$$20 \text{ ml} = V_2$$

**ANSWER:** Twenty ml of 10% acetic acid are added to 80 ml of distilled water to make 100 ml of a 2% solution of acetic acid.

### Preparation of a w/v Percentage Solution

**PROBLEM:** Prepare 500 ml of 0.85% saline.

**SOLUTION:**
1. A 0.85% solution contains 0.85 g of the solute in every 100 ml of solution.
2. Therefore, to prepare 500 ml, 5 × 0.85 g or 4.25 g of sodium chloride (NaCl) must be used.
3. To prepare the solution:
   a. Weigh out 4.25 g of NaCl
   b. Fill a 500 ml volumetric flask approximately half full with distilled water
   c. Add 4.25 g of NaCl and swirl gently to dissolve
   d. Fill the flask to the line with distilled water

### Preparation of a 1:10 Dilution

**PROBLEM:** Prepare 10 ml of a 1:10 dilution of serum using saline as the diluent.

**SOLUTION:**
1. A 1:10 dilution contains one part of a substance combined with 9 parts of a diluent to give a total of 10 parts.
2. Add 1 ml of serum to 9 ml of saline to form 10 ml of a 1:10 dilution of the serum.
3. If 50 ml were required, 5 ml of serum would be added to 45 ml saline.

# APPENDIX K
# Preparation of Reagents

Listed below are reagents which are needed in some of the procedures in this book. These reagents, and others, may also be obtained from the companies listed in Appendix L, Sources of Laboratory Supplies.

| Unit–Lesson | Reagent | |
|---|---|---|
| 2–1 | 70% alcohol | For 100 ml: 70 ml 95% ethanol<br>30 ml $dH_2O$ |
| 2–5 | RBC diluting fluids | Gower's: 12.5 g anhydrous sodium sulfate<br>33.3 ml glacial acetic acid<br>q.s. to 200 ml with $dH_2O$ |
| | | Dacie's: 5.0 g sodium citrate<br>3.0 g NaCl<br>5.0 ml Formalin<br>490.0 ml $dH_2O$ |
| 2–6 | WBC diluting fluids | 2% acetic acid: 2 ml glacial acetic acid<br>98 ml $dH_2O$ |
| | | 1% HCl: 1 ml conc. HCl<br>99 ml $dH_2O$ |
| 3–3 | New Methylene Blue stain | 0.5 g New Methylene Blue,<br>1.6 g potassium oxalate<br>q.s. to 100 ml with saline.<br>Filter before use. |

| Unit–Lesson | Reagent | |
|---|---|---|
| 3–4 | platelet diluting fluid<br>1% ammonium oxalate: | 1.0 g ammonium oxalate, q.s. to 100 ml with $dH_2O$<br>Store at 4° C. Filter before use. |
| 3–5 | Drabkin's reagent | 1 g sodium bicarbonate<br>50 mg potassium cyanide<br>200 mg potassium ferricyanide<br>q.s. to 1 liter with $dH_2O$ |
| 4–1 | Saline | 0.85 g NaCl<br>100 ml $dH_2O$ |
| 4–2 | 2–5% cell suspension | Suspend red cells in saline. Centrifuge and remove supernatant saline. Add 2 to 5 ml of the packed red cells to saline to make 100 ml. |
| 5–3 | urine control solution | 0.5 ml 30% Bovine albumin<br>300 mg glucose<br>0.5 g NaCl<br>0.5 g urea<br>10 $\mu$l whole blood<br>0.2 ml acetone<br>q.s. to 100 ml with $dH_2O$ |
| 5–3 | 20% sulfosalicylic acid | 20 g sulfosalicylic acid<br>q.s. to 100 ml with $dH_2O$ |

# APPENDIX L
## Sources of Laboratory Supplies

Supplies for the various medical laboratory procedures included in this text may be purchased from the following companies:

### Hematology

| | |
|---|---|
| Fisher Scientific<br>711 Forbes Avenue<br>Pittsburgh, PA 15219 | Scientific Division (chemicals, instruments, apparatus, supplies)<br>Education Division (kits, audio-visual software, models, charts) |
| American Scientific Products<br>1430 Waukegan Road<br>McGaw Park, IL 60085 | Laboratory supplies and equipment |
| Carolina Biological Supply Company<br>Burlington, NC 27215 | Stained blood smears, quick stains, educational materials, equipment |
| Sigma Chemical Company<br>P.O. Box 14508<br>St. Louis, MO 63178 | Biochemicals, standards, controls, diagnostic kits |
| Atlases<br>Abbott Laboratories<br>Attn: Ruth Price<br>Dept. 383<br>Abbott Park, IL 60064 | *Morphology of Human Blood Cells,* Diggs, L. W., Dorothy Sturm and Ann Bell. Abbott Laboratories, 1984. |

Urinalysis

American Scientific Products
1430 Waukegan Road
McGaw Park, IL 60085

Carolina Biological Supply Company
Burlington, NC 27215

Fisher Scientific
711 Forbes Avenue
Pittsburgh, PA 15219

Ames, Division of Miles Laboratories
Elkhart, IN 46515
— Reagents, supplies, charts, educational materials

Serology

Ortho Diagnostics, Inc.
Raritan, NJ 08869
— Blood bank products, antisera, cells

American Scientific Products
1430 Waukegan Road
McGaw Park, IL 60085
— Diagnostic kits, controls, Dade® blood banking products

Carolina Biological Supply Company
Burlington, NC 27215
— Blood typing kits and supplies

Fisher Scientific
711 Forbes Avenue
Pittsburgh, PA 15219
— Diagnostic kits, equipment, educational materials

Bacteriology

BBL Microbiology Systems
Division of Becton, Dickinson and Co.
P.O. Box 342
Cockeysville, MD 21030
— Culture media and reagents

DIFCO Laboratories
P.O. Box 1058
Detroit, MI 48232
— Culture media and reagents

American Scientific Products
1430 Waukegan Road
McGaw Park, IL 60085

Carolina Biological Supply Company
Burlington, NC 27215
— Student kits, equipment and supplies, prepared media, cultures, prepared slides

Fisher Scientific
711 Forbes Avenue
Pittsburgh, PA 15219

American Type Culture Collection
12301 Park Lawn Drive
Rockville, MD 20852
— ATCC bacterial cultures

# Index